Review of
Critical
Care
Nursing

Review of
Critical Care Nursing
CASE STUDIES AND APPLICATIONS

Sheila Drake Melander, DSN, RN, FCCM
Associate Professor of Nursing and Coordinator of the
Critical Care BSN Nursing Course
University of Southern Indiana
Supplemental Staff
Surgical Intensive Care Unit, Deaconess Hospital
Evansville, Indiana

W.B. SAUNDERS COMPANY
A Division of Harcourt Brace & Company
Philadelphia   London   Toronto   Montreal   Sydney   Tokyo

W.B. SAUNDERS COMPANY

A Division of Harcourt Brace & Company

The Curtis Center
Independence Square West
Philadelphia, Pennsylvania 19106

Library of Congress Cataloging-in-Publication Data

Melander, Sheila Drake.
    Review of critical care nursing: case studies and applcations/
Sheila Drake Melander.
        p.   cm.
    ISBN 0-7216-5537-8
    1. Intensive care nursing—Case studies. I. Title.
    [DNLM: 1. Critical Illness—nursing—case studies. 2. Critical
Care—case studies. WY 154 M517r 1996]
RT120.I5M47 1996
610.73'61—dc20
DNLM/DLC   95-36450

NOTICE

Critical care nursing is an ever-changing field. Standard safety precautions must be followed, but as new research and clinical experience broaden our knowledge, changes in treatment and drug therapy become necessary or appropriate. The editors of this work have carefully checked the generic and trade drug names and verified drug dosages to ensure that the dosage information in this work is accurate and in accord with the standards accepted at the time of publication. Readers are advised, however, to check the product information currently provided by the manufacturer of each drug to be administered to be certain that changes have not been made in the recommended dose or in the contraindications for administration. This is of particular importance in regard to new or infrequently used drugs. It is the responsibility of the treating physician, relying on experience and knowledge of the patient, to determine dosages and the best treatment for the patient. The editors cannot be responsible for misuse or misapplication of the material in this work.

THE PUBLISHER

REVIEW OF CRITICAL CARE NURSING: ISBN 0-7216-5537-8
CASE STUDIES AND APPLICATIONS

Printed in the United States of America

Last digit is the print number: 9   8   7   6   5   4   3   2

Contributors

Cinda Alexander, MSN, CCRN, CNRN
Tri-State Neurosurgical, Inc., Evansville, Indiana
Subarachnoid Hemorrhage with Aneurysm; Head Trauma Subdural Hematoma; Epidural Hematoma

Sharon West Angle, MSN, RN
Adjunct Faculty, Old Dominion University, Norfolk, Virginia; Administrative Director, Quality Improvement, Northampton Accomack Memorial Hospital, Nassawadox, Virginia
Adult Respiratory Distress Syndrome; Multiple System Organ Failure/Multiple Organ Dysfunction Syndrome

Nancy D. Blasdell, MSN, RN
Adjunct Faculty, Old Dominion University, Norfolk, Virginia
Pulmonary Contusion

Connie Cooper, MSN, RN
Instructor, Chronic Illness and Human Sexuality, School of Nursing and Health Professions, University of Southern Indiana; Member, HIV/AIDS Community Planning Group of Indiana, Evansville, Indiana
Acquired Immunodeficiency Syndrome

Anne G. Denner, MS, RN
Instructor, Department of Biology, University of Southern Indiana, Evansville, Indiana
Adrenal Crisis; Diabetic Ketoacidosis

Linda K. Evinger, MSN, RN, C–OGNP
Instructor in Nursing, University of Southern Indiana, Evansville, Indiana
Esophageal Varices

Beverly Farmer, MSN, RNC
Unit Manager, Neuro-Medical Intensive Care Unit, Deaconess Hospital, Evansville, Indiana
Syndrome of Inappropriate Antidiuretic Hormone

Gail Stamper Franks, MSN, RN

Clinical Nurse Specialist, Urology, Evansville, Indiana
Chronic Renal Failure and Renal Transplantation

Kelly A. Hertel, BSN, RNC, CCRN, CEN

Director of Pulmonary Services, Owensboro Mercy Health System, Owensboro, Kentucky
Congestive Heart Failure

Karen L. Jones, MSN, RNC

Director of Clinical Services, Cardiovascular Surgery, Inc., Evansville, Indiana
Coronary Artery Bypass Graft

Pam B. Koob, MA, MSN, RN, CCRN

Assistant Professor of Nursing, University of Southern Indiana, Evansville, Indiana
Carotid Endarterectomy

Alice Lowe, BSN, RN

Staff Nurse, Coronary Intensive Care, Deaconess Hospital, Evansville, Indiana
PTCA and Thrombolytic Therapy in Myocardial Infarction

Jamie Elizabeth Madding, BSN, RN

Instructor, Basic Life Support, and Clinical Nurse, Coronary Intensive Care, Wellborn Baptist Hospital, Evansville, Indiana
Cardiogenic Shock in Anterior Wall Myocardial Infarction

Sheila Drake Melander, DSN, RN, FCCM

Associate Professor of Nursing and Coordinator of the Critical Care BSN Nursing Course, University of Southern Indiana; Supplemental Staff, Surgical Intensive Care Unit, Deaconess Hospital, Evansville, Indiana
Adult Respiratory Distress Syndrome; Pulmonary Embolism; Pulmonary Contusion; Chronic Obstructive Pulmonary Disease with Pneumonia; PTCA and Thrombolytic Therapy in Myocardial Infarction; Coronary Artery Bypass Graft; Cardiogenic Shock in Anterior Wall Myocardial Infarction; Non-Q-Wave Myocardial Infarction; Acute Renal Failure; Multiple System Organ Failure/Multiple Organ Dysfunction Syndrome

Michael D. O'Grady, MSN, RN

Instructor of Nursing, School of Nursing and Health Professions, University of Southern Indiana, Evansville, Indiana
Gastrointestinal Tract Bleeding

Lynn Rodgers, MSN, RNC, CCRN, CNRN

Critical Care Educator, Surgical Intensive Care, Deaconess Hospital, Evansville, Indiana
Peritonitis; Sepsis/Septic Shock

Laura S. Platt Smith, MSN, RN

Home Nursing, Family Health Care, DeDeDo, Guam; formerly Instructor, DePaul School of Nursing, Norfolk, Virginia
Pulmonary Embolism; Epidural Hematoma

Ann H. White, MSN, MBA, RN, CNA

Assistant Professor, University of Southern Indiana, Evansville, Indiana
Acute Pancreatitis; Burns

Reviewers

Mary Margaret Blankenship, MSN, RN
Oral Roberts University, Tulsa, Oklahoma

Betty Nash Blevins, MSN, RN, CCRN, CS
Bluefield State College, Bluefield, West Virginia

Suzanne M. Davis, MSN, RN
Greenville Technical College, Greenville, South Carolina

Deborah A. Ennis, MSN, RN, CCRN
Harrisburg Area Community College, Harrisburg, Pennsylvania

Mary Kay Flynn, MA, RN, CCRN
Grand Canyon University, Phoenix, Arizona

Deborah Panozzo Nelson, MS, RN, CCRN
EMS Nursing Education, Tinley Park, Illinois

Barbara Pfretzschner, MSN, RN
Arapahoe Community College, Littleton, Colorado

Foreword

Almost two decades ago Knowles (1980) noted that the mission of education was to produce people who could apply their knowledge under changing conditions characterized by an explosion of knowledge and a revolution in technology. He further commented that a fundamental competence needed by all is to engage in lifelong self-directed learning. How are educators to fulfill this mission? What changes in traditional teaching strategies are needed to accomplish this task? Needed are strategies that help students learn to think, not just acquire information.

Yinger (1980) identified four major factors that affect students' ability to think: (1) knowledge and experience, (2) intellectual skills and strategies, (3) attitudes and dispositions, and (4) the thinking environment. The first three factors are internal and not amenable to teacher influence, but the fourth is external to the learner and is under the control of the teacher. A thinking environment is crucial for encouraging and supporting the internal factors. Among the various environmental influences on students' thinking, the most important are emotional and intellectual factors, which are reflected in instruction and teacher attitude.

Colgrove and colleagues (1995) characterize traditional instructional methods as "feeding the students prepackaged knowledge" and advocate a more active process of learning called *experiential learning*. This type of learning emphasizes the process of learning rather than the outcome and offers students the opportunity for direct exploration of complex concepts.

One example of experiential learning methods is the case study, which provides students with an opportunity to apply problem solving and decision making in the safe atmosphere of the classroom. Because the case study provokes critical thinking and motivates the student with active involvement, it promotes the acquisition of skills essential for a lifetime of learning.

This book of case studies in critical care nursing offers an important teaching and learning tool for faculty and students. In each case study, important concepts are emphasized, controversies in intervention are noted, and nursing management is extended beyond the critical phase of illness. An important contribution of this text is the opportunity for the faculty member to become a *facilitator* for student learning who can provide immediate feedback and challenge students to go beyond their initial response to the presented case. Linking learners with learning resources is one of the most meaningful contributions a faculty member can offer to students. This text provides an excellent mechanism for this linkage.

Marguerite R. Kinney, DNSc, RN, FAAN
Professor and Associate Director
Center for Nursing Research
School of Nursing
University of Alabama at Birmingham

References

Colgrove, S.R., Schlapman, N., & Erpelding, C. (1995). Experiential learning. In Fuszard (Ed.), Innovative Teaching Strategies in Nursing (2nd ed., pp. 9-17.) Gaithersburg, MD: Aspen.

Knowles, M.S. (1980). The Modern Practice of Adult Education: From Pedagogy to Andragogy. Chicago: Association Press.

Yinger, R.J. (1980). Can we really teach them to think? In R.E. Younger (Ed.), Fostering Critical Thinking (pp. 11-31). San Francisco: Jossey-Bass.

Preface

Review of Critical Care Nursing: Case Studies and Applications was compiled with the intent of capturing actual patient data from a critical care setting. The data were then placed in a scenario that recaptured patient events as they actually occurred. Patient scenarios were sought that represented common diagnoses seen in six body systems—respiratory, cardiovascular, renal, neurological, gastrointestinal, and endocrine—and in multisystems. The 26 chapters are grouped according to these systems for quick reference. These cases were compiled with one goal in mind, to create a tool for use with critical care students that provided a true perspective of patient needs in the critical care setting. Students could study actual patient situations and apply critical thinking skills in discussions of current treatment modalities, effectiveness of treatments and medications prescribed, alternative care options, the necessity for diagnostic tests ordered, and the impact of hemodynamic values on patient care and the "real life" necessity for hemodynamic monitoring.

The case study application text represents a different approach to education of critical care nurses. In each scenario, students follow the patient from entrance into the healthcare setting through his or her discharge from the acute care setting. Students are challenged to use critical thinking skills to accurately answer the case study questions that accompany each case and provide solutions to the patient's problem. Students can then study answers to those same questions written by the author of the chapter. Students should then be well versed in current diagnostic procedures, laboratory data required, pharmacologic needs, and treatment modalities for that particular disease entity.

This text is appropriate for the baccalaureate or graduate student and for use in the hospital setting in critical care training. The text may also serve as a review tool for nurses preparing for the CCRN examination. The answers to the case study questions provide a detailed account of the disease studied. Educators can choose the questions appropriate for the students' level or can adapt their expectations of the depth of the students' answers.

Healthcare needs are quickly changing, and we must prepare nurses to change and adapt with the healthcare system. Students who are challenged to think critically while still in the classroom setting can translate those skills into the clinical care setting to better meet the changing needs of the critically ill patient. It is hoped that this text will increase students' knowledge of the needs of the critically ill patient and enhance education in the clinical setting.

Sheila Drake Melander

Acknowledgments

I would like to express my deepest gratitude to each of the contributors to the text. Without their expertise and dedication to the profession of nursing, this text would not have been possible. I also would like to thank Dr.. Nadine Coudret, Dean of the University of Southern Indiana School of Nursing and Health Professions. Dr. Coudret has supported every effort I have made thus far in my career as an educator and truly serves as a role model and mentor. In addition, I would like to thank Amy Shively and Izetta Brakel for lending their computer skills and support, which ensured the timely completion of this text. Sincere appreciation is expressed for the excellent support received from Barbara Nelson Cullen and the staff of W.B. Saunders. Finally, I would like to thank my husband, Chuck, my 6-year-old son, Ryan, and 8-week-old son, Matthew, for their constant patience and support in this endeavor.

Sheila Drake Melander

Contents

1

Adult Respiratory Distress Syndrome

Sharon West Angle, MSN, RN
Sheila Drake Melander, DSN, RN, FCCM

CASE PRESENTATION

Postoperative Day 3

Mr. Embry, a 63-year-old, 68 kg (150 lb) white man, had undergone an anterior colon resection for rectal polyps and had an uneventful postoperative course until the evening of the third postoperative day. He was monitored with telemetry and had no unusual complaints. At 10 PM on the third postoperative day he began to complain of not feeling "right." Assessment of the patient revealed hypotension and shortness of breath. Within minutes he became confused and agitated. The shortness of breath worsened (he began gasping for air), and he experienced severe hypoxia. He was intubated and transferred to the intensive care unit (ICU).

BP	60/40	pH	7.3
HR	160 bpm	P_{CO_2}	46 mm Hg
Respirations	12–35/min	P_{O_2}	104 mm Hg
Temperature	38.8° C (101.8° F)	HCO_3^-	22 mmol/L

On arrival in the ICU he was placed on a ventilator in the synchronized intermittent mandatory ventilation (SIMV) mode.

F_{IO_2}	90%
SIMV rate	6
V_T	800 ml

1

The patient was given a 500 ml bolus of normal saline. He received dopamine (Intropin) 3 to 5 μg/kg/min for renal perfusion and was given 1 g vancomycin (Vancocin IV) intravenously (IV) every 12 hours for prophylactic staphylococcal coverage. A pulmonary artery catheter (Swan-Ganz) was inserted, and the patient's pulmonary capillary wedge pressure (PCWP) was 12 mm Hg.

Postoperative Day 4

The next morning the patient remained on ventilatory support with pressure support of 7 cm H_2O. He received IV fluids at 250 ml/h and dopamine at 7 μg/kg/min. The patient was receiving total parenteral nutrition. He has an order for morphine sulfate (Roxanol) 2 to 12 mg every hour as needed for pain or restlessness.

BP	135/70	pH	7.35
HR	140 bpm	Pco_2	46.1 mm Hg
Respirations	6–16/min	Po_2	55.5 mm Hg
Temperature	39.4° C (103° F)	HCO_3^-	25 mmol/L
Urine output	20–30 ml/h		

The patient's FIO_2 is increased from 90% to 100%; tidal volume (V_T) is 800 ml; SIMV is 6 with total respirations of 16/min. At this time a positive end expiratory pressure (PEEP) of 5 cm H_2O was added, and the patient remained on pressure support of 7 cm H_2O.

The patient was given several boluses of normal saline and continued to receive the dopamine infusion. He remained on the preceding ventilation settings. The following arterial blood gases (ABGs) were drawn 2 hours after the ventilator settings were changed:

pH	7.42
Pco_2	46.2 mm Hg
Po_2	75.2 mm Hg
HCO_3^-	28.9 mmol/L

Postoperative Day 5

PEEP is increased to 10 cm H_2O and V_T is increased to 1000 ml.

pH	7.43	BP	130/60
Pco_2	46.2 mm Hg	HR	120 bpm
Po_2	86.8 mm Hg	Respirations	10/min
HCO_3^-	30.5 mmol/L	Temperature	38.3° C (101° F)

After these changes the patient's oxygen levels gradually stabilized, and the patient was weaned from ventilatory support. The patient's urinary output also increased significantly after administration of the fluid boluses. Ten days after intubation the patient was extubated and received oxygen by nasal cannula.

Adult Respiratory Distress Syndrome

1. What is adult respiratory distress syndrome (ARDS)?

2. Discuss the pathophysiologic changes associated with ARDS.

3. What are the pathophysiologic phases of ARDS?

4. How is ARDS diagnosed?

5. What are some medical complications seen with ARDS?

6. What laboratory findings are diagnostic of ARDS?

7. What radiologic changes are seen with ARDS?

8. What changes are seen in pulmonary function studies with ARDS?

9. What clinical signs and symptoms are seen with early ARDS?

10. Tissue hypoxia is a major finding in ARDS. What assessment findings in the following systems would indicate ARDS: central nervous, cardiovascular, pulmonary, renal, gastrointestinal/hepatic, and musculoskeletal systems?

11. What is the goal of treatment in ARDS?

12. What is the principal treatment for ARDS? List and describe the types of ventilatory support available.

13. Describe nonventilator means of pulmonary support.

14. What is the role of oxygen-free radicals in ARDS?

15. What are some of the pharmacologic interventions used in ARDS?

16. What role does hemodynamic monitoring play in the management of ARDS?

17. Describe appropriate nursing diagnoses seen with ARDS.

18. What is the nurse's overall goal in caring for the ARDS patient?

QUESTIONS AND ANSWERS

Adult Respiratory
Distress Syndrome

1. What is ARDS?

ARDS refers to adult respiratory distress syndrome, which is a series of pathologic, clinical, and pathophysiologic changes that can occur with or without a preexisting pulmonary disease as a complication of some critical illness, resulting in an acute lung injury (Enger, 1989). ARDS presents as an acute onset of pulmonary disease, which is noncardiogenic in nature, caused by an increase in permeability in the pulmonary capillary bed (Enger, 1989). ARDS was first described and named by Ashbaugh, Powers, and coworkers in 1967 (Enger, 1989). It is characterized by refractory hypoxemia, tachypnea, dyspnea, and radiologic changes showing patchy scattered infiltrates that progress to a total whiteout of both lungs (Case & Sabo, 1992). ARDS is associated with a high mortality rate ranging from 60% to 90% as noted by Hudson (1990) and Vaughan and Brooks (1990).

2. Discuss the pathophysiologic changes associated with ARDS.

ARDS is described as an acute lung injury involving damage to the alveolar epithelium and pulmonary microvasculature (Vaughan & Brooks, 1990). Alterations occur, leading to a loss of integrity of the alveolar-capillary (A-C) membrane (Enger, 1989). The exact pathophysiology of ARDS is complex and not fully understood (Vaughan & Brooks, 1990). Manifestations of ARDS may not be seen immediately after a precipitating event that triggers the onset of the syndrome. Instead, ARDS develops 24 hours to 7 days after the initial injury or event (Case & Sabo, 1992).

The onset of ARDS is preceded by a major traumatic event such as multiple trauma, burns, shock, sepsis states, or any critical illness (Case & Sabo, 1992; Vaughan & Brooks, 1990). The common thread among

various etiologic events is a catastrophic stressor to the body that activates the inflammatory, immune, coagulation, and neurohormonal response systems (Vaughan & Brooks, 1990). When these systems are activated, numerous mediator substances are released, which may injure
blood vessels and lung tissue (Vaughan & Brooks, 1990).

These substances damage the endothelial capillary membrane and
the alveolar barrier. This leads to an increased permeability with a resultant interstitial edema and alveolar flooding, resulting in impaired
gas exchange and other metabolic disturbances (Enger, 1989). The injury causes a release of humoral and inflammatory products that cause
pulmonary vasoconstriction and bronchoconstriction. This contributes
to alterations in the lung and resultant problems with gas exchange in
the patient with ARDS (Vaughan & Brooks, 1990).

It is thought the precipitating clinical event responsible for triggering
ARDS determines the order of activation of blood cell and protein systems in the body, leading to a compounding of the lung abnormalities
seen with ARDS (Vaughan & Brooks, 1990). Neutrophil activation triggers or initiates an inflammatory response in the pulmonary vascular bed
(Vaughan & Brooks, 1990). Injury of lung tissue causes the neutrophils
to aggregate and adhere to the vascular wall. This activity stimulates the
release of oxygen-free radicals and stimulates the platelet activating factor (Vaughan & Brooks, 1990). This results in further alterations and injury to the vascular endothelium, causing more fluid leakage from the
vascular compartment into the lung interstitium. This leads to additional
fluid shifts and more fluid entering the lung, causing additional injury
and further stimulation of neutrophil activation (Vaughan & Brooks,
1990). Thus, a cycle is created that perpetuates the pathophysiologic
events causing ARDS.

3. What are the pathophysiologic phases of ARDS?

Enger (1989) defines four clinical phases in ARDS. These phases are
latent, acute interstitial edema, acute intraalveolar edema, and subacute
chronic. The latent phase may have a duration of several hours to several days. Unless the precipitating event is pulmonary in origin, there
may be no sign of dysfunction. However, it is during this time that
changes in the A-C membrane begin to occur (Enger, 1989).

As pulmonary capillary damage becomes evident, the patient enters
the phase of acute interstitial edema. As fluid leaks into the interstitium, swelling and reduction in compressibility occur (Enger, 1989).
Because the alveoli are less distensible, ventilation-perfusion mismatch
results and the vital capacity is impaired. The patient may exhibit signs
of restlessness or apprehension and complain of dyspnea (Enger,
1989).

As alveolar flooding begins and protein-rich fluid continues to increase, the patient enters the phase of acute intraalveolar edema (Enger,

1989). At this time surface tension is high and lung compliance is greatly reduced, leading to a compromise in gas exchange. This in turn results in intrapulmonary shunting. The patient exhibits greater agitation and shortness of breath. In addition, hypoxemia leads to persistent tachypnea and changes in mental acuity (Enger, 1989).

The subacute or chronic phase occurs if the patient does not die or recover. During this phase the acute lung injury progresses, and the patient may develop end-stage pulmonary fibrosis (Enger, 1989).

4. How is ARDS diagnosed?

The diagnosis of ARDS is usually based on the history, clinical presentation, diagnostic studies, radiologic findings, and changes in pulmonary function (Vaughan & Brooks, 1990). Usually the history includes a precipitating event or factor that serves to activate systems, leading to the lung injury that results in the development of ARDS. These events may include multiple trauma, extensive traumatic surgery, shock states, hematologic disorders, sepsis, drug overdose, aspiration, inhalation of toxins, near drowning, or radiation pneumonitis (Hudson, 1990; Shinnick, 1992). A clinical presentation suggesting ARDS includes dyspnea, tachypnea, tachycardia, restlessness, anxiety, use of accessory muscles, grunting, and labored respirations. These symptoms occur 24 hours to 7 days after the initial injury. It may also parallel the onset of a clinical sepsis (Case & Sabo, 1992; Vaughan & Brooks, 1990).

5. What are some medical complications seen with ARDS?

Sepsis and nosocomial infections involving the respiratory system are frequently seen. Pulmonary complications such as pulmonary emboli, fibrosis, barotrauma, and oxygen toxicity are often seen (Enger, 1989). Gastrointestinal hemorrhage and paralytic ileus frequently occur in patients with ARDS. Multiple organ system failure may also be a complication of this syndrome (Enger, 1989). Hematologic abnormalities such as anemia, thrombocytopenia and disseminated intravascular coagulation can occur (Enger, 1989).

6. What laboratory findings are diagnostic of ARDS?

Blood gases are the primary laboratory tests used. Hypoxemia is unresponsive to oxygen therapy (increased PEEP and increased FIO_2). The PaO_2 will be less than 55 mm Hg with an FIO_2 of more than 50%. This is due to intrapulmonary shunting (Case & Sabo, 1992). Hyperventilation leads to a decreased $PaCO_2$, causing respiratory alkalosis. Later in the course of the disease there is a buildup of CO_2, resulting in respiratory acidosis (Vaughan & Brooks, 1990). Other laboratory findings that might be present because of the pathologic process are decreased neutrophil and platelet counts (Vaughan & Brooks, 1990).

7. What radiologic changes are seen with ARDS?

Early radiologic findings show patchy scattered densities and irregular borders. As the disease progresses, there is an increase in density and size and a total whiteout of the lung (Case & Sabo, 1992).

8. What changes are seen in pulmonary function studies with ARDS?

Changes in pulmonary function are a decrease in pulmonary compliance of less than 50 ml/cm H_2O and in functional residual capacity (FRC). The decrease in FRC is secondary to microatelectasis and edema found with the lung injury (Case & Sabo, 1992). There is a right to left shunt of more than 20% of the cardiac output at 100% oxygen because of the increasing edema (Case & Sabo, 1992). Alveolar to arterial gradient increases from a normal of less than 15 to 20 mm Hg to an increase of up to 200 to 500 mm Hg with ARDS (Matus & Glennon, 1988).

9. What clinical signs and symptoms are seen with early ARDS?

Apprehension and restlessness are seen early in the course of ARDS. The patient may also complain of dyspnea. As the process continues, the patient becomes more agitated and dyspneic with changes in mental acuity (Enger, 1989).

10. Tissue hypoxia is a major finding in ARDS. What assessment findings in the following systems would indicate ARDS: central nervous, cardiovascular, pulmonary, renal, gastrointestinal/hepatic, and musculoskeletal systems?

a. Central nervous system
   (1) Agitation
   (2) Changes in mental acuity
   (3) Restlessness
b. Cardiovascular system
   (1) Right ventricular failure
   (2) Decreased cardiac output
   (3) Dysrhythmias
c. Pulmonary system
   (1) Tachypnea
d. Renal system
   (1) Decreased urine output
(Enger, 1989)

11. What is the goal of treatment in ARDS?

Treatment goals for ARDS are correction of physiologic abnormalities, limitation or suppression of alveolar inflammation, and prevention of complications (Hudson, 1990).

12. What is the principal treatment for ARDS? List and describe the types of ventilatory support available.

The main treatment for ARDS is use of mechanical ventilation. Controlled mechanical ventilation (CMV), assisted ventilation, and intermittent ventilation are types of ventilatory support. CMV is used to provide total control of the patient's respiratory rate and volume and to give the patient's muscles a chance to rest (Ashworth, 1990; Richless, 1991).

Assisted ventilation is a means of providing assistance to the patient's own breathing efforts. During the acute phase assisted ventilation is rarely used because, if the patient's ventilatory efforts fail, there is no backup (Ashworth, 1990). Assist/control mode ventilation allows for the patient to initiate each breath, and the ventilator will then assist the patient to reach a preset volume. Since the patient controls the rate with assist/control mode ventilatory support, a rapid respiratory rate is often a major problem (Ashworth, 1990; Richless, 1991).

Intermittent mandatory ventilation (IMV) is used to deliver a preset rate and volume to the patient. However, the patient may also breathe spontaneously, and the IMV is synchronized with the patient's spontaneous breathing efforts. Unfortunately, with IMV the patient may be required to increase his or her efforts to breathe spontaneously (Ashworth, 1990; Richless, 1991).

Inverse ratio ventilation (IRV) reverses the normal pattern of breathing seen with ventilatory support and causes expiration to be greater than inspiration. This allows the next breath to start before total exhalation is accomplished, allowing for more time for alveolar ventilation and less time for alveolar collapse (Juarez, 1992; Richless, 1991). IRV is uncomfortable for the patient and may require sedation or paralysis (Richless, 1991). IRV is used when the patient has an intolerance to high PEEP levels or remains hypoxemic on PEEP and conventional therapy is not working (Juarez, 1992).

Pressure support ventilation is used in conjunction with the patient's own spontaneous breathing and helps the patient overcome the work of breathing while augmenting the patient's own efforts (Ashworth, 1990). This is accomplished by augmenting the patient's volume, using a set amount of airway pressure (Richless, 1991). The advantages of pressure support ventilation are a decrease in the work of breathing and an increase in patient control and comfort (Ashworth, 1990; Richless, 1991).

13. Describe nonventilator means of pulmonary support.

Extracorporeal membrane oxygenation (ECMO) is a means of pulmonary support that does not use a ventilator. ECMO is used when the chance of recovery from ARDS is poor and as a means of decreasing the FiO_2 concentration (Dirkes, Dickinson, & Valentine, 1992). It provides external support for the lung by circulating blood through an external circulation where CO_2 is removed and oxygen is added. This process decreases the risk of barotrauma related to the increased FiO_2 and increased pressures seen when a ventilator is used. Criteria for patient selection include length of ventilatory support, reversible respiratory failure, and early initiation (Dirkes et al., 1992).

There are two types of ECMO: venoarterial and venovenous. Venoarterial ECMO is most frequently used because it does not require good cardiac function, whereas the venovenous method does. The disadvantage to the venoarterial method is the ligation of the common carotid artery and cannulation of the femoral artery. In addition, there is the risk of embolization in the arterial circulation. The venoarterial method is useful when the patient is hemodynamically unstable and requires vasoactive drugs (Dirkes et al., 1992).

14. What is the role of oxygen-free radicals in ARDS?

Oxygen-free radicals are released by activated neutrophils. Neutrophil activation causes an increase in oxygen consumption and metabolic pathway activation, resulting in a release of oxygen-free radicals. In small amounts these radicals have a bactericidal activity. However, as the neutrophil activation continues, the larger quantities of radicals cause injury to normal lung tissue (Vaughan & Brooks, 1990).

15. What are some of the pharmacologic interventions used in ARDS?

The pharmacologic agents used are dependent on the underlying processes being treated. Dopamine and dobutamine may be used to support cardiovascular dynamics through increasing cardiac output and, hence, blood pressure. Antibiotics are frequently used because of the increased risk of pulmonary infection in patients with ARDS (Vaughan & Brooks, 1990). Neuromuscular blocking agents and sedatives are also used to aid with ventilatory support.

16. What role does hemodynamic monitoring play in the management of ARDS?

Mechanical ventilation may have a great effect on cardiac output. Hemodynamic monitoring may assist in determining the effect of mechanical ventilation and PEEP on the cardiac output and arterial oxygenation (Vaughan & Brooks, 1990).

17. Describe appropriate nursing diagnoses seen with ARDS.

Nursing diagnoses vary according to which body systems are affected and which complications occur with ARDS. The most common nursing diagnoses include the following:

- ➤ impaired tissue perfusion
- ➤ alteration in cardiac output
- ➤ ineffective breathing pattern
- ➤ ineffective airway clearance
- ➤ impaired gas exchange
- ➤ alteration in nutrition
- ➤ anxiety
- ➤ alteration in communication
- ➤ high risk for infection
- ➤ high risk for impaired skin integrity

(Case & Sabo, 1992; Enger, 1989; Vaughan & Brooks, 1990).

18. What is the nurse's overall goal in caring for the ARDS patient?

The nurse's role in the care of the ARDS patient is to be aware of potential complications and through nursing assessment and interventions help to prevent complications associated with ARDS.

REFERENCES

Adult Respiratory Distress Syndrome

Ashworth, L. (1990). Pressure support ventilation. *Critical Care Nurse,* *10*(7), 20–27.

Case, S., & Sabo, C. (1992). Adult respiratory distress syndrome: A deadly complication of trauma. *Focus on Critical Care, 19*(2), 116–121.

Dirkes, S., Dickinson, S., & Valentine, J. (1992, October). Acute respiratory failure and ECMO. *Critical Care Nurse.* 39–47.

Enger, E.L. (1989). Pulmonary artery wedge pressure: When it's valid, when it's not. *Critical Care Nursing Clinics of North America, 1*(3), 603–618.

Hudson, L. (1990). The prediction and prevention of ARDS. *Respiratory Care, 35*(2), 161–173.

Juarez, P. (1992). Mechanical ventilation for the patient with severe ARDS. *Critical Care Nurse, 12*(4), 34–39.

Matus, V.W., & Glennon, S.A. (1988). Respiratory disorders. In M.R. Kinney, D.R. Packa, and S.B. Dunbar (Eds.), *AACN clinical reference for critical care nursing* (2nd ed.). St Louis: Mosby.

Richless, C. (1991). Current trends in mechanical ventilation. *Critical Care Nurse, 11*(3), 41–50.

Shinnick, M. (1992). ARDS in the postoperative cardiac surgery patient: A case study. *Critical Care Nurse, 12*(4), 12–17.

Vaughan, P., & Brooks, C. (1990). Adult respiratory distress syndrome: A complication of shock. *Critical Care Nursing Clinics of North America, 2*(2), 235–253.

2

Pulmonary Embolism

Laura S. Platt Smith, MSN, RN
Sheila Drake Melander, DSN, RN, FCCM

CASE PRESENTATION

Sandra Brown, a 35-year-old woman, was admitted to the hospital for a cholecystectomy. The admission history and physical examination revealed a healthy white woman with no history of medical problems or abnormalities except cholelithiasis and obesity. She is married and has two children. She denies taking any medications except birth control pills. Mrs. Brown's surgery is scheduled for tomorrow morning. Her preoperative diagnostic data were

BP 140/80
HR 88 bpm
Respirations 22/min
Temperature 37.1° C (98.9° F)
Hgb 15 g/dl
Hct 39%
RBCs $5.1 \times 10^6/mm^3$

WBCs $6000/mm^3$
Platelets $148,000/mm^3$
PT 13.2 s
PTT 35 s
Urine analysis normal
ECG normal sinus rhythm
CXR normal

Postoperative Day 1

Mrs. Brown tolerated the surgery without complications and was admitted to the step-down surgical unit. Vital signs remained stable. A nasogastric tube was connected to suction. A solution of 5% dextrose in 0.45% normal saline was infusing at 125 ml/h. Meperidine hydrochloride (Demerol) and hydroxyzine hydrochloride (Vistaril) were given intramuscularly every 3 to 4 hours for pain control. Mrs. Brown was informed about the need to increase her activity level and was assisted out of bed to a chair. However, Mrs. Brown stated that the pain was too intense and that she was only able to tolerate sitting up out of bed for 30 minutes.

Postoperative Day 2

Mrs. Brown's vital signs remained stable with the exception of a low-grade fever. The nasogastric tube was removed, and she began drinking clear liquids. Laboratory values remained normal with the exception of a slightly low hemoglobin count (10.8 g/dl) and hematocrit (35%). Mrs. Brown was progressing well with the exception of complaints of incisional pain and frequent requests for pain medication. When encouraged to get out of bed, her response was, "I can't get up right now. It hurts too much."

Postoperative Day 3

After morning report, the registered nurse found Mrs. Brown to be very restless and apprehensive. She was complaining of shortness of breath, chest pain that worsened on inspiration, and right calf pain. The nurse's assessment revealed crackles in the left lower lobe, labored respirations, and diaphoresis. The right calf was found to be erythematous, warm, and tender. Vital signs were

BP	160/90	Respirations	36/min
HR	124 bpm	Temperature	37.8° C (100.1° F)

Mrs. Brown was placed in a semi-Fowler position, and oxygen was started at 4 L/min per nasal cannula. The physician was notified, and stat arterial blood gases (ABGs), an electrocardiogram (ECG), and a chest x-ray (CXR) were ordered. Following are the results of these tests:

pH	7.52	SaO_2	95%
$PaCO_2$	27 mm Hg	CXR	bibasilar atelectasis
PaO_2	78 mm Hg	ECG	sinus tachycardia

A heparin bolus of 10,000 U was administered, followed by a continuous infusion of 1000 U/h. A ventilation-perfusion scan ($\dot{V}/\dot{Q}$ scan) revealed perfusion defects of the left lung with normal ventilation. Therefore a pulmonary embolism (PE) was suspected, and Mrs. Brown was transferred to the intensive care unit (ICU). A pulmonary angiogram was performed, which verified the diagnosis.

Postoperative Day 4

The next day, Mrs. Brown's respiratory distress worsened, requiring intubation and mechanical ventilation. A pulmonary artery (Swan-Ganz) catheter was inserted for hemodynamic monitoring. The following hemodynamic values were then obtained:

pH	7.58	PAWP	18 mm Hg
$PaCO_2$	24 mm Hg	PAP	38/20 mm Hg
PaO_2	60 mm Hg	PT	17.1 s
SaO_2	80%	PTT	49.2 s

Pulmonary Embolism

1. Discuss four potential origins of a PE: venous thrombosis, fat emboli, air emboli, and catheter emboli. Include a thorough discussion of the most common origin.

2. What is Virchow's triad? Describe the progression of a thrombus to a PE.

3. What alterations in pulmonary status occur as a result of PE?

4. How reflective of the diagnosis were Mrs. Brown's hemodynamic values?

5. What risk factors for PE are exhibited by Mrs. Brown?

6. What are the clinical manifestations of PE?

7. What diagnostic tests may be used in the diagnosis of PE?

8. What is the rationale for heparin therapy for Mrs. Brown? Describe three other fibrinolytic therapy modalities that may be used in the management of PE?

9. How can the nurse assist the patient in the prevention of PE?

10. What are the nursing responsibilities for the patient with PE?

11. Develop a list of nursing diagnoses appropriate for Mrs. Brown.

QUESTIONS AND ANSWERS

Pulmonary Embolism

1. Discuss four potential origins of a PE: venous thrombosis, fat emboli, air emboli, and catheter emboli. Include a thorough discussion of the most common origin.

   Venous Thrombosis

   According to Alspach (1991), a majority of pulmonary emboli originate from thrombosis in the popliteal and iliofemoral veins. The risk of PE from thrombosis in the calf veins is low; however, the risk is much higher when affected veins are above the knee (Currie, 1990).

   Fat Emboli

   Fat emboli are associated with multiple skeletal fractures and traumatic injury to the long bones and pelvis (Clochesy, Breu, Cardin, Rudy, & Whitaker, 1993). Fat globules are released from the marrow of a fractured bone into the venous circulation and may become lodged in the lung (Slye, 1991).

   Air Emboli

   Air emboli result when a large bolus of air is introduced into the venous circulation. The air entering the venous system is trapped by the forward flow of blood and lodges against the pulmonary valve (Thielen, 1990).

   Catheter Emboli

   Catheter emboli may result from excessive manipulation during insertion of a peripheral or central venous catheter. A portion of the catheter may break off and travel to the lung. Other origins of PE, although rare, include amniotic fluid emboli, septic embolism, tumor embolism, and the right atrium or ventricle emboli (Currie, 1990).

2. What is Virchow's triad? Describe the progression of a thrombus to a PE.

   According to Currie (1990), Virchow's triad identifies the three factors primarily responsible for venous thrombosis: (1) venous stasis, (2) intimal or (endothelial) vessel damage, and (3) hypercoagulability. Venous stasis is the most common cause of venous thrombosis and usually develops from immobility (Dickinson & Bury, 1989). Vascular wall damage usually occurs as a result of poorly placed intravenous lines, irritating intravenous fluids, or traumatic injury (Dickinson & Bury, 1989). Hypercoagulability may be inherited or may occur as a result of such factors as dehydration, pregnancy, and oral contraceptives (Dickinson & Bury, 1989).

Increased venous pressure, direct trauma, or sudden muscle contraction as when a person stands can dislodge the thrombus. This is most likely to occur within 72 hours of the thrombus formation (Currie, 1990). Once dislodged, the thrombus enters systemic circulation and travels through the right side of the heart, lodging in the pulmonary artery. Larger emboli may lodge in a large branch of the pulmonary artery, whereas smaller clots may block several smaller distal branches of the pulmonary vasculature (Hartshorn, Lamborn, & Noll, 1993).

3. **What alterations in pulmonary status occur as a result of PE?**

Primary Consequences

Three primary consequences in pulmonary status associated with PE include (1) increased alveolar dead space, (2) pneumoconstriction, and (3) loss of surfactant (Roberts, 1987). Alveolar dead space is an alveolar area that is ventilated but not well perfused, resulting in an elevated ventilation-perfusion ($\dot{V}/\dot{Q}$) ratio and $\dot{V}/\dot{Q}$ mismatching. As a result of $\dot{V}/\dot{Q}$ mismatching, this portion of the lung is unable to participate in gas exchange, resulting in hypocarbia (Roberts, 1987). Pneumoconstriction of the terminal bronchioles and alveolar ducts decreases the size of the alveolar dead space, a protective mechanism that shunts inspired air into functioning alveoli. However, this mechanism also increases the work of breathing for the patient (Hartshorn et al., 1993). Bronchoalveolar hypocarbia, hypoxia, humoral agents, and thrombin activation contribute to pneumoconstriction (Roberts, 1987). Pneumoconstriction leads to increased airway resistance, decreased wasted ventilation, and maldistribution of ventilation (Roberts, 1987). The third primary consequence of PE is loss of surfactant, resulting from the reduction of blood flow to the alveoli (Roberts, 1987). According to Hartshorn et al. (1993), the loss of surfactant results in (1) unequal gas distribution, (2) increased pressure within the alveoli requiring more work to inflate the alveoli, (3) alveolar collapse, and (4) atelectasis.

Secondary Consequences

Secondary consequences associated with PE include dyspnea and arterial hypoxemia (Roberts, 1987). Dyspnea is usually associated with tachypnea and results from stimulation of the intrapulmonary receptors in the alveolar-capillary wall (Roberts, 1987). Arterial hypoxemia occurs in approximately 85% to 90% of patients with PE and may result from (1) a decreased cardiac output with widened alveolar-arterial oxygen tension differences or (2) overperfusion of nonembolized lung zones that cannot be sufficiently ventilated to maintain adequate oxygenation (Roberts, 1987). Hypoxemia may also result from reperfusion of poorly ventilated lung zones on resolution of the emboli (Roberts, 1987).

4. How reflective of the diagnosis were Mrs. Brown's hemodynamic values?

Pulmonary Arterial Hypertension

According to Roberts (1987), the main hemodynamic result of a PE is pulmonary arterial hypertension. Pulmonary arterial hypertension occurs when over 50% of the pulmonary vasculature is occluded, resulting in a reduction of the available cross-sectional area (Roberts, 1987). Increased pulmonary arterial resistance, pulmonary artery pressure, and right ventricular workload result from a reduction in the cross-sectional area of the arterial bed (Roberts, 1987). As a result of the increased pulmonary arterial pressure and pulmonary resistance, the right ventricle will increase its workload to maintain cardiac output. However, the right ventricle may fail if the pulmonary artery pressure is severely increased, resulting in a decrease in cardiac output and shock (Roberts, 1987).

Pulmonary Infarction

An infrequent complication of PE is pulmonary infarction. It occurs when an embolism completely obstructs a major branch of a pulmonary artery and when other sources of oxygen from pulmonary arteries, bronchial arteries, and alveoli are inadequate for lung tissue survival (Currie, 1990). Pulmonary infarction is more common in patients with preexisting cardiopulmonary disease (Currie, 1990). According to Hartshorn et al. (1993), pulmonary infarction is manifested by alveolar hemorrhage, consolidation, and tissue necrosis and may be further complicated by lung abscesses and pleural effusion.

5. What risk factors for PE are exhibited by Mrs. Brown?

Three risk factors exhibited by Mrs. Brown were obesity, oral contraceptive use, and her recent cholecystectomy, which led to a decrease in mobility. Oral contraceptives are a risk, since estrogen increases coagulability and platelet aggregation (Hartshorn et al., 1993). Alspach (1991) identified the following additional risk factors for PE:

- history of congestive heart failure
- acute myocardial infarction
- shock
- malignancy
- polycythemia vera
- trauma
- dysproteinemia
- diabetes
- burns
- varicose veins
- previous deep vein thrombosis (DVT) or PE

Roberts (1987) identified additional risk factors to include pregnancy, age over 60 years, and pulmonary disease.

6. What are the clinical manifestations of PE?

Dyspnea is the most frequent symptom of PE and results from the development of alveolar dead space (Roberts, 1987). Pleuritic chest pain may result from atelectasis or pulmonary infarction (Roberts, 1987). Other findings include cough, hemoptysis, calf pain, syncope, palpitations, and anxiety.

The two most common physical signs of PE are tachypnea and tachycardia (Roberts, 1987). Hypotension may occur in massive PE when sympathetic stimulation is ineffective. Pneumoconstriction and loss of surfactant may lead to crackles, wheezes, and decreased breath sounds (Roberts, 1987). Also, the presence of an accentuated pulmonic heart sound indicates severe ventricular compromise. A systolic murmur resulting from the blood flow through a partially obstructed pulmonary artery may also be present (Roberts, 1987). Additional physical signs include pleural friction rub, diaphoresis, cyanosis, jugular venous distension, edema, and phlebitis (Hartshorn et al., 1993).

7. What diagnostic tests may be used in the diagnosis of PE?

The diagnosis of PE is crucial since the disease is treatable but often abruptly fatal if left undiagnosed. The diagnostic tools used include $\dot{V}/\dot{Q}$ scanning, pulmonary angiogram, ABGs, CXR, and ECG.

$\dot{V}/\dot{Q}$ Scan

When PE is clinically suspected, the first diagnostic test to be completed should be a $\dot{V}/\dot{Q}$ scan (Currie, 1990). According to Currie (1990), perfusion defects with normal ventilation indicate PE in 90% of patients. However, false-positive results do occur. Bell and Simons (cited in

Stratton, 1990) revealed that 83% of $\dot{V}/\dot{Q}$ scans were erroneously reported as positive. According to Currie (1990), a negative $\dot{V}/\dot{Q}$ scan is a reliable method for ruling out PE with minimal risk to the patient.

Pulmonary Angiography

According to Alspach (1991), pulmonary angiography is the most definitive diagnostic test for PE. The test is used to validate the results of the $\dot{V}/\dot{Q}$ scan. However, angiography is invasive and requires injection of a contrast media directly into the pulmonary arteries. According to Currie (1990), pulmonary angiography is indicated when the diagnosis of PE remains in doubt such as in a nondiagnostic $\dot{V}/\dot{Q}$ scan. It is also indicated when thrombolytic or surgical therapy is necessary or when anticoagulation therapy is contraindicated (Currie, 1990). Positive results from an angiogram will show a filling defect or cutoff of blood flow of the affected pulmonary vessels (Clochesy et al., 1993). Potential complications include cardiac perforation, arrhythmias, and allergic reactions to dye. However, the complication rate is only 4% (Currie, 1990).

Arterial Blood Gases

ABG analysis may be helpful but not definitive for the diagnosis of PE. According to Currie (1990), hypoxemia is present in up to 88% of patients. However, Po_2 is not a specific indicator of PE, as it is decreased in many other clinical conditions. According to Alspach (1991), ABG findings may indicate respiratory alkalosis as a result of hyperventilation and an increased alveolar-arterial (A-a) gradient. It is used as a guide with oxygen or ventilation therapy and to determine acid-base balance.

Chest x-ray

As with ABGs, a CXR may be useful in the diagnosis of PE but is not used to make a definitive diagnosis. According to Clochesy et al. (1993), CXR findings include an elevated hemidiaphragm, atelectasis, infiltration, pleural effusion, a wedge-shaped density in the periphery, or an enlarged pulmonary artery. However, CXR findings may also be normal. It is necessary to corroborate findings of $\dot{V}/\dot{Q}$ scans with a CXR within 12 hours of the $\dot{V}/\dot{Q}$ scan to rule out other pathology (Stratton, 1990).

Electrocardiogram

According to Hartshorn et al. (1993), ECG findings are usually normal with PE unless a massive pulmonary embolism has occurred. Potential ECG changes include sinus tachycardia, nonspecific T-wave changes, right axis deviation, and a right bundle branch block (Clochesy et al., 1993). The ECG provides supportive information and can help to rule out a myocardial infarction (Currie, 1990).

Since PE is frequently related to venous thrombosis, an evaluation of the leg veins must be included in the diagnostic process. The studies may include venography, radiofibrinogen leg scan, radiovenography, and Doppler ultrasound scan. A diagnosis of deep venous thrombosis (DVT) does not necessarily confirm the diagnosis of PE; however, it may impact the therapeutic plan (Currie, 1990).

8. **What is the rationale for heparin therapy for Mrs. Brown? Describe three other fibrinolytic therapy modalities that may be used in the management of PE?**

Anticoagulant Therapy

Intravenous heparin, an anticoagulant, has been identified as the treatment of choice for PE or DVT (Currie, 1990). By enhancing the effect of antithrombin III to inactivate coagulation factors IXa and Xa, heparin can prevent progress of the thrombus or embolus and can decrease the incidence of recurrent PE (Currie, 1990). After a loading dose, a maintenance infusion of heparin is started to maintain a partial thromboplastin time (PTT) of 1.5 to 2 times normal. Heparin is usually given for 7 to 10 days. In Mrs. Brown's case, the second set of clotting times indicates that the dose of heparin is nontherapeutic and that there is a need for adjustment. PTT levels should be evaluated daily to maintain a therapeutic level of heparin.

According to Hartshorn et al. (1993), warfarin (Coumadin) is usually started on the fourth or fifth day of heparin therapy to maintain a prothrombin time (PT) of 1.5 to 2 times normal. Warfarin prevents thrombus progression and permits fibrinolysis by suppression of factors II, VII, IX, and X (Currie, 1990). Contraindications to anticoagulant therapy include active bleeding, subarachnoid hemorrhage, recent brain, eye, or spinal surgery, or malignant hypertension (Currie, 1990).

Three other medical therapeutic options include thrombolytic therapy, inferior vena caval interruption, and pulmonary embolectomy.

Thrombolytic Therapy

According to Clochesy et al. (1993), thrombolytic therapy with agents such as streptokinase and urokinase is indicated for patients with severe hemodynamic compromise. According to Vermilya (1989), thrombolytic agents are capable of lysis of the pulmonary thrombus, but in 1989 no studies had shown a decrease in mortality among patients with PE who were treated with these agents. Two major weaknesses of thrombolytic therapy include the cost and the increased risk of bleeding involved with the treatment (Hartshorn et al., 1993).

Inferior Vena Cava Interruption

Inferior vena cava (IVC) interruption should be used in those patients in whom anticoagulation therapy is contraindicated, when there is recurrent PE or complications from thrombolytic therapy, and for prevention of further PE (Currie, 1990). Ligation, clips, or filters can be used. However, the Greenfield filter, which is placed transvenously under fluoroscopy, is often preferred (Currie, 1990). The complication rate for inferior vena caval filters is low. However, venous stasis sometimes does occur. IVC interruption will prevent recurrences of major PE but will not prevent minor recurrences or emboli originating from sites other than the lower extremities (Currie, 1990).

Pulmonary Embolectomy

Pulmonary embolectomy may be used in the patient with massive PE unresponsive to other therapies. An embolectomy may be performed as a life-saving technique in patients who have become severely hemodynamically unstable. However, the surgery may also be used in the treatment of chronic thromboembolic pulmonary hypertension. In this case, the mortality rate is significantly higher when the patient's pulmonary artery pressure exceeds 30 mm Hg (Buchalter, Groves, & Zorn, 1992). Pulmonary embolectomy is most often completed via median sternotomy with cardiopulmonary bypass. It is suggested that at the time of surgery an IVC interruption be completed to prevent recurrent emboli (Buchalter et al., 1992).

9. How can the nurse assist the patient in the prevention of PE?

The first step in preventing PE is to identify those patients at risk for developing a DVT or PE. Once these patients are identified, the nurse can help prevent PE by instituting ambulation and range of motion exercises soon after surgery. According to Hartshorn et al. (1993), intermittent pneumatic compression stockings may be effective in prevention in that they increase venous flow. Patients must be taught the following measures for prevention of PE: (1) avoiding pillows below the knee; (2) avoiding crossing the legs; (3) changing positions frequently and increasing mobility; and (4) using elastic, gradient, or pneumatic compression stockings. According to Currie (1990), pharmacologic agents suitable for prophylactic use include low-dose heparin, oral anticoagulants, and dextran.

10. What are the nursing responsibilities for the patient with PE?

As a result of hypoxia and ischemia from PE, the patient will experience chest pain and anxiety. Placing the patient in a semi-Fowler position will promote lung expansion and improve ventilation and perfusion (Dickinson & Bury, 1989). The patient should be encouraged to remain in bed and to avoid unnecessary activities with the intent of decreasing myocardial oxygen demand. ABGs must be monitored for hypoxemia and respiratory alkalosis or acidosis. Good pulmonary hygiene may be required if secretions are interfering with airway clearance. Oxygen should be used to decrease ischemia and increase tissue oxygenation. A narcotic analgesic may also be used to decrease pain and anxiety.

Assessment of intake and output is important, as the changes in alveolar membrane permeability may result in an increase in pulmonary congestion (Hartshorn et al., 1993). The increase in pulmonary artery resistance may also increase the risk of pulmonary edema and congestive heart failure; therefore the nurse must monitor for jugular vein distension, peripheral edema, dysrhythmias, and tachypnea (Hartshorn et al., 1993). Intubation and mechanical ventilation may be required in more severely ill patients to promote tissue oxygenation.

If a large portion of the pulmonary vasculature bed is obstructed, the patient may go into shock. Therefore the nurse is responsible for monitoring for signs of shock such as tachycardia, hypotension, and decreased cardiac output.

Once the crisis has resolved, the patient must be taught the signs, symptoms, and risk factors associated with the development of a thrombus. The patient will most likely receive maintenance doses of an oral anticoagulant such as warfarin (Coumadin). Therefore it is necessary to review the medication's purpose and side effects such as bleeding. The nurse is also responsible for monitoring PT and PTT levels in the presence of anticoagulant therapy in addition to assessing for signs of bleeding (Dickinson & Bury, 1989).

11. Develop a list of nursing diagnoses appropriate for Mrs. Brown.

According to Hartshorn et al. (1993) the following list of nursing diagnoses is appropriate for the patient with PE:

- ➤ activity intolerance
- ➤ anxiety
- ➤ decreased cardiac output
- ➤ ineffective breathing patterns
- ➤ ineffective family coping
- ➤ impaired gas exchange
- ➤ potential fluid volume excess
- ➤ potential for injury
- ➤ knowledge deficit
- ➤ pain
- ➤ alteration in tissue perfusion

Pulmonary Embolism

Alspach, J. G. (Ed.). (1991). *American Association of Critical Care Nurses: Core curriculum for critical care nursing* (4th ed.). Philadelphia: Saunders.

Buchalter, S. E., Groves, R. H., & Zorn, G. L. (1992). Surgical management of chronic pulmonary thromboembolic disease. *Clinics of Chest Medicine, 13*(1), 17–21.

Clochesy, J. M., Breu, C., Cardin, S., Rudy, E. B., & Whitaker, A. A. (1993). *Critical care nursing.* Philadelphia: Saunders.

Currie, D. L. (1990). Pulmonary embolism: Diagnosis and management. *Critical Care Nurse Quarterly, 13*(2), 41–49.

Dickinson, S. P., & Bury, G. M. (1989). Pulmonary embolism: Anatomy of a crisis. *Nursing, 4,* 34–41.

Hartshorn, J., Lamborn, M., & Noll, M. L. (1993). *Introduction to critical care nursing.* Philadelphia: Saunders.

Roberts, S. L. (1987). Pulmonary tissue perfusion altered: Emboli. *Heart and Lung, 16*(2), 128–137.

Slye, D. A. (1991). Orthopedic complications: Compartment syndrome, fat embolism syndrome, and venous thromboembolism. *Nursing Clinics of North America, 26*(1), 113–131.

Stratton, D. A. (1990). Ventilation-perfusion scintigraphy in diagnosis of pulmonary thromboembolism. *Focus on Critical Care, 17*(4), 287–293.

Thielen, J. B. (1990). Air emboli: A potentially lethal complication of central venous lines. *Focus on Critical Care, 17*(5), 374–383.

Vermilya, S. K. (1989). Future indications for thrombolytic therapy with tissue plasminogen activator. *Journal of Emergency Nursing, 15*(2), 204–206.

3

Pulmonary Contusion

Nancy D. Blasdell, MSN, RN
Sheila Drake Melander, DSN, RN, FCCM

CASE PRESENTATION

Mr. Fields, a 54-year-old man, was not wearing his seat belt when he fell asleep at the wheel and hit a bridge abutment head on at approximately 35 miles per hour. He was arousable at the scene, slightly disoriented, and was able to follow commands. Mr. Fields complained of chest and back pain. Oxygen at 2 L via nasal cannula and two peripheral lines were started before the patient was transported to the nearest hospital. On arrival at the emergency department, he was alert and cooperative but anxious. He was able to communicate without difficulty. Mr. Fields complained of right-sided chest pain (stated as rib pain); he had marked ecchymosis with medial to lateral progression. Following are diagnostic data on admission:

BP	176/94	K+	3.1 mmol/L
HR	138 bpm	Hgb	12.0 g/dl
Respirations	32/min and slightly labored	Hct	36.3 vol/dl
Temperature	37.2° C (99° F)	WBCs	10,500/mm³

pH	7.43*
Po₂	108 mm Hg
Pco₂	37 mm Hg

*Arterial blood gases (ABGs) with patient on 2 L oxygen by nasal cannula

The chest x-ray (CXR) revealed four fractured ribs on the right side and two fractured ribs on the left side. A fractured right femur was also identified. Findings from computed tomographic (CT) scans of the head, chest, and abdomen were negative, and findings from the electrocardiogram (ECG) were normal except for a sinus tachycardia. Physical examination revealed symmetric chest expansion, a midline trachea, bruising of the right chest and flank, and some facial bruising. Auscultation of the lungs revealed fine crackles in the right lung and clear breath sounds in the left lung field. The CXR revealed a right pulmonary contusion. Mr. Fields was transferred to the telemetry unit for monitoring.

Physician's Orders:

D5 in 0.45 NS at 75 ml/h
Clear liquids
Accurate intake and output
Cefazolin 1 g every 8 hours

Meperidine (Demerol) 50 mg intramuscularly was ordered for pain every 4 hours.

Mr. Fields was taught incentive spirometry and used it every hour faithfully. Mr. Fields received education regarding the extent of his injuries and the potential dangers they may present. Mr. Fields progressed well and was discharged on the second day.

QUESTIONS

Pulmonary Contusion

1. What is the mechanism of injury resulting in a pulmonary contusion?

2. What is the pathophysiology of a pulmonary contusion?

3. How does a pulmonary contusion affect respiratory function?

4. What diagnostic methods are required for the diagnosis and monitoring of pulmonary contusion?

5. What is the nurse's responsibility in the diagnosis of pulmonary contusion?

6. Why is the automatic application of pneumatic antishock garments to trauma victims prohibited?

7. What is the most common complication of pulmonary contusion?

8. List the most common antibiotic treatment for the following organisms causing pneumonia: *Streptococcus pneumoniae, Staphylococcus aureus* (methicillin sensitive and methicillin resistant), *Haemophilus influenzae, Klebsiella pneumoniae, Pseudomonas aeruginosa, Mycoplasma pneumoniae, Legionella, Branhamella catarrhalis,* group B streptococcus, *Chlamydia psittaci, Francisella tularensis, Coxiella burnetii, Yersinia pestis, Bacillus anthracis,* and *Bacteroides fragilis.*

9. List 10 types of treatment for a patient who has a flail chest.

10. Name seven nursing interventions for a patient with a pulmonary contusion.

11. As the nurse is discharging Mr. Fields, what discharge instructions would be appropriate?

12. What nursing diagnosis might be appropriate for the care of a patient diagnosed with pulmonary contusion?

QUESTIONS AND ANSWERS

Pulmonary Contusion

1. What is the mechanism of injury resulting in a pulmonary contusion?

Pulmonary contusions are typically a result of a blunt trauma and can be potentially life threatening. The blunt forces causing pulmonary contusions are largely from motor vehicle accidents, falls, accidents, farming, physical alterations, cardiopulmonary resuscitation, and falling objects (Sahd, 1991). This type of injury frequently accompanies multiple injuries and rarely is isolated (Sahd, 1991).

2. What is the pathophysiology of a pulmonary contusion?

Disruption in the pulmonary vasculature allows blood to enter the alveoli and interstitium (Luchtefeld, 1990). The symptoms of pulmonary contusion typically are insidious but progressive in nature (Luchtefeld, 1990). Therefore, with knowledge of the mechanism of injury one should suspect a pulmonary contusion and demonstrate astute assessment skills. Interstitial edema begins early and within 24 hours can be massive, resulting in perfusion without ventilation, which leads to intrapulmonary shunting and hypoxemia (Luchtefeld, 1990). Hypoxemia refractory to increases in oxygen is a sign of intrapulmonary shunting (Luchtefeld, 1990).

3. How does a pulmonary contusion affect respiratory function?

Blunt chest trauma usually bruises the lung; however, pulmonary tears or lacerations may be seen (Sahd, 1991). The area of injury may be localized or generalized and is typically seen with rib fractures and flail chest (Sahd, 1991). The initial injury results in hemorrhage and alveolar edema, with general inflammation seen throughout the surrounding areas of injury (Sahd, 1991). Disruption in the alveolar-capillary unit results in the following: hypercapnia, increased pulmonary blood flow, systemic hypoxia, and ventilation-perfusion imbalance (Sahd, 1991). Although pulmonary contusion is typically a secondary diagnosis, the need for close monitoring, physical assessment, and identification of subtle changes is extremely important (Sahd, 1991).

4. What diagnostic methods are required for the diagnosis and monitoring of pulmonary contusion?

Physical findings may include ecchymosis at the site of impact, guarding of the site, hemoptysis, dull percussion, and moist crackles (Sahd, 1991). Other findings include dyspnea; tan, bloody, or clear sputum; decreased level of consciousness; tachypnea; tachycardia; decreased capillary refill; and restlessness (Luchtefeld, 1988). When pulmonary contusion occurs with flail chest, subcutaneous emphysema, paradoxical chest movement, and increased pain are also normal occurrences (Luchtefeld, 1990).

According to Sahd (1991), the hallmark sign of pulmonary contusion is arterial and venous hypoxemia following chest trauma. Several tissue oxygenation measures can be used to identify pulmonary contusion and to monitor the patient's progress in addition to the partial pressure of oxygen in arterial and venous blood (PaO_2 and PvO_2). The hemoglobin saturation of venous blood (SvO_2) will identify changes in tissue oxygenation and perfusion at the cellular level before any changes are seen clinically. Arterial and venous oxygen content (CaO_2 and CvO_2) are necessary to calculate some measures of cardiac output and estimate intrapulmonary shunting (Sahd, 1991). The alveolar-arterial oxygen difference ($PA–aO_2$) identifies pulmonary diffusion capacity and is a reliable indicator of pulmonary contusion (Sahd, 1991). A low PaO_2, wide PA-aO_2, and radiologic changes confirm the presence of pulmonary contusion (Sahd, 1991).

Radiologic changes within 6 hours of injury typically show patchy, irregular areas of consolidation to complete consolidation of one or both lungs reflecting intraalveolar hemorrhage (Sahd, 1991). The lung will appear larger because of edema and will push the diaphragm down. The CXR lags behind the pathophysiology by several hours, indicating a greater injury than is apparent on x-ray (Sahd, 1991). CT scan is one of the most accurate methods for assessing pulmonary damage in trauma (Sahd, 1991). The CT scan can identify small tears and lacerations by allowing transverse sections of the lung to be studied (Sahd, 1991).

5. What is the nurse's responsibility in the diagnosis of pulmonary contusion?

The diagnosis of pulmonary contusion is dependant on physical examination findings, tissue oxygenation measures, and CXR and CT results (Clochesy, Breu, Cardin, Rudy, & Whittaker, 1993; Sahd, 1991).

The diagnosis is often delayed until signs of complications occur as a result of associated injuries and because of lack of radiographic changes and external evidence of injury (Sahd, 1991). Inspection, auscultation, history taking, and monitoring of laboratory and diagnostic data allow the nurse to identify potential future changes in the patient's condition, since signs and symptoms may not develop for 24 to 48 hours (Clochesy, et al., 1993; Sahd, 1991).

6. **Why is the automatic application of pneumatic antishock garments to trauma victims prohibited?**

   As a result of an elevation of blood pressure a fresh clot may become easily dislodged by the pulse wave in the pneumatic antishock garment (Huggins, 1990). Also, a possible abrupt increase in blood pressure from return of volume to the central circulation may occur in conjunction with an acute increase in afterload (Huggins, 1990).

7. **What is the most common complication of pulmonary contusion?**

   Pneumonia is the most common complication due to decreased lung bacterial clearance (Hammond, 1990). Prevention is best achieved through surveillance for infection by daily CXR, white blood cell (WBC) count, vital signs, and sputum culture (Hammond, 1990).

   According to Hammond (1990), physical evidence is not always present in the chest trauma patient. A thorough history and evaluation of clinical states is essential. Signs and symptoms include ineffective cough, hemoptysis, increasing shortness of breath, and increasing respirations. Interventions should be geared toward maintaining ventilation and restricting fluids.

8. **List the most common antibiotic treatment for the following organisms causing pneumonia: *Streptococcus pneumoniae*, *Staphylococcus aureus* (methicillin sensitive and methicillin resistant), *Haemophilus influenzae*, *Klebsiella pneumoniae*, *Pseudomonas aeruginosa*, *Mycoplasma pneumoniae*, *Legionella*, *Branhamella catarrhalis*, group B streptococcus, *Chlamydia psittaci*, *Francisella tularensis*, *Coxiella burnetii*, *Yersinia pestis*, *Bacillus anthracis*, and *Bacteroides fragilis*.**

   The common treatments for organisms causing pneumonia are listed in Table 3–1.

9. **List 10 types of treatment for a patient who has a flail chest.**

   Moore, Mattox, and Feliciano (1991) state that flail chest is common with severe thoracic injury. The authors point out that flail chest is "an unstable segment of the normally rigid chest wall that moves sep-

Table 3–1 Antibiotics Commonly Used to Treat Pneumonia

Organism	Antibiotic
Streptococcus pneumoniae	Penicillin Alternate: erythromycin
Staphylococcus aureus (methicillin sensitive)	Oxacillin Alternate: vancomycin
Staphylococcus aureus (methicillin resistant)	Vancomycin Alternate: trimethoprim-sulfamethoxazole
Haemophilus influenzae	Ampicillin Alternate: trimethoprim-sulfamethoxazole
Klebsiella pneumoniae	Cefazolin with gentamicin Alternate: ceftizoxime with amikacin
Pseudomonas aeruginosa	Ticarcillin with gentamicin Alternate: piperacillin with tobramycin
Mycoplasma pneumoniae	Erythromycin Alternate: doxycycline
Legionella	Erythromycin with or without rifampin Alternate: rifampin
Branhamella catarrhalis	Trimethoprim-sulfamethoxazole Alternate: erythromycin
Group B *Streptococcus*	Penicillin Alternate: erythromycin
Chlamydia psittaci	Doxycycline Alternate: chloramphenicol
Francisella tularensis	Gentamicin Alternate: doxycycline
Coxiella burnetii	Doxycycline Alternate: chloramphenicol
Yersinia pestis	Streptomycin Alternate: doxycycline
Bacillus anthracis	Penicillin Alternate: doxycycline
Bacteroides fragilis	Penicillin Alternate: metronidazole

Adapted from McDonnell, K., Fahey, P., & Segal, M. (1987). *Respiratory intensive care.* Boston: Little, Brown & Co.

arately and in an opposite direction from the rest of the thoracic cage during the respiratory cycle."

Moore et al. (1991) suggest that treatment should include the following:

1. mechanical ventilation and endotracheal intubation
2. normal saline IV or lactated Ringer's solution
3. maintenance volume of a balanced crystalloid solution
4. antibiotics and steroids
5. aggressive pulmonary physiotherapy and suctioning
6. incentive spirometry
7. early mobilization

   8. air humidification
   9. intermittent positive pressure breathing
   10. therapeutic fiberoptic bronchoscopy to suction retained secretions and treat atelectasis

10. Name seven nursing interventions for a patient with a pulmonary contusion.

Sahd (1991) stated that nursing care is critical; the nurse should

   1. maintain PEEP setting on ventilation and maintain patient's arterial blood gases
   2. turn the patient to provide adequate ventilation
   3. position the patient with unilateral injury with the injured side up to improve ventilation-perfusion
   4. observe airway for obstruction, clots, or bloody mucus
   5. administer frequent suctioning with the use of saline irrigation of the endotracheal tube
   6. use the semi-Fowler position to assist in inspiratory capacity by decreasing the pressure of the abdominal organs on the diaphragm
   7. control pain, since pain decreases the capacity of inspiration and the volume of the respiration

11. As the nurse is discharging Mr. Fields, what discharge instructions would be appropriate?

Discharge instructions for the pulmonary contusion patient must include information regarding potential change in respiratory status. The patient should be instructed to report immediately to their primary physician any change in respiratory status such as tightness in the chest or difficulty breathing deeply. It is crucial that patients understand that these signs may be signals for impending respiratory difficulties that have developed as a result of their trauma.

12. What nursing diagnosis might be appropriate for the care of a patient diagnosed with pulmonary contusion?

Nursing diagnoses appropriate for the care of the patient diagnosed with pulmonary contusion include the following:

➤ ineffective airway clearance related to decreased pulmonary compliance
➤ impaired gas exchange related to interstitial hemorrhage
➤ ineffective breathing pattern related to decreased pulmonary compliance
➤ anxiety related to unusual muscular effort required for breathing
➤ activity intolerance related to hypoxemia

Pulmonary Contusion

Clochesy, J. M., Breu, C., Cardin, S., Rudy, E., & Whittaker, A. A. (Eds.). (1993). *Critical care nursing*. Philadelphia: Saunders.

Hammond, S. (1990). Chest injuries in the trauma patient. *Nursing Clinics of North America, 25*(1), 1–10.

Huggins, B. (1990). Trauma physiology. *Nursing Clinics of North America, 25*(1), 1–10.

Luchtefeld, W. B. (1990). Pulmonary contusion. *Focus on Critical Care, 17*(6), 482–488.

Moore, E., Mattox, K., & Feliciano, D. (1991). *Trauma* (2nd ed.). Norwalk, CT: Appleton & Lange.

Sahd, L. R. (1991). Pulmonary contusion: The hidden danger in blunt chest trauma. *Critical Care Nurse, 2*(6), 46–57.

Thelan, L. A., Davie, J. K., & Urden, L. D. (1994). *Textbook of critical care nursing: Diagnosis and management*. St. Louis: Mosby–Year Book.

4

Chronic Obstructive Pulmonary Disease with Pneumonia

Sheila Drake Melander, DSN, RN, FCCM

CASE PRESENTATION

Mr. Stevens, a 62-year-old retired coal miner, has been experiencing a productive cough off and on for approximately 3 years. He decided to come to the emergency department because he has experienced difficulty in his breathing pattern on exertion. He stated that he has experienced several bouts of chest colds during the past few years, but this time he stated he "can't seem to shake this round." His wife stated that he is allergic to penicillin.

Mr. Stevens stated during his history that he has smoked two packs of cigarettes a day for 25 years. Crackles were noted in the lower bases of his lungs with an occasional expiratory wheeze. He also stated that he had been running a low-grade fever for approximately 2 to 3 days and had experienced chills and general weakness. CXR disclosed some consolidation in the right lower lobe. Bronchography revealed nonuniform tapering of airway. Following are additional diagnostic data:

BP	158/98	WBCs	20,000/mm^3
HR	107 bpm	Hct	56%
Respirations	32/min	Gram's stain	Negative
Temperature	38.9° C (102° F)		

pH	7.25
Po$_2$	52 mm Hg*
Pco$_2$	54 mm Hg
HCO$_3^-$	30 mmol/L

*On room air.

As a result of Mr. Stevens' arterial blood gas (ABG) levels, he was placed on a Venturi mask at 28% oxygen. His ABGs then were

pH	7.42
P_{O_2}	58 mm Hg
P_{CO_2}	48 mm Hg
HCO_3^-	30 mmol/L

On the basis of the above data, Mr. Stevens was diagnosed with chronic obstructive pulmonary disease (COPD) with an acute exacerbation of chronic bronchitis. Sputum cultures revealed a gram-positive organism, *Streptococcus pneumoniae*. Mr. Stevens received erythromycin after a secondary diagnosis of pneumonia was made. He also received theophylline at this time.

Mr. Stevens responded to the antibiotic and bronchodilator therapy. He was discharged 3 days later.

QUESTIONS

Chronic Obstructive Pulmonary Disease with Pneumonia

1. Discuss the pathophysiology involved in the diagnosis of COPD.

2. Mr. Stevens was diagnosed with chronic bronchitis. This is one of the medical diagnoses associated with COPD. Discuss chronic bronchitis and the other two medical diagnoses that belong to the COPD group.

3. Were Mr. Stevens' presenting symptoms among the classic signs and symptoms elicited by patients diagnosed with COPD? Compare and contrast symptomatology associated with bronchitis and emphysema.

4. Why is Mr. Stevens' temperature of concern?

5. Why was a Venturi mask chosen as the route of administration for oxygen therapy?

6. Was the organism cultured from Mr. Stevens a common finding in COPD patients?

7. Why was Mr. Stevens given erythromycin?

8. What are the contributing factors for the development of pneumonia in Mr. Stevens' case? List other contributing factors along with signs and symptoms associated with pneumonia not present in Mr. Stevens' case.

9. What diagnostic tests are significant in the determination of a diagnosis of pneumonia?

10. Discuss medical management for the patient diagnosed with pneumonia.

11. What is the goal of therapy with theophylline, and what special considerations exist with this treatment for Mr. Stevens?

12. What is the clinical significance of the pH reading, and what is the appropriate range of the Po_2 in the patient diagnosed with COPD?

13. Why were steroids not ordered for Mr. Stevens?

14. Were Mr. Stevens' laboratory results consistent with those expected in patients diagnosed with COPD and pneumonia?

15. What other pulmonary function tests would have assisted in the diagnosis of Mr. Stevens' COPD?

16. Had Mr. Stevens' condition deteriorated and had he not responded to the bronchodilator and antibiotic therapy, what considerations concerning ventilatory management would be important?

17. Discuss the occurrence of pneumonia patients diagnosed with COPD.

18. What teaching considerations are of special concern for Mr. Stevens before his discharge?

QUESTIONS AND ANSWERS

Chronic Obstructive Pulmonary Disease with Pneumonia

1. **Discuss the pathophysiology involved in the diagnosis of COPD.**

   As stated by Clochesy, Breu, Cardin, Rudy, and Whittaker (1993) and Hartshorn, Lamborn, and Noll (1993), COPD refers to a group of chronic diseases that obstruct airflow within the airways or the lung parenchyma:

   - chronic bronchitis
   - emphysema
   - asthma

   Both of the preceding references agree that COPD usually presents as a gradual decline in function but that an acute episode of respiratory failure can occur at any time because of patients' lack of respiratory reserve. As described by Hartshorn et al. (1993), dyspnea and hyperventilation are early signs of respiratory compromise in the patient diagnosed with COPD.

   Several factors have been cited in the pathogenesis of COPD:

   - tobacco
   - air pollution
   - occupational exposure (coal miners, metal molders, workers handling stone, glass, or clay products, those who work with cotton or grain dust, fire fighters, workers exposed to asbestos)
   - genetics

2. **Mr. Stevens was diagnosed with chronic bronchitis. This is one of the medical diagnoses associated with COPD. Discuss chronic bronchitis and the other two medical diagnoses that belong to the COPD group.**

Chronic Bronchitis

Chronic bronchitis is described as chronic cough and sputum production that is present for most days during at least 3 consecutive months for not less than 2 successive years (Clochesy et al., 1993).

Pathophysiology: Production of mucus increases because of the enlargement of the bronchial mucous gland and an increase in the number of goblet cells. Other changes include inflammation of the bronchial and bronchiolar walls, loss of cilia, and the presence of mucous plugs. Physiologic changes are related to the narrowed airways. Chronic bronchitis is a disease of the central airways, and approximately 80% of the measurable airway resistance is in the central airways.

Bronchography shows the degree of tapering of the airway. The tapering is nonuniform, and the airway wall surfaces and outpouchings are irregular. It is believed that these changes account for the increased airway resistance seen in bronchitis. Functionally, this resistance results in inspiratory and expiratory air flow obstruction, overinflation of the alveoli, and abnormal distribution of ventilation. The narrowed airway leads to overinflation of the alveoli with increased total lung capacity (TLC), increased residual volume (RV), and decreased vital capacity (VC) (Clochesy et al., 1993; Hartshorn et al., 1993).

Emphysema

Emphysema can be defined as abnormal enlargement of the air spaces distal to the terminal bronchioles, accompanied by nonuniformity in the pattern of respiratory airspace enlargement and destruction of the alveolar walls (Clochesy et al., 1993; Hartshorn et al., 1993).

Genetics: One cause of emphysema is a deficiency of a serum protein called α_1-protease inhibitor. Patients with decreased circulatory levels in their blood are predisposed to early development of emphysema. Two cells are seen in the inflammatory responses in the lungs (alveolar macrophages and polymorphonuclear leukocytes [PMNs]). These cells manufacture elastase, the enzyme capable of breaking down elastin. PMNs are believed to be the major source of elastase in the lung. Most people also have an elastase *inhibitor* in the lung, which allows a balance between elastase and its inhibitor. When this balance is disturbed, either by an increase in elastase or a decrease in the inhibitor, damage to the alveolar walls occurs, resulting in emphysema (Clochesy et al., 1993; Hartshorn et al., 1993).

Pathology: Emphysema destroys the alveolar walls and enlarges the air spaces distal to the terminal bronchioles. The portion of the lung distal to the terminal bronchioles—the acinus—comprises the functional units of the lung.

The loss of airway support contributes to airway narrowing because airways collapse on expiration. This loss of alveolar wall and reduction in elastic recoil also contribute to increased lung compliance, decreased driving pressure on expiration and subsequent hyperinflation, and increased RVs. Ultimately the surface area available for gas exchange decreases, causing alterations in diffusing capacities and ventilation-perfusion abnormalities. These abnormalities lead to the hypoxemia seen in emphysema (Clochesy et al., 1993; Hartshorn et al., 1993).

Asthma

Asthma is a chronic disease of variable severity characterized by airway hyperactivity and airway narrowing of a reversible nature caused by bronchospasms. The bronchospasms cause air trapping, ventilation-perfusion mismatching, prolonged expiration acidosis, hypercapnia, and cough production of thick sputum. The lungs become stiff and overinflated and thus increase the workload of breathing. Intrathoracic pressure increases, thus decreasing venous return and cardiac output (Alspach, 1991; Hartshorn et al., 1993).

3. **Were Mr. Stevens' presenting symptoms among the classic signs and symptoms elicited by patients diagnosed with COPD? Compare and contrast symptomatology associated with bronchitis and emphysema.**

Bronchitis Clinical Manifestations
- onset varies; symptoms usually insidious
- cough and sputum production
- symptomatic in the 40s and 50s
- disability from the disease in the late 50s and early 60s
- history of frequent chest colds
- increased purulent sputum production
- dyspnea that worsens as the disease progresses
- infections exacerbate the disease
- later in the disease may be severe derangements in the ventilation-perfusion ratios
- characterized as a "blue bloater"
- low minute volumes
- development of arterial hypoxemia and hypercapnia
- patients usually stocky or obese
- central and peripheral cyanosis
- wheezing may be present
- crackles (rales) may be present because of secretions
- pulmonary hypertension
- cor pulmonale
- polycythemia
- hypoxemia and hypercapnia with compensated respiratory acidosis

Emphysema Clinical Manifestations

- signs and symptoms vary
- progressive expiratory flow obstruction and overinflation
- dyspnea with exertion at the beginning; as disease progresses, dyspnea at rest
- some patients have slow progression; others rapidly become markedly disabled
- advanced cases show enlargement of anteroposterior diameter of the chest, dorsal kyphosis, elevated ribs, and wide costal angle (barrel chest)
- thin physique with muscle wasting
- acyanotic unproductive minimal cough
- in later stages patient shows signs and symptoms of right ventricular failure (cor pulmonale)
- use of accessory muscles for breathing
- patients may breathe through pursed lips with prolonged expiration ("pink puffers")
- percussion shows increased resonance (hyperresonance) because of the increased lung volumes
- decreased, difficult to hear breath sounds
- distant heart sounds due to barrel chest
- expiratory wheezes may be present
- normal ABGs in mild to moderate emphysema; in advanced cases the PO_2 is commonly decreased, and PCO_2 increases
- hypoxemia greatest during sleep

Frequently, emphysema patients are seen in the intensive care unit (ICU) as a result of infection, heart failure, pulmonary embolism, pneumothorax, bronchospastic episodes, gastrointestinal tract bleeding, or metabolic abnormalities. Some patients require medical attention because they changed the dosages of their medications without physician knowledge. Other patients are unable to maintain their medication regimen because of coughing, nausea, or vomiting. These patients sometimes require a change in their oxygen dosage, which may also trigger acute respiratory failure (Hudak, Gallo, & Lohr, 1986).

Common Findings in ICU

- cough and fatigue
- mental confusion
- irritability and lethargy
- accessory muscle use
- tachycardia
- hypoxia
- crackles, wheezes, or stridor or consolidation
- cor pulmonale

- oxygen saturation greater than 70% (This is OK if patient has an adequate cardiac output.)

Because of increased pulmonary vascular pressure, COPD patients have increased pulmonary artery systolic, diastolic, and mean pressures (Alspach, 1991; Clochesy et al., 1993; Hartshorn et al., 1993). The usual clinical findings for COPD:

- significant and progressive reduction in expiration of air flow as measured by the forced expiratory volume (FEV)
- varying degrees of exertional dyspnea
- chronic cough and sputum production
- decreased ABGs, hypoxemia, and hypercapnia with compensated respiratory acidosis
- polycythemia

The bottom line becomes

- the degree of air flow obstruction as measured by FEV
- the age of the patient at the time of diagnosis
- the degree of reversibility
- the rate of change in the FEV over time (Hodgkin & Petty, 1987)

A higher prevalence of COPD is reported in men, and mortality rates are related to socioeconomic status. It is estimated that as many as 35% of ICU patients are patients with COPD ("Task Force Report," 1980).

4. Why is Mr. Stevens' temperature of concern?

Carbon dioxide and oxygen consumption increase as much as 10% for each degree Fahrenheit rise in temperature; thus treatment for an elevated temperature is recommended to prevent additional strain on the respiratory system (Chin & Pesce, 1983).

5. Why was a Venturi mask chosen as the route of administration for oxygen therapy?

The Venturi mask allows for precise delivery of oxygen. This is extremely important for the COPD patient because of the hypoxic drive. The goal of oxygen therapy is to keep the $PaO_2 \leq 60$ mm Hg and the $PaCO_2$ at a level to maintain pH within normal limits (Clochesy et al., 1993).

6. Was the organism cultured from Mr. Stevens a common finding in COPD patients?

The most common form of pneumonia is due to aspiration of gastric or oropharyngeal secretions into the lower respiratory tract. Bacterial pneumonia commonly is caused by Streptococcus pneumoniae, a gram-positive coccus. It is spread through droplets or airborne nuclei and carries a 50% mortality rate for patients who are debilitated (Rytel, 1983).

Nosocomial pneumonia is a concern for the hospitalized patient. The Centers for Disease Control and Prevention (CDC) reported in 1986 that nosocomial pneumonia (gram-negative organisms) was the second most frequently reported hospital-acquired infection.

7. **Why was Mr. Stevens given erythromycin?**

Mr. Stevens' wife stated that the patient was allergic to penicillin, which according to Katzung (1992) is the drug of choice, with erythromycin listed as the drug of second choice.

8. **What are the contributing factors for the development of pneumonia in Mr. Stevens' case? List other contributing factors along with signs and symptoms associated with pneumonia not present in Mr. Stevens' case.**

Contributing factors in Mr. Stevens' case were the frequent bouts with chest colds. Crackles were noted in the lower bases of the lung and an occasional expiratory wheeze. Mr. Stevens also ran a low-grade fever for 2 to 3 days and had an elevated white blood cell (WBC) count, general weakness, and chills. The sputum culture of Streptococcus pneumoniae confirmed the diagnosis of pneumonia. Chest x-ray (CXR) also revealed consolidation in the lower lung bases.

As noted by Clochesy et al. (1993), the following have been identified as contributing factors for the development of and signs and symptoms associated with pneumonia:

Contributing Factors for Development of Pneumonia
- tracheal intubation
- decreased level of consciousness (LOC) (allowing for aspiration)
- underlying chronic lung disorder
- endotracheal intubation (bypasses upper airway and host defense mechanisms)
- suctioning (creates mechanical irritation or injury to the mucosa, predisposing the lungs to inoculation and colonization of bacteria)

Signs and Symptoms of Bacterial Pneumonia
- sudden onset including shaking, chills, and fever of 38.9° to 40.6° C (102° to 105° F)
- cough initially dry; becomes productive, rusty in color early then yellow green (rusty early because of a mixture of red blood cells (RBCs) and inflammatory cells in infected alveoli)

- malaise, weakness
- headache, myalgia
- cyanosis (depending on the degree of respiratory compromise)
- if elderly, altered mental state
- coarse inspiratory rales
- friction rub may be present
- pleuritic chest pain
- CXR shows either lobar consolidation or scattered interstitial infiltrates

9. What diagnostic tests are significant in the determination of a diagnosis of pneumonia?

The following tests are necessary in the diagnosis of pneumonia:

- vital signs
- blood cultures
- sputum cultures (avoid collecting saliva; may have colonization)
- CXRs
- ABGs
- electrolytes
- electrocardiogram (ECG)
- hemoglobin (Hgb) and hematocrit (Hct)

Therapy is based on results obtained from Gram's stain and sputum cultures (Clochesy et al., 1993; Hartshorn et al., 1993).

10. Discuss medical management for the patient diagnosed with pneumonia.

Any patient admitted to the hospital is a candidate for pneumonia; prevention is the number one priority. The following criteria must be considered in the management of the patient diagnosed with pneumonia (Clochesy et al., 1993; Hartshorn et al., 1993):

- identification of risk factors and susceptible patient populations
- aseptic technique including handwashing and handling of respiratory equipment to prevent cross contamination to susceptible patients
- antibiotic therapy
- humidified oxygen
- chest physical therapy
- frequent TCDB
- assessment of airway protective mechanisms (cough, gag, and swallowing reflexes)
- head of bed elevated to decrease gastric reflux, facilitate swallowing, and postural drainage

- careful and frequent assessment of temperature, heart rate, respirations, chest sounds, and CXR, respiratory effort, and use of accessory muscles with breathing
- suctioning
- assessment of patient's total volume fluid status
- monitor fluid and electrolytes
- bronchodilators

11. What is the goal of therapy with theophylline, and what special considerations exist with this treatment for Mr. Stevens?

Therapeutic blood levels of the theophylline compounds must be monitored closely in COPD patients. Smokers tend to metabolize theophylline *faster* than nonsmokers, and patients with liver or cardiac disease metabolize theophylline *slower;* so dosages must be individualized.

The goal with theophylline therapy is to maintain a blood level of 10 to 20 µg/ml (Clochesy et al., 1993; Hartshorn et al., 1993).

12. What is the clinical significance of the pH reading, and what is the appropriate range of the Po_2 in the patient diagnosed with COPD?

Normal values for the COPD patient

- Pao_2 <60 mm Hg
- $Paco_2$ >50 mm Hg

As stated by Clochesy et al. (1993), pH is the key to diagnosis. A severely acidotic range ≤ 7.25 is often given as the marker for acute respiratory failure with increases in carbon dioxide and decreases in oxygen. The goal of oxygen therapy is to keep Pao_2 between 55 and 65 mm Hg. In this range saturation of hemoglobin is optimal without disruption of the "hypoxic drive" stimulus. Oxygen for the COPD patient is delivered by Venturi masks, nasal cannulas, rebreathing masks, and mechanical ventilation.

COPD increases pulmonary vascular pressures (pulmonary artery systolic [PAS] and pulmonary artery diastolic [PAD]) and the pulmonary artery pressure is 5 to 20 mm Hg higher than the pulmonary capillary wedge pressure (PCWP). (Normally these two readings are within 1 to 2 mm Hg of each other). Mechanical ventilators generate falsely elevated readings, and this is especially true when positive end expiratory pressure (PEEP) is used.

13. Why were steroids not ordered for Mr. Stevens?

The use of steroids remains controversial. Practitioners use this classification more in the care of the asthma patient than with patients diagnosed with chronic bronchitis. Whenever steroids are used, patients should be monitored for side effects of short-term therapy, such as hyperglycemia.

Steroids such as methylprednisolone (Solu-Medrol) are used intravenously for 1 to 2 days, followed by oral prednisone ordered in increasingly lower doses until a maintenance dose is reached. Aerosol steroids have not proven effective (Clochesy et al., 1993; Hartshorn et al., 1993).

14. **Were Mr. Stevens' laboratory results consistent with those expected in patients diagnosed with COPD and pneumonia?**

Usual Laboratory and Diagnostic Findings

Po_2	decreased
Pco_2	normal or elevated
recoil of lung	normal
Hct	often elevated
cor pulmonale	increased neck vein distension, enlarged liver, and edema; common α_1-antiprotease phenotype

Chest X-ray Films

CXRs usually are normal in uncomplicated chronic bronchitis. Classic findings seen in later stages are flattening of the diaphragm, hyperlucency, decreased vascular markings, widening of the rib spaces, and increased anteroposterior diameter (reflects hyperinflation).

Arterial Blood Gases

ABG levels may be normal in mild to moderate emphysema. In advanced cases the most common abnormality is decreased Po_2. Pco_2 levels may be normal or increased, especially when seen with infection (Clochesy et al., 1993).

15. **What other pulmonary function tests would have assisted in the diagnosis of Mr. Stevens' COPD?**

Pulmonary Function Tests

- increased RV and functional residual capacity
- decreased VC
- increased TLC
- decreased diffusing capacity
- increased FEV and maximal midexpiratory flow rate (MMFR)
- flow volume loop showing caved appearance

Pulmonary function tests with spirometry usually demonstrate normal findings. These may show an increased RV and mild reduction in VC consistent with the degree of hyperinflation (Clochesy et al., 1993; Hartshorn et al., 1993).

16. **Had Mr. Stevens' condition deteriorated and had he not responded to the bronchodilator and antibiotic therapy, what considerations concerning ventilatory management would be important?**

Ventilatory Management

Using a ventilator for the COPD patient allows the patient to rest and allows for deep suctioning. The problem with ventilator use with this patient population is the difficulty in weaning COPD patients from the ventilator.

Weilitz (1991) states that when a patient is weaned from the ventilator, three areas must be monitored: oxygenation, carbon dioxide elimination, and mechanical efficiency. The author states that some general guidelines for weaning may be helpful to the clinician:

- oxygen concentration of less than 50%
- PEEP of less than 5 cm H_2O
- respiratory rate of less than 30 breaths per minute
- minute ventilation of less than 10 L/min (volume of air patient breathes at rest)
- low dynamic static pressures (compliance of at least 35 cm H_2O)
- adequate ABG levels with the above guidelines

Weilitz (1991) further states that current clinical practice uses T-pieces or continuous positive airway pressure (CPAP), alternating with full ventilator support such as synchronized intermittent mandatory ventilation (SIMV) or assist control. Pressure support is another mechanism for decreasing ventilator use while offering consistent internal alveoli support.

17. **Discuss the incidence of pneumonia patients diagnosed with COPD.**

According to Lynch (1993), pneumonia occurs in 10% to 40% of intubated patients requiring mechanical ventilation for more than 24 hours and carries with that a mortality of 30% to 70%. Lynch also states that any changes on CXR can be subtle and that establishing a specific cause may be difficult. Sputum cultures may be misleading, but resistant gram-negative pathogens such as *Pseudomonas aeruginosa* are the most prevalent, occurring in 20% to 30% of pneumonia cases in mechanically ventilated patients.

Lynch states that although not all pneumonia requires combination antibiotic therapy, pneumonia due to *Pseudomonas, Serratia, Acinetobacter,* or *Xanthomonas* does require it. In these cases Lynch suggests either antipseudomonal penicillin or a third-generation cephalosporin and aminoglycoside.

Pneumococcal pneumonia may take some time to resolve, with consolidation in the lungs taking up to 6 weeks to clear. CXR of the patient with pneumococcal pneumonia will reveal consolidation manifested by dullness to percussion and increased fremitus (palpable vibrations transmitted through the bronchopulmonary system to the chest wall when the patient speaks). Mortality is related more often to concomitant host disease than to the type of gram-negative organism.

Staphylococcal pneumonia has an insidious onset in the chronically ill. High fever and chills may last up to 1 week in severe cases despite the use of antibiotics. Cough with blood-tinged sputum and tachypnea with cyanosis occur early in the course of the disease. Gram-negative bacterial pneumonia has a highly variable course. It may progress slowly or rapidly over a few days. Patients will have a fever, a productive cough of purulent sputum, and pleuritic chest pain.

A vaccine is available for pneumococcal pneumonia. It is recommended prophylactically for high-risk groups, including the elderly and those with COPD, congestive heart failure, renal failure, alcoholism, cirrhosis, splenic dysfunction or splenectomy, Hodgkin's disease, myeloma, or other immunocompromised states. The vaccine should be given only once to adults to avoid significant adverse reactions. Influenza vaccines are also available (Lynch, 1993).

18. What teaching considerations are of special concern for Mr. Stevens before his discharge?

As stated by Clochesy et al. (1993), patients with advanced pulmonary disease who stop smoking at age 65 years have an increased survival rate over those patients who continue to smoke. Other areas that need to be addressed with the patient before discharge are

- good hydration and sputum mobilization
- prevention of and avoidance of exposure to infection
- annual prophylactic multivalent influenza vaccines and a one-time pneumococcal pneumonia vaccine
- avoidance of exposure to sudden temperature changes
- patient's understanding of bronchodilation therapy, normal blood levels, and diet management
- referral of patient to a support group

Chronic Obstructive Pulmonary Disease with Pneumonia

Alspach, J. G. (Ed.). (1991). *Core curriculum for critical care nursing.* Philadelphia: Saunders.

Centers for Disease Control and Prevention (1986). Nosocomial infection surveillance, 1984. *Surveillance Summaries, 35,* 17–29.

Chin, R., & Pesce, R. (1983). Practical aspects in management of respiratory failure in chronic obstructive pulmonary disease. *Critical Care Quarterly, 6*(2), 1–21.

Clochesy, J. M., Breu, C., Cardin, S., Rudy, E. B., & Whittaker, A. A. (1993). *Critical care nursing.* Philadelphia: Saunders.

Hartshorn, J., Lamborn, M., & Noll, M. L. (1993). *Introduction to critical care nursing.* Philadelphia: Saunders.

Hodgkin, J., & Petty, T. (1987). *Chronic obstructive pulmonary disease: Current concepts.* Philadelphia: Saunders.

Hudak, C., Gallo, B., & Lohr, T. (1986). *Critical care nursing: A holistic approach.* Philadelphia: Lippincott.

Katzung, B. (1992). *Basic and clinical pharmacology.* Norwalk, CT: Appleton & Lange.

Lynch, J. (1993). Combination therapy vs. monotherapy for ventilator-associated pneumonia. *Society of Critical Care Medicine 1993 Educational Symposium Highlights,* pp. 11–12.

Rytel, M. (1983). Pneumococcal pneumonia: Diagnosis and management. *Journal of Respiratory Disease, 4*(9), 80–87.

Task force report on epidemiology of respiratory diseases (1980). (NIH Publication No. 81-2019). Washington, DC: U.S. Department of Health and Human Services.

Weilitz, P. B. (1991). Weaning from mechanical ventilation: Old and new strategies. *Critical Care Nursing Clinics of North America, 3*(4), 585–590.

5

PTCA and Thrombolytic Therapy in Myocardial Infarction

Alice Lowe, BSN, RN
Sheila Drake Melander, DSN, RN, FCCM

CASE PRESENTATION

Mr. Smith, a 54-year-old man, began having chest pain 1 hour after lunch while at work. He described the pain as a "grabbing pressure" located mid-sternally. He rated the pain at "about a 4" on a scale of 1 to 10. He stated that the pain radiated down his left arm and through to his back. On admission after transportation to the emergency department (ED) via ambulance, Mr. Smith was pale and diaphoretic and complained of shortness of breath. He denied nausea or vomiting. He was diagnosed in the ED with unstable angina, and myocardial infarction (MI) was ruled out. He had experienced chest pain for 1 hour on arrival in the ED at 12:59 PM.

The patient reports no previous episodes of chest pain or pressure. He has smoked two packs of cigarettes daily for 25 years. His mother died of Alzheimer's disease and his father died of cancer. There is no family history of heart disease.

On initial examination, the patient did not exhibit jugular venous distension (JVD), the carotid arteries were 2+/4 without bruits, and point of maximum impulse (PMI) was located at the fifth intercostal space midclavicular line. Normal S_1 and S_2 sounds were auscultated with an S_4 present. No S_3 sounds or murmurs were heard. There were vesicular lung sounds with scattered wheezes, but no crackles were heard. No edema was present and bowel sounds were normal.

Admission diagnostic data were

BP	140/90
Respirations	32/min
HR	92 bpm and regular
Temperature	36.9° C (98.5° F)
SaO$_2$	95% on oxygen 4 L/min per nasal cannula
Height	173 cm
Weight	104 kg

The 12-lead ECG findings at 12:59 PM were
- normal sinus rhythm (NSR) with frequent premature ventricular contractions (PVCs) and 3–4 beat runs of ventricular tachycardia (VT)
- ST elevation in leads I, aVL, and V$_2$-V$_6$ (3 to 4 mm)
- ST depression in leads III and aVF
- Q waves in V$_1$ through V$_4$

Chest x-ray (CXR) revealed slight cardiomegaly with mild congestive heart failure (CHF).

The echocardiogram findings were
- trileaflet aortic valve with normal opening
- normal mitral configuration with normal opening of mitral valve in diastole and normal coaptation in systole
- right atrium and right ventricle normal
- thin layer pericardial effusion (mostly posterior)
- anterior septal and infraapical akinesia with small, mildly dyskinetic apex
- left ventricular ejection fraction (LVEF) 25% to 30%
- mild mitral valve regurgitation

Tables 5–1 and 5–2 show the cardiac enzyme levels and laboratory data for Mr. Smith at admission and at various times following.

In the ED, Mr. Smith's chest pain was unrelieved after three sublingual nitroglycerin (NTG) (Tridil) tablets. Morphine sulfate (Roxanol) 5 mg intravenous push (IVP) was administered, resulting in a small decrease in pain.

Table 5–1   Cardiac Enzyme Levels

	Admission (12:59 PM)	Day of Admission (6:17 PM)	Day 1 (2:50 AM)
Creatine kinase (CK) (U/L)	254	7357	5638
Lactate dehydrogenase (LDH) (U/L)	509	1849	4055
CK-MB (%)	10	>300	>300

Table 5–2   Laboratory Data

		Postadmission		
Laboratory Test	Day of Admission	Day 1	Day 2	Day 3
WBCs ($\times 10^3/mm^3$)	12.9	19.6	14.4	12.7
Hgb (g/dl)	15.9	13.4	13.4	13.2
Hct (%)	47.4	40	38.1	37.9
Platelets ($\times 10^3/mm^3$)	244	216	166	165
BUN (mg/dl)	13	11	15	14
Creatinine (mg/dl)	1.2	1	1	1.1
K^+ (mmol/L)	4.3	3.3	3.7	3.3
Cholesterol (mg/dl)	288	182	194	186
AST (SGOT) (U/L)	36	653	635	72
Triglycerides (mg/dl)	271	109	121	134
Glucose (mg/dl)	162	152	145	120

After evaluation of the initial laboratory results, presenting symptoms, and the ECG, the diagnosis of an extensive anterolateral myocardial infarction (MI) was made. Mr. Smith was assessed for contraindications to thrombolytic therapy. The patient was considered a candidate for thrombolytic therapy, and tissue plasminogen activator (tPA) was started immediately using front-loaded dosing technique. An NTG (Tridil) drip (50 mg/250 ml 5% dextrose in water [D_5W]) was begun at 20 μg/min (6 ml/h). A 100 mg bolus of lidocaine (Xylocaine) was given, and a lidocaine drip (2 g/500 ml D_5W) was started at 30 ml/h (2 mg/min). A heparin (Calciparine) bolus of 8000 U was given, and a drip was hung at 10 ml/h (1000 U/h). Metoprolol tartrate (Lopressor) 25 mg and an enteric aspirin were given. The patient was then transferred to the coronary intensive care unit (ICU).

In the coronary care unit (CCU) Mr. Smith's chest pain returned at a rating of 7. After 1.5 hours of tPA his blood pressure was 96/60. A sublingual NTG was given, but the pain did not decrease. The ECG showed no change. Mr. Smith was sent to the catheterization laboratory for an emergency cardiac catheterization and possible percutaneous transluminal coronary angioplasty (PTCA).

Cardiac catheterization showed 90% blockage of the left anterior descending artery (LAD), and an emergency rescue angioplasty (PTCA) was performed.

Mr. Smith continued having chest pain throughout the procedure. A total of 23,000 U of heparin was given IVP, and 500,000 U of urokinase was given intracoronary. Mr. Smith became hypotensive, tachycardic, cool, pale, and diaphoretic. His SaO$_2$ dropped to 86%, and he was placed on a 100% nonrebreather mask.

Arterial blood gases (ABGs) on admission day at 8:40 PM with 100% oxygen via nonrebreather mask were

pH   7.37
P_{CO_2} 45.1 mm Hg
P_{O_2} 38.7 mm Hg
HCO_3^- 25.8 mmol/L
Base   0.5
Sa_{O_2} 86%

A dopamine (Intropin) infusion was started at 2 µg/kg/min and was gradually increased to 4 µg/kg/min. A dobutamine (Dobutrex) drip was started at 5 µg/kg/min. The PTCA was successful with a residual stricture of the LAD at 30%. A pulmonary artery (Swan-Ganz) catheter was placed to monitor for CHF and cardiogenic shock. An intraaortic balloon pump (IABP) was placed to stabilize Mr. Smith's BP, decrease the workload of the heart, and improve cardiac output.

On return to the CCU, Mr. Smith was pain free. His vital signs and hemodynamic readings were

BP	133/59	Right atrium	10 mm Hg
HR	90 bpm	Pulmonary artery systolic	42 mm Hg
Sa_{O_2}	99%	Pulmonary artery diastolic	22 mm Hg
ECG	NSR	Mean pulmonary artery pressure	31 mm Hg
		Pulmonary artery wedge pressure	22 mm Hg

ECG Day of Admission (6 PM)
- NSR, T wave inverted in aVR
- ST elevated in leads I, aVL, and V_2 through V_6 (1 to 2 mm)

ECG Postadmission Day 1 (6:50 AM)
- NSR, ST almost baseline
- T wave inverted in aVR

ECG Postadmission Day 2
- NSR, ST almost baseline
- Q waves in V_2 through V_6
- aVR T wave now upright

Mr. Smith's IABP and pulmonary artery catheter were removed on day 2. On day 3 his dopamine, dobutamine, and NTG drips were tapered. He was released to the cardiac progressive step-down unit on day 4 and released to home on day 6. He was instructed in outpatient cardiac rehabilitation and a prudent diet. He was sent home with prescriptions for diltiazem (Cardizem) 30 mg t.i.d., captopril (Capoten) 6.25 mg t.i.d., and prn NTG tablets.

QUESTIONS

PTCA and Thrombolytic Therapy in Myocardial Infarction

1. Describe angina pectoris and discuss the difference between angina pectoris and unstable angina.

2. Define coronary artery disease (CAD) and discuss associated major risk factors.

3. Describe an MI and its effects on the heart and lifestyle.

4. List the symptoms of an AMI.

5. What is the significance of the following heart sounds: S_3, S_4, and murmur?

6. What do crackles auscultated during lung sound assessment signify?

7. Discuss the use of cardiac enzymes and their normal values. What laboratory values would be indicative of an MI for Mr. Smith?

8. What is the significance of Mr. Smith's ST changes?

9. What are the desired pharmacologic effects of NTG?

10. Discuss the pharmacologic effects of morphine.

11. What was the rationale for using a lidocaine (Xylocaine) drip?

12. Discuss the pharmacologic actions of heparin and the indications for use with the MI patient.

13. Describe what a β-blocker is and the rationale for Mr. Smith's receiving this medication.

14. Mr. Smith was sent home with a prescription for diltiazem (Cardizem). Why would a heart patient be given a calcium channel blocker?

15. tPA is a thrombolytic agent. Discuss the effect of a thrombolytic and why it was used.

16. What are the contraindications for thrombolytics?

17. What is PTCA? What does the procedure involve?

18. What made Mr. Smith a candidate for a PTCA? What are the potential contraindications for a patient receiving a PTCA?

19. What is cardiogenic shock? What symptoms did Mr. Smith exhibit?

20. What are the therapeutic effects of dopamine (Intropin) at low doses and at moderate doses? How do these effects differ at high doses?

21. What are the therapeutic effects of dobutamine (Dobutrex)? Why would dopamine and dobutamine be used together?

22. What do the readings from the pulmonary artery (Swan-Ganz) catheter tell the nurse about Mr. Smith?

23. What advantage does an IABP after coronary artery bypass graft (CABG) have for Mr. Smith?

24. What significance does the IABP have in relation to the tPA and urokinase given previously?

QUESTIONS AND ANSWERS

PTCA and
Thrombolytic Therapy
in Myocardial Infarction

1. **Describe angina pectoris and discuss the difference between angina pectoris and unstable angina.**

   Angina pectoris is a state of transient myocardial ischemia without cell death (Alspach, 1991). Ischemia causes the membranes of the myocardial cells, white blood cells, and platelets to become increasingly permeable. Potassium, serotonin, and histamine are released from these cells into the circulation, where they stimulate the nerve fibers responsible for the sensation of pain. These nerve fibers are also stimulated by lactic acid created by the anaerobic metabolism occurring in the hypoxic myocardial tissues. In the spinal cord, cardiac pain fibers stimulate sensory nerves from other body areas, resulting in the radiation of chest pain to the neck, jaw, shoulders, and so on (Mims, 1990).

   ### Etiology Factors for Angina Pectoris
   Atherosclerotic heart disease, hypertension, aortic valve disease, anemia, dysrhythmia, thyrotoxicosis, shock, CHF, and coronary artery spasm are the etiologic factors associated with angina pectoris.

   ### Precipitating Factors for Unstable Angina
   Physical activity, ingestion of a large meal, and recumbent positions may precipitate nocturnal angina, cold exposure, and anxiety (Alspach, 1991).

   Unstable angina is chest pain triggered by an unpredictable degree of exertion or emotion. The attacks characteristically increase in number, duration, and intensity. Unstable angina may also be a change in a previously established stable pattern of angina or a new onset of severe angina. It is usually more intense and described as pain rather than discomfort. The pain usually lasts longer than 30 minutes and may awaken the patient from sleep. The symptoms may only be partially relieved by rest or nitrates (Thelan, Davie, & Urden, 1994).

2. **Define coronary artery disease (CAD) and discuss associated major risk factors.**

CAD affects the arteries that supply blood to the heart muscle. It is caused most often by atherosclerosis, which is the gradual buildup of fatty deposits (mainly cholesterol) on the inner lining of the artery walls. Atherosclerosis progressively narrows the artery and decreases the blood flow. The disease may involve the arteries in many different areas of the body, including the heart (leading to a heart attack) and the brain (leading to a stroke). When the blood flow is severely reduced by atherosclerosis, a clot can form as blood trickles and sludges through the narrowed vessel, causing a sudden, complete stoppage of blood flow. The process of atherosclerosis usually begins at an early age. Significant disease may be present in some individuals before age 20 years. Long before the function of the heart is affected, there is a period without symptoms; the narrowing progresses slowly. Risk factor changes may halt or slow the process of atherosclerosis (American Heart Association [AHA], 1991).

Heredity: CAD Tends to Run in Families.

Age: CAD is more prevalent in older age groups. The incidence of MI increases with age (Alspach, 1991).

Gender: CAD is more prevalent in men than in women (Alspach, 1991). In men an acute myocardial infarction (AMI) is uncommon before the age of 40 years, but 45% of all events occur before the age of 65 years. CAD is the leading cause of death in women older than 45 years, believed to be due to the decrease in estrogen. One in three women has some form of cardiovascular disease, and 73% of acute events occur after age 65 years (AHA, 1991).

Race: The American Heart Association (1991) reports that African-Americans are twice as likely as Caucasians to develop CAD. It is believed this difference may be due to hypertension in the African-American race, cultural differences, and diet. But in a study performed by Keil, Sutherland, Knapp, Lackland, Gazes, and Tyroller (1993), there were no significant differences between African-Americans and Caucasians in coronary mortality rates, although there were significant differences in coronary mortality rates between men and women. Both African-American and Caucasian women fared better than men.

Major Risk Factors That Can Be Controlled or Modified

Hypertension: Systolic BP is more than 160 mm Hg, or a diastolic BP is more than 95 mm Hg.

Diabetes Mellitus: Patients with diabetes mellitus are two times more likely to develop CAD than those without diabetes mellitus.

Cigarette Smoking: Smokers have a two to six times higher risk of death from CAD than nonsmokers.

Hyperlipidemia: High levels of triglycerides and low-density and very low-density lipoproteins are associated with an increased risk of CAD.

Contributing Factors

Obesity: Morbid obesity has been shown to be positively associated with an increased risk of CAD. In addition, it also contributes to the development of hypertension and diabetes.

Sedentary Lifestyle: It is controversial as to whether a sedentary lifestyle is a risk factor by itself; however, studies do show a low positive relationship between inactivity and CAD.

Stress: It was previously believed that the type A personality was twice as prone to CAD as compared with others. Current studies are now challenging this theory (Alspach, 1991).

3. Describe an MI and its effects on the heart and lifestyle.

An MI is defined as necrosis of the cells of an area of the heart muscle occurring as a result of oxygen deprivation, caused by obstruction of the blood supply (Miller & Keane, 1991). The hemodynamic significance of plaques is not usually apparent until 70% of the arterial cross-sectional area has been compromised. At that time symptoms may result during times of increased myocardial oxygen demand (e.g., exertion, a heavy meal, anxiety) because of inadequate oxygen supply. Until recently, AMI was thought to occur when the atheromatous plaque grew large enough to totally occlude the coronary artery. It is now recognized that physiologic events cause disruption of the intima covering the plaque (Riegel, 1993). Infarction results from the mechanical obstruction caused by thrombosis, plaque rupture, dissection, and sometimes spasm (Hartshorn, Lamborn, & Noll, 1993; Miller & Keane, 1991; Riegel, 1993).

Other causes of MI are related to a sudden increased unmet need for blood supply to the heart, as in restriction of blood flow through the aorta in aortic stenosis (Miller & Keane, 1991).

Prolonged acute ischemia lasting 30 to 45 minutes causes irreversible cellular damage and muscle death (necrosis). Permanent deterioration of contractile function occurs in the necrotic or infarcted area of the myocardium (Hartshorn et al., 1993).

Recovery from AMI is difficult; approximately 88% of patients experience emotional distress and family turmoil after AMI. Many patients fail to return to work when physiologically capable of doing so (Riegel, 1993).

4. List the symptoms of an AMI.

Pain: The pain associated with AMI is usually described as an uncomfortable pressure, squeezing, fullness or tightness, aching, crushing, constricting, oppressive, heavy, or burning sensation (AHA, 1991; Hartshorn et al., 1993; Riegel, 1993).

Location: Pain is generally located in the midsternal chest area behind the breastbone. It may spread to one or both shoulders, arms, jaw, neck, or through to the back (AHA, 1991; Riegel, 1993).

Duration: The discomfort of a heart attack will usually last longer than 30 minutes, it may come and go and is usually not relieved with rest or sublingual NTG tablets. Other symptoms include shortness of breath, diaphoresis, weakness, nausea and vomiting, and a general feeling of doom (AHA, 1991; Riegel, 1993).

5. What is the significance of the following heart sounds: S_3, S_4, and murmur?

Cardiac auscultation often reveals muffled heart sounds that become clearer as healing progresses. A fourth heart sound (S_4) immediately preceding the first heart sound is almost unique with an acute infarction and is heard best between the left sternal border and the apex. The S_4 reflects atrial contraction and is heard because the left atrium is contracting against a noncompliant left ventricle with an elevated left ventricular end-diastolic pressure (LVEDP) (Riegel, 1993).

A third heart sound (S_3) can be heard in patients with (1) large transmural infarcts and extensive left ventricular (LV) dysfunction, (2) decreased contractile strength, (3) hypertensive crisis, or (4) a ventricular septal defect (Riegel, 1993).

A murmur is caused by turbulent blood flow through incompetent or stenotic cardiac chambers. The presence of a murmur can signify disease of any of the four valves. Most common are aortic or mitral valve diseases. A new, high-pitched holosystolic, blowing murmur at the cardiac apex may be the first sign of mitral valve regurgitation secondary to papillary muscle dysfunction. If the murmur is loud, harsh, and radiating in all directions from the apex, the papillary muscle or chordae tendineae may have ruptured (Thelan et al., 1994).

6. What do crackles auscultated during lung assessment signify?

Crackles heard during lung auscultation suggest left ventricular failure (LVF) or decreased LV compliance and can be used to estimate prognosis (Killip classification of patients with AMI from the 1960s from Riegel, 1993):

Class I absence of crackles over the lung fields and absence of S_3 (mortality 8%)

Class II crackles over 50% or less of the lung fields or the presence of an S_3 (mortality 30%)

Class III crackles over more than 50% of the lung fields, frequently pulmonary edema (mortality 44%)

Class IV shock (mortality 80% to 100%)

7. Discuss the use of cardiac enzymes and their normal values. What laboratory values would be indicative of an MI for Mr. Smith?

Three enzymes are released into the blood during AMI:

(1) CK: creatine kinase
(2) LDH: lactate dehydrogenase
(3) AST (SGOT): aspartate aminotransferase (serum glutamic-oxaloacetic transaminase)

CK, formerly creatine phosphokinase (CPK), is composed of three isoenzymes: MM, found in both skeletal and cardiac muscle; BB, found in brain and kidney; and MB, found in cardiac muscle. CK-MB is the primary diagnostic enzyme for AMI (Hartshorn et al., 1993; Riegel, 1993).

LDH is an intracellular enzyme that is widely distributed in the tissues of the body, particularly in the kidney, heart, skeletal muscle, brain, liver, and lungs (Fischbach, 1992). Increases in the reported value usually indicate cellular death, and leakage of the enzyme from the cell. LDH remains elevated longer than CK or AST; therefore, it can be useful in the late diagnosis of MI. AST is the third cardiac enzyme that becomes elevated with myocardial damage. AST is present in many tissues of the body such as the liver, skeletal muscles, renal tissue, red blood cells, the brain, pancreas, and lung tissue. Because it is fairly prevalent throughout the body and there is no identifiable isoenzyme specific to cardiac damage, this test tends to be not as specific and not as highly significant as the other two serum enzyme studies (Hartshorn et al., 1993).

CK values normally range from 40 to 180 U/L (lower for women). Isoenzyme CK-MB levels should be less than 5% when analyzed by standard methods (Riegel, 1993). LDH normal values range from 95 to 200 U/L. AST normal is 7 to 12 U/L (Fischbach, 1992; Hartshorn et al., 1993). Table 5–3 shows Mr. Smith's enzyme levels.

Table 5–3   Enzyme Levels

Enzyme	Initial Rises	Peak	Return to Baseline
CK	4–8 h	24 h	3–4 d
LDH	24–48 h	3–6 d	8–14 d
AST	8–12 h	18–36 h	3–4 d

On admission, Mr. Smith's CK was 254 U/L, his LDH was 509 U/L, and his CK-MB was 10%. The CK was more than the normal of 180 U/L, the LDH was more than 200 U/L, and the CK-MB was more than 5%. These enzyme levels suggest AMI. The enzyme readings are never definitive for an MI by themselves but must be viewed in context with the ECG and the patient's presenting symptoms.

8. What is the significance of Mr. Smith's ST changes?

The ST segment represents the resting phase between ventricular depolarization and repolarization. Thus, it is normally neutral or isoelectric, that is, near baseline on the ECG. ST segment shifts (elevations or depressions) associated with myocardial cell injury may be the result of an inability of the affected cells to maintain their normal intracellular polarity during the resting phase (Purcell & Haynes, 1984).

The T wave represents repolarization of the myocardium and is normally positive (upward deflection) in all of the 12 leads except V_1 and sometimes III and V_2. In addition to T wave inversion, the QT interval may be prolonged, reflecting longer repolarization. T wave inversion associated with AMI may persist for several days and is associated with ischemia (Purcell & Haynes, 1984).

Although ventricular depolarization is described as a QRS complex in any lead, it is not normal for every lead to have a Q, R, and S wave. Any initial negative (downward) deflection during a QRS complex is labeled a Q wave. The first positive deflection (upright) is the R, and the following negative deflection is the S.

Pathologic Q waves are >0.04 seconds deep and usually >0.03 seconds wide. Q waves normally occur in leads III and aVF and are likely to disappear with deep inspiration or position change (Purcell & Haynes, 1984).

An AMI Evolves in Three Stages

(1) *Ischemia:* Ischemia results from a temporary interruption of the myocardial blood supply (*ECG interpretation: Clinical skillbuilders,* 1990). It is the least acute stage of tissue hypoxia and is often reversible with little or no permanent cell death if prompt intervention increases blood supply to the myocardium or reduces oxygen demand (Purcell & Haynes, 1984). Its characteristic ECG change is T wave inversion, a result of altered tissue repolarization. ST segment depression also may occur (*ECG interpretation: Clinical skillbuilders,* 1990).

(2) *Injury:* Injury to myocardial cells results from a prolonged interruption of blood flow. Its characteristic ECG change, ST segment elevation, reflects altered depolarization. Usually, an elevation >1 mm is significant (*ECG interpretation: Clinical skillbuilders,* 1990).

(3) *Necrosis:* Infarction results from an absence of blood flow to myocardial tissue, leading to necrosis. The ECG shows pathologic
Q waves, reflecting abnormal depolarization in damaged tissue or
absent depolarization in scar tissue. A pathologic Q wave has a
duration of 0.04 seconds or an amplitude measuring at least one
third the height of the entire QRS complex (*ECG interpretation:
Clinical skillbuilders, 1990*).

Inferior MI (Leads II, III, and aVF)

The right coronary artery (RCA) supplies the inferior myocardium and
lower third of the interventricular septum. Infarction of these surfaces is
best reflected in the inferior leads. Because the infarcted tissue on the inferior surface no longer depolarizes, opposing forces become dominant, and
current traveling away from the positive pole is visible as a new Q wave.

Lateral MI (Leads I, aVL, V_5, and V_6)

The circumflex artery and the diagonal branches of the LAD supply the
lateral myocardium. Infarction in this area is best seen in leads I, aVL,
V_5, and V_6.

Anterior MI (Leads V_1 Through V_6)

The LAD supplies the anterior ventricular myocardium and upper two
thirds of the septum. Infarction in this area is best seen in leads V_1 through
V_6. The result is smaller or absent R waves. Loss of R waves in V_2 through
V_4 indicates necrosis of the anteroseptal surface; loss of R waves in V_2
through V_6 indicates extensive anterior or anterolateral infarction.

Posterior MI (V_1 and V_2)

The mid- and posterior marginal branches of the circumflex artery supply the posterior wall of the heart. The process of infarction here can
sometimes be seen in leads V_1 and V_2 as

- ST segment depression
- reversal of the T wave polarity
- initial R wave upswing that is wider than normal

Mr. Smith's STs are elevated in leads I, aVL, and V_2 through V_6. This
would signify that he is having anterolateral injury. The Q waves in
leads V_1 through V_4 could be from a previous silent MI or could represent some necrosis in the anterior portion of the myocardium. The
ST depression in leads III and aVF signify reciprocal changes.

9. What are the desired pharmacologic effects of NTG?

The main therapeutic action of nitrates is to reduce oxygen demand
and increase oxygen supply. Nitrates increase capacity of the systemic

venous bed (increase venous capitance), "trapping" blood in the veins and decreasing blood return to the heart, thereby reducing preload). Nitrates relax vascular smooth muscle, thus reducing blood pressure by generalized vasodilation. Both of these actions lower peripheral resistance against which the heart must pump. The workload of the heart is diminished, and the oxygen need of the myocardium drops (Spencer, Nichols, Lipkin, Sabo, & West, 1989). Hemodynamic effects include decreased pulmonary artery wedge pressure (PAWP) and LV end-diastolic and end-systolic volumes. Decreases in preload generally lead to an increase in cardiac output. Nitrates also decrease systemic arterial pressure and afterload, which may result in hypotension. Tachycardia and hypotension can both increase infarct size. In patients with AMI with systolic BP of more than 95 mm Hg, nitrates can be used to decrease ischemia, lessen pain, and facilitate cardiac output by decreasing resistance to ejection or afterload.

At low to moderate doses NTG works on the venous system, increasing venous capacity. At high doses it exerts venous and arterial effects.

10. Discuss the pharmacologic effects of morphine.

Relief of pain and ischemia is a high priority. Morphine sulfate is the drug of choice for the pain associated with AMI. In addition to its analgesic properties, morphine exerts favorable, although mild, hemodynamic effects by increasing venous capitance (thereby reducing venous return and preload) and by reducing systemic vascular resistance (thereby reducing the impedance to LV emptying or afterload). The result of both effects is a reduction in myocardial oxygen demand. Additionally, relief of pain alleviates anxiety and, thus, excretion of catecholamines (AHA, 1990).

11. What was the rationale for using a lidocaine (Xylocaine) drip?

Prophylactic lidocaine is no longer recommended for AMI; however, dysrhythmias are common with reperfusion of the myocardium. PVCs are so common that they are thought to represent markers of successful reperfusion. Accelerated idioventricular rhythm or ventricular tachycardia (VT) may occur without warning. Therefore, prophylactic lidocaine is sometimes begun when administration of the thrombolytic agent is started. Toxic effects of lidocaine may include drowsiness, slurred speech, hallucinations, and seizures (Thelan et al., 1994). Mr. Smith's ECG showed PVCs and VT before thrombolytics were started. Therefore, treatment with lidocaine was strongly recommended to prevent further ectopy.

12. Discuss the pharmacologic actions of heparin and the indications for use with the MI patient.

Heparin is an anticoagulant; it inhibits activated factors IX, X, XI, and XII, which are involved in the conversion of prothrombin to thrombin, thereby reducing clot formation (Spencer et al., 1989). Heparin potentiates the effects of antithrombin III. In low doses it prevents the conversion of prothrombin to thrombin. Higher doses neutralize thrombin, preventing the conversion of fibrinogen to fibrin and thus thrombus formation and extension of existing thrombi (Deglin & Vallerand, 1991). Heparin is started with thrombolytic therapy to prevent clots from forming.

13. Describe what a β-blocker is and the rationale for Mr. Smith's receiving this medicine.

Examples of commonly used β-blockers are atenolol (Tenormin), metoprolol (Lopressor), nadolol (Corgard), and propranolol (Inderal).

β-Blockers have been shown to interrupt evolving infarcts, limit infarct size, and decrease the incidence of ventricular dysrhythmias by decreasing oxygen demand. These agents are effective in reducing ischemic pain, presumably because of changes in cardiac index, stroke index, heart rate, BP, tension-time index, and free fatty acid production, all of which affect myocardial oxygen consumption. β-Blockers are contraindicated in patients with heart failure, hypotension, bradycardia, heart block, and bronchial asthma (Riegel, 1993).

β-Adrenergic receptor blocking agents compete with sympathetic (adrenergic) neurotransmitters (epinephrine and norepinephrine) for β-adrenergic receptor sites.

β_1-Adrenergic receptor sites are located chiefly in the heart, where stimulation results in increased heart rate, contractility and AV conduction.

β_2-Adrenergic receptors are found mainly in bronchial and vascular smooth muscle and the uterus. Stimulation of β_2-adrenergic receptors produces vasodilation, bronchodilation, and uterine relaxation.

β-Blockers may be relatively selective. β_1-Blockers are cardioselective and work mainly on blocking adrenergic receptors in the heart. Examples of these β-blockers are metoprolol (Lopressor), atenolol (Tenormin), and acebutolol (Sectral). β_2-Blockers are noncardioselective, blocking both β_1- and β_2-adrenergic receptors. Examples are propranolol (Inderal), nadolol (Corgard), and timolol (blocadren).

β-Blockers are used in the management of hypertension, angina pectoris, tachyarrhythmias, hypertrophic subaortic stenosis, migraine headaches (prophylaxis), and MI (prevention).

Lopressor (metoprolol) is a cardioselective β-blocker. Its side effects are bronchospasm, CHF, and decreased HR. β-Blockers should not be used for an HR less than 50 bpm (Deglin & Vallerand, 1991). One protocol recommends metoprolol in three 5 mg intravenous boluses for AMI. Following each bolus, vital signs must be assessed for 2 to 5 minutes. Any HR less than 60 bpm or a systolic BP of less than 100 mm Hg signals the end of the protocol (Riegel, 1993).

14. Mr. Smith was sent home with a prescription for diltiazem (Cardizem). Why would a heart patient be given a calcium channel blocker?

Examples of calcium channel blockers include diltiazem (Cardizem), nifedipine (Procardia), and verapamil (Calan). Calcium channel blockers inhibit the influx of extracellular calcium ions across the membranes of cardiac and smooth muscle cells, decreasing myocardial contractility and oxygen demand, and dilate coronary arteries and peripheral arterioles. This decreases systemic BP, total peripheral resistance, and afterload of the heart. Platelet aggregation may be inhibited and bleeding prolonged (*Nursing 94: Drug handbook,* 1994; Spencer et al., 1989).

Calcium channel blockers are used in the management of mild to moderate hypertension and chronic stable angina. Calcium channel blockers should not be used for systolic BP less than 90 mm Hg or HR less than 60 bpm.

15. tPA is a thrombolytic agent. Discuss the effect of a thrombolytic and why it was used.

The administration of a thrombolytic agent will result in the lysis of the acute thrombus, thus recanalizing the obstructed coronary artery and restoring blood flow to the affected myocardium (Thelan et al., 1994). The most effective treatment for limiting infarct size is thrombolysis. Because 80% to 90% of AMIs are the result of thrombus, early reperfusion of ischemic and jeopardized myocardium can supply needed oxygen to the threatened myocardium if it is implemented soon after the onset of symptoms (Riegel, 1993). The earlier therapy is implemented, the lower the mortality. At this time three major thrombolytic agents are available in the United States: streptokinase, urokinase, and tissue plasminogen activator (tPA).

Activase (tPA) is an enzyme with a strong binding affinity for fibrin. It converts fibrin-bound plasminogen to plasmin on the clot surface. It is a naturally occurring human protein with identical amino acid sequence produced via rDNA technology. The half-life of tPA is 5 minutes (Busman, David, Housholder, Majoros, & Moccia, 1992).

Eligibility Criteria for Patients Receiving Thrombolytics (Thelan et al., 1994)

- less than 6 hours from onset of chest pain
- ST segment elevation on ECG

- ischemic chest pain of 30 minutes duration
- chest pain unresponsive to sublingual NTG or nifedipine (Procardia)
- less than 75 years of age (may vary)
- no conditions that may predispose to hemorrhage

Front Loading tPA

- 15 ml IVP immediately
- 50 ml/h x 30 min
- 35 ml/h x 60 min
- 20 ml NS added to bag and infused at 35 ml/h to empty all of tPA out of the bag

Standard tPA

- 10 ml IVP
- 50 ml/h x 1 h
- 20 ml/h x 2 h
- 20 ml NS to bag at 20 ml/h

16. What are the contraindications for thrombolytics?

- recent (within 2 months) surgery, especially intracranial or intraspinal, or trauma
- intracranial neoplasm, aneurysm, or arteriovenous malformation
- history of stroke
- uncontrolled hypertension systolic BP more than 180 mm Hg or diastolic BP more than 110 mm Hg
- active internal bleeding
- any known bleeding disorder (e.g., hemophilia)
- predisposition to hemorrhage (e.g., thrombocytopenia)
- recent hemorrhage or active internal bleeding
- gastrointestinal tract or genitourinary tract bleeding within 10 days
- over 75 years of age (may vary) or recent cardiopulmonary resuscitation (CPR) (Riegel, 1993)

17. What is PTCA? What does the procedure involve?

A percutaneous transluminal coronary angioplasty (PTCA) involves the use of a balloon-tipped catheter that when advanced through an atherosclerotic coronary lesion can be intermittently inflated for the purpose of dilating the stenotic area and improving blood flow through it. The mechanism of dilation was originally thought to be plaque compression that resulted in the immediate expression of plaque contents or its redistribution within the vessel wall. However, it is now believed that the stretching of the vessel wall by the high balloon inflation pressures fractures the plaque that narrows the vessel lumen (Thelan et al.,

1994). Waller (1989) suggests that the major mechanism of human coronary angioplasty is "breaking," "cracking," "splitting," or "fracturing" of atherosclerotic plaque.

Angioplasty Via Balloon

A PTCA is performed in the cardiac catheterization laboratory by means of fluoroscopy. Introducer sheaths are commonly inserted percutaneously into the femoral artery. The patient is systemically heparinized to prevent clots from forming on or in any of the catheters. A special guiding catheter designed to engage the coronary ostia is inserted through the arterial sheath and advanced in a retrograde manner through the aorta. NTG or a calcium channel blocker may be given at this time to prevent coronary artery spasm and maximize coronary vasodilation during the procedure. A guidewire is then advanced down the coronary artery and negotiated across the occluding atheroma. The balloon catheter is advanced over this guidewire and positioned across the lesion. The balloon is inflated and deflated repetitively until evidence of dilation is demonstrated on angiogram. It is believed that the stretching of the vessel wall with high balloon inflation pressures fracture the plaque that narrows the vessel lumen (Thelan et al., 1994).

The introducer sheaths are left in place for several reasons. First the intravenous infusion of heparin is continued for 6 to 24 hours following PTCA to prevent clot formation on the roughened endothelium at the site of dilation. Therefore removal of the sheaths during this time would predispose to bleeding. Second, it allows for rapid vascular access should redilation become necessary. However, the arterial sheath must be attached to a continuous heparinized saline flush, and intravenous fluids must be infused through the venous sheath to maintain luminal patency (Thelan et al., 1994). Although the technique of balloon angioplasty has been highly successful, the procedure has been plagued with two major problems at the site of angioplasty: (1) early closure and (2) late closure (restenosis) (Waller, 1989).

New techniques used to prevent restenosis are pyroplasty, stents, laser, and atherectomy. Pyroplasty may also be referred to as thermal angioplasty. The heat is used to "weld" intraluminal flaps after angioplasty. This may prevent or at least delay the smooth muscle response in the development of intimal fibrous hyperplasia (Waller, 1989). A stent is a permanent, noncollapsible tube usually made of stainless steel. Balloon expansion of the stent within the vessel dilates the stent beyond its elastic limits and secures it in place (Hontz, Tripp, & Kline, 1991). A laser light can be transmitted through a fiberoptic bundle with enough pulsed energy to ablate atheroma. This technique is limited to date by inadequate delivery systems, a high frequency of vessel perforation and thrombosis, and the creation of small recanalized channels (Waller, 1989). In atherectomy a cutting instrument, a circular blade rotating at a high speed, is pressed against the diseased part of the vessel by an inflated balloon (Waller, 1989).

18. What made Mr. Smith a candidate for a PTCA? What are the potential contraindications for a patient receiving a PTCA?

Indications for a PTCA are patients with single-vessel disease or multiple-vessel disease, chronic stable angina, angina following coronary artery bypass grafting, recent-onset as well as postinfarction unstable angina, and AMI. Patients who are asymptomatic but demonstrate evidence of ischemia during treadmill testing may be considered candidates for elective PTCA (Thelan et al., 1994).

Mr. Smith was a candidate for a PTCA because his pain recurred after he was treated with tPA. The current recommendation is that intravenous thrombolysis be administered immediately following the onset of symptoms. Catheterization and possible PTCA should be performed prior to discharge. Any recurrence of symptoms following patient stabilization, e.g., return of chest pain following 2 hours or more of a stable period, requires immediate catheterization (Riegel, 1993).

19. What is cardiogenic shock? What symptoms did Mr. Smith exhibit?

Cardiogenic shock occurs in 10% of AMI patients and is associated with a mortality of 85% to 100%. The onset and severity of cardiogenic shock are directly associated with the amount of damaged myocardium. The majority of patients with shock have lost approximately 40% of the LV pump function (Alspach, 1991; Thelan et al., 1994). Clinical presentation of cardiogenic shock is manifested by decreased perfusion, pallor, diaphoretic, mottled appearance, decreased or absent urine output, obtundation, and tachycardia (Alspach, 1991; Thelan et al., 1994). BP is less than 90 mm Hg. Respiratory rate is normal. Invasive hemodynamic monitoring is essential for these patients. Prognosis can be estimated using arterial blood lactate levels (a by-product of anaerobic metabolism), cardiac output, and arterial pressure, in that order (Alspach, 1991).

Mr. Smith was in cardiogenic shock when his systolic BP was 80 to 90 mm Hg. His skin was cool, pale, and diaphoretic. His SaO_2 was 86%, and he was tachycardic.

20. What are the therapeutic effects of dopamine (Intropin) at low doses and at moderate doses? How do these effects differ at high doses?

Dopamine (Intropin) is a catecholamine that stimulates dopaminergic β_1-adrenergic receptors. Fifty percent of its effect is due to release of stored norepinephrine from sympathetic fibers (Jones, 1994). It stimulates the sympathetic nervous system. At low doses (0.5 to 2 $\mu g/kg/min$) it improves renal, brain and mesenteric perfusion.

At moderate doses (3 to 10 µg/kg/min) it has a positive inotropic effect (increases the force and velocity of myocardial systolic contraction). This improves the pumping efficiency of the heart, resulting in increased cardiac output, more complete emptying of the cardiac chambers, and a reduction in elevated ventricular end-diastolic pressure and venous pressures (Spencer et al., 1989).

At high doses (>10 µg/kg/min) dopamine has pure alpha effects; that is, high doses of dopamine increase renal vasoconstriction and peripheral resistance. The vasoconstriction increases systemic vascular resistance, decreases urinary output, and increases oxygen demands of the heart (Deglin & Vallerand, 1991; Spencer et al., 1989). Adverse reactions to dopamine include tachycardia, angina, palpitations, nausea, vomiting, diarrhea, and headache. Also at high doses it can extend the MI because oxygen consumption is greater than supply. Extravasation of intravenous dopamine solution may cause severe vasoconstriction and tissue damage. If extravasation occurs, use of phentolamine (Regitine) at the site counteracts the effects (Spencer et al., 1989).

21. What are the therapeutic effects of dobutamine (Dobutrex)? Why would dopamine and dobutamine be used together?

Dobutamine (Dobutrex) stimulates β_1-adrenergic receptors with relatively minor effects on heart rate and peripheral blood vessels (Deglin & Vallerand, 1991). It does not cause release of endogenous norepinephrine (Spencer et al., 1989). Dobutamine is used to increase cardiac output in treatment of persons with inadequate cardiac contractility. It increases cardiac output without vasoconstriction or a significant increase in heart rate. Adverse effects include arrhythmias, tachycardia, palpitations, and hypertension (Deglin & Vallerand, 1991; Spencer et al., 1989).

22. What do the readings from the pulmonary artery (Swan-Ganz) catheter tell the nurse about Mr. Smith?

Bedside hemodynamic monitoring via flow-directed balloon-tipped pulmonary artery catheter allows for continuous bedside hemodynamic monitoring so that vascular tone, myocardial contractility, and fluid balance can be assessed and effectively managed. It can measure

- right atrial pressure (RAP) through the proximal port of the catheter. The RAP is a determinant of right ventricular end-diastolic pressure (RVEDP), which reflects venous return to the right side of the heart.
- central venous pressure (CVP), which reflects pressure in the great veins. It is used to monitor blood volume, RV function, and central venous return.
- right ventricular pressures.

Table 5–4   Normal Hemodynamic Readings

	RA	RV	PAP	PCWP
Systolic		20–30 mm Hg	20–30 mm Hg	
Diastolic		0–5 mm Hg	10–20 mm Hg	
Mean	2–6 mm Hg	2–6 mm Hg	10–15 mm Hg	4–12 mm Hg

- pulmonary artery pressure (PAP) and pulmonary capillary wedge pressure (PCWP), which are measured through the distal port.

PAP reflects left- and right-sided heart pressures. Pulmonary artery systolic pressure (PAS) represents pressure produced by the right ventricle. The pulmonary artery diastolic pressure (PAD) reflects LVEDP and is used as a measure of LV function and diastolic filling pressures, hence preload. The PCWP is a reflection of left atrial pressures and is used to assess LV filling pressure (LVEDP) (Alspach, 1991). Normal hemodynamic readings are shown in Table 5–4.

23. What advantages does an IABP after coronary artery bypass graft (CABG) have for Mr. Smith?

An IABP is a displacement device. The balloon works on the principle of counterpulsation that is in opposition to systole. When the heart is in systole, the balloon is deflated; when the heart is in diastole, the balloon is inflated. The balloon inflation displaces blood proximally toward the aortic arch to perfuse coronary arteries and distally toward the renal arteries and periphery. This supportive action decreases the heart's workload by reducing afterload and improves the supply of oxygen to the myocardium by increasing perfusion back through the coronary arteries during diastole (Stolarik & Kay, 1992).

Counterpulsation with the IABP is another intervention used to treat decreases in cardiac output following an AMI. Phased pulsation augment coronary perfusion pressure during diastole and deflation throughout systole to facilitate ventricular emptying. In this way, the IABP augments oxygen supply and decreases oxygen demand by minimizing afterload. The IABP is used primarily in treatment of hemodynamically unstable patients, particularly those in cardiogenic shock (Riegel, 1993). The IABP is used for afterload reduction, whereas positive inotropic agents are used to increase ventricular contractility (Thelan et al., 1994).

24. What significance does the IABP have in relation to the tPA and urokinase given previously?

Mr. Smith is at high risk of bleeding from his sheath sites after PTCA. He will return from the cardiac catheterization laboratory with a sheath remaining in his right groin, and the IABP catheter usually is threaded through this insertion site. There is a high potential for bleeding at this site because of the infusion of tPA and urokinase. A compression device such as a Fem-O-Stop or a C-Clamp may be used on his groin to hold pressure if bleeding develops.

References

PTCA and Thrombolytic Therapy in Myocardial Infarction

Alspach, J. G. (1991). *AACN's core curriculum for critical care nursing* (4th ed.). Philadelphia: Saunders.

American Heart Association. (1990). *Textbook of advanced cardiac life support*. Dallas: Author.

American Heart Association. (1991). *1991 heart and stroke facts*. Dallas: Author.

Busman, D., David, S. M., Housholder, S. D., Majoros, K. A., & Moccia, J. M. (1992, July). *Clot combat: Strategic planning for optimal outcomes*. Symposium conducted by Genetech, Evansville, IN.

Deglin, J. H., & Vallerand, A. Z. (1991). *Nurse's med deck* (2nd ed.). Philadelphia: F. A. Davis.

ECG interpretation: Clinical skillbuilders. (1990). Springhouse, PA: Springhouse.

Fischbach, F. (1992). *A manual of laboratory diagnostic tests* (4th ed.). Philadelphia: J. B. Lippincott.

Hartshorn, J., Lamborn, M. L., & Noll, M. L. (1993). *Introduction to critical care nursing*. Philadelphia: Saunders.

Hontz, R. A., Tripp, M. D., & Kline, L. P. (1991). Stents keep occluded vessels open. *RN, 54*(3), 50–54.

Jones, K. (1994, March). Advanced drug management of the cardiac surgery patient. In *The heart of cardiovascular nursing*. Symposium conducted by the American Heart Association at Evansville, IN.

Keil, J. E., Sutherland, S. E., Knapp, R. G., Lackland, D. T., Gazes, P. C., & Tyroller, H. A. (1993). Mortality rates and risk factors for coronary disease in black as compared with white men and women. *New England Journal of Medicine, 329*(2), 73–78.

Miller, B. F., & Keane, C. B. (1991). *Encyclopedia and dictionary of medicine, nursing, and allied health* (5th ed.). Philadelphia: Saunders.

Mims, B. C. (1990). *Case studies in critical care nursing*. Baltimore: Williams & Wilkins.

Nursing 94: Drug handbook. (1994). Springhouse, PA: Springhouse.

Purcell, J. A., & Haynes, L. (1984, May). Using the EKG to detect MI. *American Journal of Nursing, 84,* 627–642.

Riegel, B. (1993). Patients with myocardial infarction. In Clochesy, J. M., Breu, C., Cardin, S., Rudy, E. B., & Whittaker, A. A. (Eds.). *Critical care nursing* (pp. 302–320). Philadelphia: Saunders.

Spencer, R. T., Nichols, L. W., Lipkin, G. B., Sabo, H. M., & West, F. M. (1989). *Clinical pharmacology and nursing management* (3rd ed.). Philadelphia: J. B. Lippincott.

Stolarik, A. H., & Kay, M. C. (1992). Managing an intra-aortic balloon pump. *Critical Care Choices*, 24–29.

Thelan, L. A., Davie, J. K., & Urden, L. D. (1994). *Textbook of critical care nursing: Diagnosis and management.* St. Louis: Mosby–Year Book.

Waller, B. F. (1989). Crackers, breakers, stretchers, drillers, scrapers, shavers, burners, welders, and melters—The future treatment of atherosclerotic coronary artery disease? A clinical morphologic assessment. *Journal of American College of Cardiology*, 13, 969–987.

6

Coronary Artery Bypass Graft

Karen L. Jones, MSN, RNC
Sheila Drake Melander, DSN, RN, FCCM

CASE PRESENTATION

Mr. Howard, a 57-year-old man, had a 3 month history of progressive typical anginal chest pain. He reported that the symptoms first occurred with heavy exertion and involved what he described as a "heaviness" in his chest. The symptoms were promptly relieved with rest. Over the past weeks he had been experiencing increasingly frequent episodes of chest pain and diaphoresis. The episodes had become more prolonged, and he had experienced one episode of pain occurring at rest following a heavy meal. Mr. Howard was moderately obese and had a 20 year history of hypertension, which had been under treatment. Other risk factors in Mr. Howard's history include hypercholesterolemia (350 mg/dl), which he was attempting to treat with dietary modifications, and a 30-year, two pack a day smoking history, which continued up to the present time. Mr. Howard had undergone prior surgery for a bilateral inguinal hernia repair, cholecystectomy, and arthroscopic surgery on his left knee. He also gave a history of problems with gastric reflux and was currently taking cimetidine (Tagamet).

Mr. Howard was evaluated by his family physician after a prolonged episode of chest pain. The results of an electrocardiogram (ECG) were unremarkable; however, in view of the progression of his symptoms he was referred to a cardiologist. Mr. Howard underwent a stress treadmill examination with a thallium scan. The stress test was terminated after 3.2 minutes because of the development of anterior chest pain. This pain was promptly relieved with sublingual nitroglycerin. The thallium scan revealed two areas of reversible defects in the anterior wall of the left ventricle. The decision was made to proceed with cardiac catheterization to further delineate the extent of disease. Cardiac catheterization revealed the following:

- Severe triple vessel coronary artery disease was found with significant left main stenosis of 70%.

  Left anterior descending coronary artery (LAD) 99% obstruction
  Right coronary artery (RCA) 90% (dominant) obstruction
  First obtuse marginal ramus (OM1) 80% obstruction

- The mitral and aortic valves both appeared normal and were without significant stenosis or regurgitation. The left ventricular end-diastolic pressure was 7 mm Hg before injection and 14 mm Hg after dye injection. The left ventricular ejection fraction was estimated to be within the normal range at 55%.

- Mild to moderate hypokinesia was seen in the anterior wall. The left internal mammary artery was found to be of good caliber and available for a conduit.

Because of the critical stenosis of the left main coronary artery and the presence of severe triple vessel disease, angioplasty was ruled out. Urgent coronary artery revascularization was scheduled for the following morning with bypass grafts proposed to the LAD, diagonal artery, RCA, circumflex coronary artery (Cx), and OM1. Immediately after the catheterization Mr. Howard developed severe (9 out of 10 on pain scale) anterior chest pain with radiation to the left arm. He became diaphoretic, and his systolic blood pressure fell to 90 mm Hg. He was stabilized with intravenous (IV) nitroglycerin and an infusion of dobutamine (Dobutrex) (3 μg/kg/min). Because of the left main stenosis an intraaortic balloon pump (IABP) was inserted via the left femoral artery. Excellent augmentation was obtained with a 2:1 setting, and all pain was relieved. The following morning cardiac surgery was performed, using the left internal mammary artery to bypass the LAD, with separate saphenous vein grafts placed to the LAD diagonal artery, OM1, and RCA. Atrial and ventricular pacing wires were placed. The IABP was left in place and functioned before and after the bypass. The surgery was uneventful, and Mr. Howard was admitted to the open heart recovery area 4 hours after initiation of anesthesia.

On admission to the open heart recovery area the following data were obtained:

BP	110/70 (via arterial line)
HR	110 bpm (sinus tachycardia rate)
Respirations	10/min on ventilator with IMV 10
Temperature	35.1° C (95.2° F)
PAP	25/8/18 mm Hg (systolic, diastolic, MAP)
PCWP	7 mm Hg
Cardiac index	2.3 L/min/m² (cardiac output: 4.2 L/min)
SVR	1500 dyne/s/cm⁻⁵
CXR	confirmed correct placement of pulmonary artery (Swan-Ganz) catheter, endotracheal tube, and nasogastric tube

Laboratory Data

Hgb   10.3 g/dl
Hct   31%
Glucose 220 mg/dl
K^+ 3.2 mmol/L

Ventilator Setting

IMV   10
V_T 1000 ml
F_{IO_2} 90%
PEEP   5 cm

Arterial Blood Gases

pH   7.38
P_{O_2} 96 mm Hg
P_{CO_2} 24 mm Hg
HCO_3^- 16 mmol/L
Sa_{O_2} 96%

Lines

- Right radial arterial line
- Pulmonary artery (Swan-Ganz) catheter in the right subclavian vein
- Endotracheal tube (oral)
- Nasogastric tube via the left nare to low continuous suction
- Peripheral IV via no. 19 angiocath in left forearm
- Chest tube in mediastinum has drained 150 ml since placement
- Foley catheter
- IABP

Urinary Output

- Produced 300 ml urine during bypass
- 250 ml since termination of bypass

Drips

- Dobutamine (Dobutrex) 5 µg/min
- Nitroglycerin 15 µg/min

Coronary Artery Bypass Graft

1. Discuss the pathophysiology of coronary artery atherosclerosis. Include a discussion of risk factors associated with the development of this disease. How does Mr. Howard fit the profile of the "typical" coronary artery bypass graft (CABG) patient?

2. Explain the purpose of thallium scanning and include a discussion of Mr. Howard's findings and how this led to the decision to proceed with cardiac catheterization.

3. What are the indications for coronary artery bypass surgery? Why was angioplasty not considered an option for Mr. Howard? What would be the relative risk of CABG in Mr. Howard?

4. Discuss the significance of left main coronary artery stenosis.

5. An IABP was used for Mr. Howard. Discuss the mode of action of the IABP and the reason for its use in this case.

6. Compare and contrast the use of the internal mammary artery and saphenous vein as conduits in CABG surgery. What are the relative benefits and concerns associated with each?

7. Explain the purpose of the pulmonary artery (Swan-Ganz) catheter in this patient. Include in the discussion normally expected parameters. What are the potential complications associated with its use?

8. Describe the reason for use of dobutamine and nitroglycerin in this patient. How do each of these drugs affect volume, preload, contractility, and afterload? Discuss the parameters used in titrating these drugs.

9. Analyze the hemodynamic findings as presented and discuss therapy adjustments that might be necessary.

10. Based on the arterial blood gas results, are the ventilator settings correct? If not, what alterations would you recommend and why? What complications might be expected as a consequence of Mr. Howard's smoking history?

11. Describe the cardiopulmonary bypass machine and discuss myocardial protection during surgery. What are the potential complications associated with the bypass machine?

12. What is the expected postoperative chest tube drainage in the CABG patient? Discuss autotransfusion as it relates to CABG patients.

13. List appropriate nursing diagnoses that might be used in planning care for the CABG patient.

14. In the post-CABG patient, discuss lifestyle modifications that might be necessary. What is the importance of a cardiac rehabilitation program in the recovery of the patient?

QUESTIONS AND ANSWERS

Coronary Artery Bypass Graft

1. **Discuss the pathophysiology of coronary artery atherosclerosis. Include a discussion of risk factors associated with the development of this disease. How does Mr. Howard fit the profile of the "typical" coronary artery bypass graft (CABG) patient?**

Arteriosclerosis produces a hardening of the arteries or thickening of the arterial walls. Arteriosclerosis is generally characterized by lipid deposits that can progress to partial or total obstruction of the lumen wall. Coronary arteries are particularly susceptible to atherosclerosis, which is most frequently seen in patients with a history of smoking, sedentary lifestyle, and high-fat diets. The atherosclerotic lesion or plaque consists of an elevated area of fatty streaks, which are muscle cells filled with lipids and secondary deposits of calcium salts and blood products. An elevated level (above 200 mg) of cholesterol is associated with an increased risk for development of coronary artery disease (National Institutes of Health [NIH], 1989).

Risk factors can be divided into two categories: modifiable and unmodifiable. Unmodifiable risk factors are uncontrollable and include age over 55 years, gender (men have a greater incidence than women until menopause), family history of coronary artery disease, hyperlipidemia, race (African-Americans have a higher incidence than Caucasians), and diabetes. Modifiable risk factors are controllable and include hypertension (BP > 140/90), smoking, increased low-density lipoprotein (LDL) levels, obesity, stress, and sedentary lifestyle (Castelli et al., 1986; Wenger, 1985).

Mr. Howard's history fits the "typical" profile for the CABG patient. He is moderately obese and has a 20 year history of hypertension. He also has hypercholesterolemia with a laboratory value of 350 mg/dl, which he states he is attempting to modify through his diet. Mr. Howard also has a 30 year two pack per day smoking history and a positive family history for coronary atherosclerosis.

2. **Explain the purpose of thallium scanning and include a discussion of Mr. Howard's findings and how this led to the decision to proceed with cardiac catheterization.**

Thallium 201 is the radioactive isotope used in conjunction with either a treadmill stress ECG or bicycle ergometer to differentiate between ischemia and infarction. Thallium scanning will reveal wall motor defects and evaluate heart pump performance during increased oxygen demand. When the thallium is injected during peak exercise, normal myocardium will have greater activity than abnormal myocardium, thus cold spots indicate decreased or absent blood flow. Ischemia is indicated by thallium scan results that are abnormal during exercise but that return to normal 4 hours after exercise. If the scan results are positive for infarction, they will remain abnormal even after the patient has rested. If a patient has normal results from a thallium stress study, the need for a cardiac catheterization may be eliminated (Fischbach, 1992).

Mr. Howard's stress thallium scan was terminated after 3.2 minutes because of the development of anterior chest pain. The scan revealed two areas of reversible defects in the anterior wall of the left ventricle. Because of the test results it was necessary to proceed with the cardiac catheterization for further evaluation of cardiac disease.

3. **What are the indications for coronary artery bypass surgery? Why was angioplasty not considered an option for Mr. Howard? What would be the relative risk of CABG in Mr. Howard?**

The following indicators for coronary artery bypass surgery were stated by Gray and Matloff (1990, p. 15) and Clochesy, Breu, Cardin, Rudy, and Whittaker (1993, p. 386):

- chronic stable angina refractory to medical therapy
- significant left main coronary occlusion (> 50%)
- triple vessel coronary artery disease
- left ventricular dysfunction or proximal LAD disease
- unstable angina
- left ventricular failure (congestive heart failure or cardiogenic shock)
- after thrombolytic therapy, in presence of critical triple vessel disease
- postinfarction angina with multivessel disease
- in patients with nonmechanical cardiogenic shock; if patient is stabilized, acute left ventricular aneurysm
- in association with mechanical defects such as ventricular septal defects, mitral regurgitation (intermittent and persistent), and cardiac rupture with tamponade

Mr. Howard was diagnosed with severe triple vessel disease with significant left main stenosis, both of which indicate the need for CABG and rule out the need for angioplasty.

4. Discuss the significance of left main coronary artery stenosis.

The left main coronary artery supplies the apex, part of the lateral wall, the anterior wall, and two thirds of the septum. Because of the amount of myocardium that is dependent on blood supply from the left main coronary artery, significant stenosis of the artery or the proximal LAD places the myocardium at increased risk for myocardial infarction. Prompt surgical intervention in patients with left main coronary artery disease has been effective in increasing their 3 year survival rates to 85% or 90% compared to medical treatment rates of 65% to 69% (CASS, 1984; Rahimtoola, 1985).

5. An IABP was used for Mr. Howard. Discuss the mode of action of the IABP and the reason for its use in this case.

The IABP is used to increase coronary artery perfusion and support the failing coronary circulation. Indications for use of the IABP are:

a. Left ventricular failure after cardiac surgery
b. Unstable angina refractory to medications
c. Recurrent angina
d. Complications of acute myocardial infarction
   (1) cardiogenic shock
   (2) papillary muscle dysfunction
   (3) ventricular septal defect
   (4) refractory ventricular dysrhythmias (Thelan, Davie, Urden, & Lough, 1990, p. 340)

The IABP inflates during diastole and deflates prior to systole. Balloon inflation is timed by using the dicrotic notch, which denotes the closure of the aortic valve. The inflation forces blood forward and backward simultaneously to increase coronary perfusion and decrease afterload. The forward flow increases perfusion to the organs and the periphery, whereas the backward flow forces an increased amount of blood into the coronary arteries. The sudden deflation reduces the pressure in the aorta and decreases afterload, which lessens the workload of the heart (Hartshorn, Lamborn, & Noll, 1993).

The IABP was implemented in this case after the catheterization, when Mr. Howard developed severe chest pain and his systolic pressure dropped to 90 mm Hg. Because of Mr. Howard's severe left main coronary artery stenosis, the IABP did assist in increasing coronary artery perfusion, decreasing his afterload, and lessening the workload of the heart. Once the IABP was instituted, all pain was relieved.

6. **Compare and contrast the use of the internal mammary artery and saphenous vein as conduits in CABG surgery. What are the relative benefits and concerns associated with each?**

   The most commonly used conduits, or vessels, today are the saphenous vein and the internal mammary (or internal thoracic) artery. Both conduits have been individually used successfully in surgical revascularization and in combination when multiple graft sites were necessary. The patency rate for saphenous vein grafts at 1 year is 98% but falls to 81% at 10 years. Advantages for use of the saphenous vein include technical ease, decreased harvest time, and flexibility of the vein.

   The internal mammary artery is viewed by many as the graft of choice for bypass of the LAD (Loop et al, 1986). Use of both internal mammary arteries in younger patients enhances revascularization results and increases survival rates and graft longevity (Green, 1989). As reported by Loop et al. (1986), the internal mammary patency rate at 10 years is 96%. The absence of valves minimizes luminal turbulence, which reduces the risk of occlusion by thrombosis. Angiography has validated the ability of the internal mammary artery to dilate in response to increased demand (Green, 1989). Limitations include increased time needed for harvesting of the graft, increased bleeding, and increased postoperative chest wall discomfort (Jansen & McFadden, 1986).

7. **Explain the purpose of the pulmonary artery (Swan-Ganz) catheter in this patient. Include in the discussion normally expected parameters. What are the potential complications associated with its use?**

   Postoperative hemodynamic monitoring is needed for the CABG patient so that vascular tone (preload and afterload), myocardial contractility, cardiac output, and volume or fluid balance may be monitored at the bedside. This is accomplished through use of a pulmonary artery (Swan-Ganz) catheter. Postoperatively, patients may exhibit a low cardiac output because of preexisting heart disease or prolonged time on the cardiopulmonary bypass machine. In most patients reduced preload is the cause of the reduced cardiac output. Also high systemic vascular resistance or increased afterload from vasoconstriction can result in decreased cardiac output. Through use of the pulmonary artery (Swan-Ganz) catheter parameters can be assessed, and early intervention can be pursued to correct any postoperative problems (Thelan et al., 1990).

   The balloon-tipped pulmonary artery (Swan-Ganz) catheter allows for measurements of the following: (1) right atrial pressure (RAP) or central venous pressure through use of the proximal port, which represents the right ventricular end-diastolic pressure (RVEDP) and reflects venous return to the right side of the heart, and (2) central venous pressure (CVP), which indicates pressure from the great veins and also the RAP and is used to monitor right ventricle function, central venous return, and blood volume. Normal values for CVP vary from individual to individual; therefore, it is important to monitor the trend in CVP along with the clinical picture. As a general rule values of 2 to 8 cm H_2O are considered within normal limits. The pulmonary artery (Swan-Ganz) catheter also measures (1) right ventricle pressures (RVP), (2) pulmonary artery pressures (PAP), and (3) pulmonary capillary wedge pressures (PCWP), which are measured through the distal port. Pulmonary artery systolic (PAS) represents pressures that are produced by the right ventricle. The pulmonary artery diastolic (PAD) reflects left ventricular end-diastolic pressure (LVEDP) and is used as a measure of diastolic filling and left ventricular function or preload. The PCWP reflects the left atrial pressures and is used in the assessment of left ventricular filling (LVEDP). Left atrial pressure (LAP) measurement is achieved through percutaneous insertion of a catheter directly into the left atrium during cardiac surgery and brought out of the chest wall to be connected to pressure monitoring devices. This provides a continuous display of left atrium pressures, which can be used instead of inflating the balloon on the Swan to obtain a PCWP. LAP is the most accurate measurement of left ventricular preload and in the normal heart is the same as the LVEDP. Increased levels may be due to decreased contractility, tachydysrhythmias, fluid overload, and mitral stenosis or regurgitation. Decreased levels may be due to hypovolemia, indicating hemorrhage postoperatively (Alspach, 1991). See Table 6–1.

8. **Describe the reason for use of dobutamine and nitroglycerin in this patient. How do each of these drugs affect volume, preload, contractility, and afterload? Discuss the parameters used in titrating these drugs.**

   Dobutamine (Dobutrex) is a synthetic catecholamine with mostly a β_1 effect. Dobutamine is more effective than dopamine at increasing myocardial contractility. It increases stroke volume and cardiac output by increasing contractility and also decreases systemic vascular resistance and reduces the PCWP. Dobutamine is very effective in the treat-

Table 6–1   Normal Hemodynamic Readings

CVP   4–13 cm H_2O
LAP   4–12 mm Hg

	RAP	RVP	PAP	PCWP
Systolic		20–30 mm Hg	20–30 mm Hg	
Diastolic		0–5 mm Hg	10–20 mm Hg	
Mean arterial	2–6 mm Hg	2–6 mm Hg	10–15 mm Hg	4–12 mm Hg

ment of heart failure, especially in patients who are hypotensive and cannot tolerate vasodilator therapy. Dobutamine does not have the renal vasodilating effect of dopamine, except indirectly as an effect of increased cardiac output. At low doses dobutamine can decrease blood pressure, especially if the patient is volume depleted. A major advantage of dobutamine is the effect on reducing the PCWP or left ventricular preload, which is especially important in postsurgical patients. Many physicians combine this drug with dopamine to maximize the renal blood flow and reduce the PCWP. An arterial line should be used to assess blood pressure. It should be infused via a volumetric infusion pump. Normal dosage is 2.5 to 20 µg/kg/min and should be titrated on the basis of hemodynamic parameters (Alspach, 1991).

Nitroglycerin (Tridil) is a nitrate and direct smooth muscle relaxant. This drug produces smooth muscle relaxation, which causes decreased peripheral vascular resistance. Hypotension may occur as a result of peripheral vasodilation. Patients may complain of headaches from the cerebral vasodilation. This pooling of blood in the systemic circulation decreases venous return and decreases preload. It is indicated for left ventricular failure, postcardiac surgery, hypertension, angina pectoris, and congestive heart failure. Patients should have an arterial line so that continuous blood pressure readings may be obtained. Nitroglycerin should be infused via a volumetric infusion pump for accuracy and safety. Usually, the IV is started at 5 µg/min and titrated to the lowest amount that produces the desired effect. This drug should not be stopped suddenly but weaned from the patient by reducing the flow rate 5 to 10 µg every 15 minutes. During the weaning process the patient should be constantly observed for return of ischemic symptoms or hypertension.

9. **Analyze the hemodynamic findings as presented and discuss therapy adjustments that might be necessary.**

The hemodynamic parameters that would be of concern are the increased heart rate at 110 bpm, blood pressure of 110/70, PCWP of 7 mm Hg, cardiac index of 2.3 L/min/m² BSA, SVR of 1500 dyne/s/cm⁻⁵, and the temperature of 35.1° C (95.2° F). These data indicate that the patient is "dry" and cold. When the patient begins to warm up after surgery, the vasodilation coupled with volume depletion could possibly cause the patient to "bottom out" hemodynamically. Administration of plasma expanders, such as albumin, and possibly an increase in the rate of IV fluids should be instituted at this time.

10. **Based on the arterial blood gas results, are the ventilator settings correct? If not, what alterations would you recommend and why?**

What complications might be expected as a consequence of Mr. Howard's smoking history?

Mr. Howard's pH is leaning toward the acidotic range even though he is currently within normal limits. His PCO_2 is a little low, as well as his HCO_3; to prevent hyperventilation, incrementally increasing the positive end expiratory pressure (PEEP) to 7.5 cm H_2O, and to 10 cm H_2O if needed, while monitoring the blood pressure would improve Mr. Howard's ventilation. According to the successful use of the PEEP, the FIO_2 may be decreased from 90% to 80%. Arterial blood gases should be obtained in 1 hour to evaluate the patient's response to these changes.

Mr. Howard's extensive history of smoking may increase the difficulty level of weaning Mr. Howard from the ventilator postoperatively. He could develop increased secretions, which could alter oxygen exchange. Close monitoring of Mr. Howard's arterial blood gases, vital signs, and airway secretions may be necessary.

11. **Describe the cardiopulmonary bypass machine and discuss myocardial protection during surgery. What are the potential complications associated with the bypass machine?**

The cardiopulmonary bypass machine provides a mechanism to divert the patient's blood from the arrested heart's right atrium through a membrane or a bubble oxygenator. Once in the oxygenator, carbon dioxide is given off and oxygen is bound to hemoglobin through diffusion. Once arterialized with oxygen, the blood is returned to the systemic circulation through the aorta. This diversion creates a bloodless, motionless area in which to operate. The patient is systemically heparinized prior to initiation of the bypass pump to prevent clotting within the bypass circuit (Clochesy et al., 1993).

Myocardium protection during bypass surgery has been a concern from the inception of this surgery. Experience has shown that the key to myocardium preservation is continuous myocardium hypothermia. This decreases the need for oxygen. A balance must be struck between heat escaping and heat entering the tissues, especially during cross clamping of the aorta. To prevent tissue injuries from warm venous blood entering the heart chambers, cold cardioplegia and topical cooling measures are used. Intermittent infusion of cardioplegic solution approximately every 20 to 30 minutes after the initial dose for diastolic arrest is necessary for the maintainence of myocardial hypothermia and cardioplegic arrest. Whether a cooling jacket, topical measures, or cardioplegia is used, myocardial hypothermic temperatures should remain between 12° and 20° below normal to provide adequate protection (Clochesy et al., 1993; Gray & Matloff, 1990). Potential complications from the use of the cardiopulmonary bypass are outlined as probable causes and effects in Table 6–2.

12. What is the expected postoperative chest tube drainage in the CABG patient? Discuss autotransfusion as it relates to CABG patients.

Gray and Matloff (1990) state that an excess of 250 to 300 ml of chest tube drainage during the first 2 hours after bypass surgery would be reason to reenter the chest to assess the situation. Normal chest tube drainage should be no more than 100 to 150 ml/h. One of the dangers of increased bleeding is cardiac tamponade.

Autotransfusion is a mechanism in which the patient's own blood can be collected, filtered, and reinfused to minimize complications from usage of blood from donors or the blood bank system. Heparin or re-

Table 6–2   Potential Complications of Cardiopulmonary Bypass

Causes	Effects
Third space losses, postoperative diuresis, sudden vasodilation (drugs, rewarming)	Intravascular fluid deficit (hypotension)
Decreased plasma protein concentration, increased capillary permeability	Third space losses (weight gain, edema) and subsequent relative hypovolemia
Hypothermia, increased systemic vascular resistance, prolonged cardiopulmonary bypass pump time, preexisting heart disease, inadequate myocardial protection	Myocardial depression (decreased cardiac output)
Systemic heparinization, mechanical trauma to platelets, depressed release of clotting factors from liver as a result of hypothermia	Coagulopathy (bleeding)
Decreased surfactant production, pulmonary microemboli, interstitial fluid accumulation in the lungs	Pulmonary dysfunction (decreased lung mechanics and impaired gas exchange)
Red blood cell damage in pump circuit	
Decreased insulin release, stimulation of glycogenolysis	Hemolysis (hemoglobinuria) Hyperglycemia (rise in serum glucose)
Intracellular shifts during bypass, postoperative diuresis secondary to hemodilution	Hypokalemia and hypomagnesium
Inadequate cerebral perfusion, microemboli to the brain	
Catecholamine release and systemic hypothermia causing vasoconstriction	Neurologic dysfunction
	Hypertension

Data from Thelan, L., Davie, J., Urden, L., & Lough, M. (1990). *Critical care nursing: Diagnosis and management* (2nd ed.). St. Louis: Mosby–Year Book.

gional anticoagulants such as citrate phosphate dextrose (CPD) or acid phosphate dextrose (APD) are added to the autotransfusion collection system. The blood may then be reinfused to the patient as whole blood or packed red blood cells. Potential complications are coagulation problems, air embolism, hemolysis, cardiac tamponade, and sepsis. Autotransfusion is a common procedure after open heart surgery and is accomplished through use of mediastinal drainage systems. When using these systems as autotransfusion mechanisms, it is necessary to remove all air and add a filter that will remove all clots before returning the blood to the patient (Hartshorn et al., 1993).

13. List appropriate nursing diagnoses that might be used in planning care for the CABG patient.

➤ decreased cardiac output
➤ ineffective airway clearance
➤ ineffective breathing pattern
➤ impaired gas exchange
➤ altered tissue perfusion
➤ activity intolerance
➤ self-care deficit
➤ altered body temperature, hypothermia
➤ acute pain
➤ altered sensory-perceptual deficit
➤ altered thought processes
➤ anxiety
➤ fear
➤ powerlessness
➤ self-concept disturbance
➤ high risk for sexual dysfunction
➤ fluid volume deficit
➤ high risk for fluid volume overload
➤ high risk for infection
➤ impaired swallowing
➤ impaired tissue integrity
➤ altered oral mucous membranes
➤ high risk for constipation
  (Gordon, 1987)

14. In the post-CABG patient, discuss lifestyle modifications that might be necessary. What is the importance of a cardiac rehabilitation program in the recovery of the patient?

Patients who have had CABG surgery must maintain the regimen of care prescribed by their physicians after they leave the hospital. Nurses in the critical care unit begin instructing the patient in the regimen, and this process continues in the step-down units until the patient is discharged. Compliance is stressed in the areas of diet, exercise, medications, stress reduction, control of hypertension, and smoking cessation. As stated by Rankin, Hennein, and Keith (1994), risk modification and continued medical therapy are necessary after CABG, since atherosclerotic involvement of saphenous vein grafts is a long-term major complication. Lipid abnormalities must be treated through drug administration or diet to reduce the chance of reoperation for coronary artery disease.

Spouses or significant others should be included in all teaching sessions whenever possible. Patients and families should be linked to a support group, if possible. Cardiac rehabilitation must continue after discharge, since it provides a built-in support group to assist in the maintenance of new lifestyle modifications. Frequently, rehabilitation facilities provide support groups for spouses of CABG patients to emphasize food preparation (low-fat, low-cholesterol, low-sodium diets) or exercise. Spousal support groups can be effective in dealing with fears and concerns of the group members. Continuing cardiac rehabilitation once the patient is discharged from the hospital is the key to recovery for the CABG patient (Clochesy et al., 1993). Gray and Matloff (1990) state that participation in an inexpensive rehabilitation program involving simple calisthenics and graduated walking has been shown to significantly increase employment rates after surgery.

Coronary Artery Bypass Graft

Alspach, J. (1991). *American Association of Critical Care Nurses core curriculum for critical care nursing* (4th ed.). Philadelphia: Saunders.

CASS Principle Investigators. (1984). Myocardial infarction and mortality in the coronary artery surgery study (CASS) randomized trial. *New England Journal of Medicine, 310*(12), 750–758.

Castelli, W. et al. (1986). Incidence of coronary heart disease and lipoprotein cholesterol levels: The Framingham study. *JAMA, 256*(20).

Clochesy, J., Breu, C., Cardin, S., Rudy, E., & Whittaker, A. (1993). *Critical care nursing*. Philadelphia: Saunders.

Fischbach, F. (1992). *A manual of laboratory and diagnostic tests*. New York: J. B. Lippincott Company.

Gordon, M. (1987). *Nursing diagnosis: Process and application*. New York: McGraw-Hill.

Gray, R., & Matloff, J. (1990). *Medical management of the cardiac surgical patient*. Baltimore: Williams & Wilkins.

Green, G. (1989). Use of internal thoracic artery for coronary artery bypass grafting. *Circulation, 79*(6, Suppl. 1), 1–33.

Hartshorn, J., Lamborn, M., & Noll, M. (1993). *Introduction to critical care nursing*. Philadelphia: Saunders.

Jansen, K., & McFadden, P. (1986). Postoperative nursing management in patients undergoing myocardial revascularization with the internal mammary artery bypass. *Heart and Lung, 15*(1), 48–51.

Loop, F., et al. (1986). Influence of the internal mammary artery graft on 10 year survival and other cardiac events. *New England Journal of Medicine, 314*, 1–6.

National Institutes of Health. (1989). *Report of the expert panel on the detection, evaluation, and treatment of high blood cholesterol in adults* (NIH Publication No. 89-2925). Bethesda, MD: Author.

Rahimtoola, S. (1985). A perspective on the 3 large multicenter randomized clinical trials of CABG for chronic stable angina. *Circulation, 72*(Suppl. 5), 123–135.

Rankin, J., Hennein, H., & Keith, F. (1994). The heart: 1. Acquired disease. In current *Surgical diagnosis and treatment*. Norwalk, Conn: Appleton & Lange.

Thelan, L., Davie, J., Urden, L., & Lough, M. (1990). *Critical care nursing: Diagnosis and management* (2nd ed.). St. Louis: Mosby–Year Book.

Wenger, N. (1985). *Exercise and the heart*. Philadelphia: F. A. Davis.

7

Cardiogenic Shock in Anterior Wall Myocardial Infarction

Jamie Elizabeth Madding, BSN, RN
Sheila Drake Melander, DSN, RN, FCCM

CASE PRESENTATION

Mrs. Adams, a 50-year-old white woman, presented to the emergency department at 6:30 AM with a 2 hour history of crushing substernal chest pain radiating to the jaw, back, and subxiphoid area. She was mildly diaphoretic and slightly short of breath and complained of nausea. Lungs had bibasilar wheezes on auscultation. Heart sounds revealed the presence of an S_3 heart sound and no murmurs. Initial chest x-ray showed no abnormalities. Initial vital signs were

BP	136/98
HR	120 bpm
Respirations	28/min
Temperature	37° C (98.6° F)

The patient had a history of angina pectoris for an undetermined period of time. However, she revealed that for the past 3 weeks she has experienced substernal pain radiating to the back on the frequency of every hour with episodes of crescendo pain. Pain was relieved with nitroglycerin sublingual (SL). There is a family history of a brother dying from a myocardial infarction (MI) and a sister with a history of three MIs. The patient smokes one pack of cigarettes a day. Currently, she takes the following medication:

Current Medications
- propranolol hydrochloride (Inderal) 80 mg q.d.
- diltiazem (Cardizem CD) 120 mg q.d.

A peripheral IV was started with 5% dextrose and water (D_5W) at a keep open rate. The patient was given morphine sulfate (Roxanol) intravenously and started on oxygen at 6 L via nasal cannula. A Foley catheter was placed.

ECG Changes

The initial 12-lead ECG revealed early Q waves in leads V_2 to V_6 and involving leads II, III, and aVF.

7 AM

The patient experienced several short runs of ventricular tachycardia (VT) and was given a 1 mg/kg bolus of lidocaine, after which a drip was started at 2 mg/min. Admission laboratory specimens were drawn for electrolytes, complete blood count, and enzymes. Laboratory data results were as follows:

WBCs	13.9/mm^3	Glucose	117 mg/dl
Hgb	14 g/dl	BUN	6 mmol/L
Hct	41.8%	Creatinine	0.9 mg/dl
NA$^+$	141 mmol/L	LDH	182 U/L
K$^+$	4 mmol/L	AST (SGOT)	38 U/L
Cl$^-$	103 mmol/L	CK	110 U/L
CO$_2$	24 mmol/L		

A tissue plasminogen activator (tPA) infusion was started and nitroglycerin patch applied, and the patient was transferred to the intensive care unit (ICU). A heparin drip of 20,000 U/L D_5W was started at 50 ml/h. A second set of vital signs was taken:

BP	90/60
HR	120 bpm
Respirations	28/min

A second ECG revealed a left bundle branch block.

8 AM

The patient experienced pain relief and occasional premature ventricular contractions (PVCs). An echocardiogram revealed an interoapical dyskinesia with the entire septum, apex, anterior wall, and inferoapical segments being kinetic. The ejection fraction was 20%. A pulmonary artery (Swan-Ganz) catheter was inserted.

10 AM

At 10 AM enzyme and arterial blood gas levels were determined:

AST	500 U/L	pH	7.261
LDH	1186 U/L	P$_{CO_2}$	52.1 mm Hg
CK	1900 U/L	P$_{O_2}$	45.1 mm Hg
CK-MB	2.5%	HCO$_3^-$	22.4 mmol/L

The patient was placed on 60% oxygen via face mask, and vital signs and hemodynamic values were taken:

BP	100/60	PCWP	12 mm Hg
HR	130 bpm	CO	4 L/min
Respirations	30/min	CI	2 L/min/m²
		SVR	1200 dyne/s/cm⁻⁵

2 PM

The patient complained of increased shortness of breath. There were rales throughout all lung fields. She experienced increasing restlessness. Chest x-ray revealed increasing congestive heart failure with pulmonary edema. Vital signs and hemodynamic values were taken.

BP	100/60	PCWP	20 mm Hg
HR	130 bpm	CO	2.5 L/min
Respirations	36/min	CI	1.5 L/min/m²
Urine output	20 ml/h × 2 h	SVR	1800 dyne/s/cm⁻⁵

The patient received dopamine (Intropin) at 5 µg/kg/min and dobutamine (Dobutrex) at 2 µg/kg/min.

3 PM

The dobutamine was discontinued, and maintenance doses of dopamine were given to maintain blood pressure at 100 mm Hg systolic.

8 PM

The patient experienced increased shortness of breath and restlessness. She was given 40 mg of furosemide (Lasix) intravenously. Vital signs and enzymes were

BP	80/60	AST	1044 U/L
HR	120 bpm	LDH	1719 U/L
Respirations	30/min	CK	1248 U/L

Both the patient and family refused the initiation of intubation and mechanical ventilation. The patient was given another 40 mg of furosemide intravenously. The dopamine drip was continued with the order to titrate to maintain systolic blood pressure of 100 mm Hg, and the dobutamine drip was restarted at 2 µg/kg/min.

10:30 PM

By 10:30 PM Mrs. Adams' vital signs had changed to the following:

BP	110/60
HR	110 bpm
Respirations	30/min

The patient continued to receive dopamine to maintain blood pressure. The patient still refused ventilatory support. By 11:30 PM the urine output had increased to 150 ml/h, and the following rates were being maintained:

Dopamine   6 µg/kg/min
Dobutamine   2 µg/kg/min
HR   110 bpm
Respirations   26/min

The patient was breathing easier and was less restless and more alert.

Day 2

The morning of the second day of her hospital stay, Mrs. Adams' diagnostic data had changed as follows:

AST	1076 U/L	BP	100/60
LDH	2324 U/L	HR	110 bpm
CK	6408 U/L	Respirations	34/min
CK-MB	3.5%	PCWP	13 mm Hg
		CO	3 L/min
		CI	2 L/min/m^2

The transient left bundle branch block was gone, and the urine output was 100 ml/h. The drips remained unchanged.

Day 3

In the morning of the third day the patient did not experience chest pain, and vital signs were as follows:

BP   100/60
HR   110 bpm
Respirations   24/min

In the evening of the third day the patient experienced a run of symptomatic VT unresponsive to lidocaine. A procainamide bolus was given, and a procainamide drip was started at 3 mg/min. The patient received digoxin (Lanoxin) with the following regimen:

Digoxin 0.5 mg IV now
Digoxin 0.25 mg IV in 6 h
Digoxin 0.25 mg IV in 12 h
Digoxin 0.25 mg PO q.d.

Day 4

By the morning of the fourth day the patient had no further episodes of VT, and lidocaine and procainamide drips were continued. In the evening of the fourth day the patient experienced a run of sustained VT (7 minutes), followed by an intermittent atrioventricular (AV) block. A transvenous external pacemaker was inserted. A bretylium drip was begun at 1 mg/min, and the procainamide was discontinued. The lidocaine drip was discontinued.

Day 5

By the morning of the fifth day Mrs. Adams' vital signs had once again changed:

BP   100/60
HR   83 bpm
Respirations 22/min

An S_3 heart sound was audible to auscultation. The patient continued to receive dopamine. She was in a normal sinus rhythm. No pacing had been required. The patient then agreed to be transferred to a tertiary center for electrophysiology studies.

QUESTIONS

Cardiogenic Shock in Anterior Wall Myocardial Infarction

1. Discuss the pathophysiology of acute myocardial infarction (AMI).

2. How is a diagnosis of AMI determined?

3. Discuss transmural vs. nontransmural MI and the significance in terms of an anterior wall MI. What is the prognosis for a patient with anterior wall MI?

4. What complications are frequently seen following an MI? What are the most common complications seen with an anterior wall MI?

5. What type of rhythm changes may be commonly seen with an anterior wall MI?

6. What are the treatment goals for an AMI patient?

7. Discuss the role of nitrates and β-blockers in the AMI patient.

8. Discuss the role of thrombolytic therapy in an AMI patient. Include indications and contraindications for use of thrombolytics.

9. What are some of the risks of thrombolytic therapy following reperfusion?

10. Discuss nursing implications for the AMI patient.

11. Discuss nursing implications for patients receiving thrombolytic therapy.

12. Define cardiogenic shock and common causes associated with cardiogenic shock.

13. What is the prognosis for the patient with cardiogenic shock?

14. Discuss the pathophysiologic process involved in cardiogenic shock.

15. What changes are seen in the hemodynamic parameters in the patient with cardiogenic shock?

16. Discuss the role of preload and afterload in the management of cardiogenic shock.

17. Discuss the role of inotropic agents and vasodilators in cardiogenic shock.

18. Discuss the purpose of volume infusion in cardiogenic shock.

19. What types of mechanical support devices may be used in cardiogenic shock and why?

20. What are nursing implications for the patient in cardiogenic shock?

QUESTIONS AND ANSWERS

Cardiogenic Shock in Anterior Wall Myocardial Infarction

1. **Discuss the pathophysiology of acute myocardial infarction (AMI).**

   AMI is the sudden development of ischemia resulting in necrosis of myocardial tissue. In the majority of cases it is the result of severe atherosclerotic narrowing of one or more of the coronary arteries. Coronary thrombosis, coronary artery spasm, platelet aggregation, and rupture of atherosclerotic plaque cause occlusion of coronary arteries (American Heart Association [AHA], 1992). The anterior wall of the left ventricle is supplied by the left anterior descending coronary artery (LAD). When infarction occurs, there are three zones of tissue: necrotic, injured, and ischemic. Once myocardial tissue dies, it never rejuvenates. Injured and ischemic tissue, however, if supplied with oxygen and allowed to rest, may recover. Infarcted tissue does not contract, nor does it conduct electrical impulses along the normal pathways. Thus, electrical instability with lethal arrhythmias may occur, as well as a decreased ejection fraction (EF) and cardiac output (CO).

2. **How is a diagnosis of AMI determined?**

   The clinical presentation of AMI patients includes chest pain lasting more than 30 minutes. The pain is typically retrosternal but may radiate down the ulnar aspect of the left hand or involve the neck, jaw, teeth, shoulders, and intrascapular region. The pain may be confused with indigestion. It is important to note that 20% to 60% of infarctions are symptomless. Patients experiencing AMI are usually extremely uncomfortable, restless, anxious, and distressed. Approximately 50% of patients experience hypotension or bradycardia, and 50% of those with anterior infarcts experience hypertension and tachycardia. In congestive heart failure, patients may be short of breath with frothy, pink sputum and jugular venous distension. Cardiac auscultation may show extra heart sounds, including S_4. In addition, S_4 heard immediately preceding S_1 is reflective of a noncompliant left ventricle. The S_3 sound is heard after S_2 and is found in patients with large transmural infarcts and extensive left ventricular dysfunction. It also occurs with mitral regurgitation due to papillary muscle dysfunction. Transient pericardial friction rubs may also be auscultated, as they occur in 7% to 20% of AMI cases (Clochesy, Breu, Cardin, Rudy, & Whittaker, 1993).

A diagnosis of AMI is made through a variety of studies. Although electrophysiologic changes are usually present on a 12-lead ECG, they are not always immediately present or easily detected. Normal results from an ECG alone do not rule out the possibility of cardiac dysfunction. ECG changes are evolutionary. T wave inversion occurs with ischemia due to altered repolarization. Injury causes elevation of the ST segment (elevation increases with more acute injury). Q waves occur with necrosis and are significant when they are one fourth the size of the R wave. ST elevation and T wave inversion will resolve over time; however, the Q wave always remains (Hanisch, 1991).

Laboratory tests include creatine kinase (CK), lactate dehydrogenase (LDH), their isoenzymes (CK-MB and LDH_1), and aspartate aminotransferase (AST), which has taken the place of serum glutamic-oxaloacetic transaminase (SGOT) in most hospitals because it is more cardiac specific. The initial rise of the CK-MB occurs in 4 to 8 hours, peaks in 24 hours, and returns to normal in 3 to 4 days. LDH levels rise in 24 to 48 hours, peak in 3 to 6 days, and return to normal in 8 to 14 days. AST levels rise in 6 to 12 hours, peak in 36 hours, and return to baseline in 5 to 7 days (Thompson, McFarland, Hirsch, Tucker, & Bowers, 1989).

An echocardiogram is often used to confirm the infarction. Echocardiograms enable the physician to determine the extent of the MI by showing wall motion irregularities, structural damage, and EF.

In the case of this patient, the clinical presentation was typical of AMI. The patient had experienced over 2 hours of substernal, crushing chest pain that radiated to the jaw, back, and subxiphoid area. The patient was also diaphoretic and short of breath and complained of nausea. Heart sounds revealed the presence of an S_3. The 12-lead ECG showed Q waves in leads V_2 to V_6 and involvement in leads II, III, and aVF, indicating an anterior wall MI and inferior wall MI. The CK at 8:00 AM was 1900 U/L, LDH 1186 U/L, AST 500 U/L, and CK-MB 2.5%. These levels were all significantly elevated and indicated extensive damage to the myocardium. The echocardiogram revealed a significantly reduced EF of 20% and an anteroapical dyskinesia affecting the entire septum, apex, and anterior wall, whereas inferoapical segments were kinetic.

3. **Discuss transmural vs. nontransmural MI and the significance in terms of an anterior wall MI. What is the prognosis for a patient with anterior wall MI?**

There are two types of infarction: transmural and nontransmural (or subendocardial). A transmural MI involves a larger portion of the heart with necrosis extending from the epicardium to the endocardium. A nontransmural MI involves a smaller portion of the heart and is usually within the subendocardial wall of the left ventricle, the ventricular septum, and papillary muscles (AHA, 1992). Mrs. Adams experienced a transmural MI, demonstrated by her laboratory studies, 12-lead ECG, and echocardiogram.

The prognosis of patients with an anterior wall MI is significantly worse than that of patients with an inferior wall MI (Hanisch, 1991). The rationale is unclear. It could be the result of the site or the size of the MI. Patients with an anterior wall MI generally have more myocardial damage than those with inferior wall infarction. Because the left ventricle is involved, the likelihood of heart failure or cardiogenic shock is much greater in anterior wall MI.

4. **What complications are frequently seen following an MI? What are the most common complications seen with an anterior wall MI?**

Complications following an AMI include the following, in order of occurrence: arrhythmias, heart failure, infarct expansion, left ventricular mural thrombus, pericarditis, cardiogenic shock, left ventricular aneurysm, and other structural defects (Clochesy et al., 1993).

Mrs. Adams experienced some very life-threatening complications of AMI. The arrhythmias she experienced included VT and AV block. She experienced heart failure, as was noted by her dyspnea, crackles in all lung fields, and chest x-ray, which depicted pulmonary edema. The most serious complication Mrs. Adams experienced was cardiogenic shock.

5. **What type of rhythm changes may be commonly seen with an anterior wall MI?**

Arrhythmias commonly seen with an anterior wall MI include sinus tachycardia, PVCs, premature atrial contractions, atrial tachycardia, atrial flutter, and atrial fibrillation. Intraventricular conduction disturbances include right and left bundle branch blocks, and Mobitz II block progressing to complete AV block often occurs (Hanisch, 1991).

Mrs. Adams experienced numerous rhythm disturbances. She had PVCs, several episodes of VT, a left bundle branch block, and an AV block that required a pacemaker.

6. What are the treatment goals for an AMI patient?

The goals for an AMI patient are to limit the size of the infarct, support the heart during the shock, relieve pain, and manage arrhythmias. Other goals include providing education concerning the diagnosis and necessary lifestyle changes needed to prevent another infarct in the future (Clochesy et al., 1993).

7. Discuss the role of nitrates and β-blockers in the AMI patient.

Nitrates are frequently used in treating AMI patients. Nitroglycerin dilates the large coronary arteries, prevents vasospasm, and increases coronary collateral blood flow to the ischemic myocardium. Sublingual nitroglycerin decreases left ventricular filling pressure without significantly lowering systemic vascular resistance. Intravenous nitroglycerin reduces both left ventricular filling pressure and systemic vascular resistance, which may result in hypotension. Nitroglycerin must be administered cautiously, as a 10% reduction in blood pressure may cause compromised coronary artery perfusion and aggravate myocardial ischemia (AHA, 1992).

β-Blockers such as propranolol (Inderal) and metoprolol (Lopressor) are used to decrease the effects of circulating catecholamines by blocking their ability to bind to β-adrenergic receptors. The desired effect is to reduce heart rate and blood pressure. A less desirable effect, however, is the decrease in myocardial contractility. β-Blockers also are used to control arrhythmias and may be given when recurrent VT or fibrillation occur. The use of β-blockers with AMI is controversial. Some studies have suggested a decrease in infarct size and mortality if they are administered early after the onset of AMI; however, their routine use is not recommended (AHA, 1992).

Mrs. Adams received nitroglycerin, in the form of a transdermal patch, when the tPA was begun. She had received propranolol 80 mg q.d. at home.

8. Discuss the role of thrombolytic therapy in an AMI patient. Include indications and contraindications for use of thrombolytics.

Thrombolytics are the most effective treatment for limiting infarct size according to Clochesy et al. (1993). This is because 80% to 90% of AMIs are the result of a thrombus. If oxygen is able to reach ischemic tissue, the tissue can recover.

Thrombolytics should be initiated within 6 hours of symptom onset. The earlier therapy is initiated, the lower the mortality. Thrombolytics seem most effective in patients younger than 65 years experiencing their first anterior wall MI. Contraindications include recent hemorrhage,

history of a stroke, recent major surgery or trauma, severe hypertension, dental extraction, pregnancy or recent delivery, and advanced age
(Clochesy et al., 1993, p. 315).

Mrs. Adams received thrombolytic therapy in the form of tPA. She
had experienced pain for approximately 2 hours and was only 50 years
of age. Thus, Mrs. Adams had no obvious contraindications.

9. What are some of the risks of thrombolytic therapy following reperfusion?

Cellular edema due to ischemia may prevent restoration of flow at
the microvascular level, even when the thrombus is dissolved. Reperfusion may increase the swelling and inhibit oxygenation of the ischemic
myocardium. Another cause of cellular reperfusion injury may be oxygen-free radicals (Clochesy et al., 1993).

The second major risk of reperfusion is dysrhythmias. PVCs are often
a sign of successful reperfusion. Sinus bradycardia, VT, and accelerated
idioventricular rhythms may occur (Clochesy et al., 1993). Mrs. Adams
experienced reperfusion arrhythmias in the form of occasional PVCs.

10. Discuss nursing implications for the AMI patient.

Nursing implications for an AMI patient are based completely on the
nursing process. AMI patients need continuous assessment of their
physical status, including lung and heart auscultation, pain level, heart
rhythm, laboratory results, and hemodynamic status.

The assessment data are organized and nursing diagnoses are for-
mulated. The diagnoses include the following (Thompson et al., 1989):

> ➤ altered comfort: pain related to myocardial ischemia
> ➤ altered cardiac output: decreased related to reduced contractility
>   due to mechanical and electrical dysfunction
> ➤ activity intolerance related to pain, imbalance between oxygen
>   supply and demand, medications, and illness state
> ➤ ineffective individual and family coping related to fear of death
>   and the critical care environment

Planning involves establishing goals such as relieving pain, decreasing myocardial oxygen demand and increasing supply to meet the demands, maintaining an optimal cardiac output, and enabling the patient
and family to develop coping methods to deal with this crisis.

Implementation of nursing interventions to meet the goals is the
next stage of the nursing process. Nursing interventions include administering oxygen and pain medications such as morphine, limiting
patient activity during the initial infarction stage and progressively increasing activity as the patient's status improves, and administering inotropic and vasoactive drugs such as dobutamine, dopamine, and an-

tiarrhythmics as ordered. For the diagnosis of ineffective coping, the interventions include patient education and advocacy for the patient and family within the critical care environment.

Evaluation is the final stage in the nursing process. In the AMI patient evaluation is integrated with intervention. Because the patient is critically ill, one must evaluate the effectiveness of interventions as one administers them, altering the course of care as necessary. Outcomes are evaluated for achievement, and the care plan is modified as necessary.

11. Discuss nursing implications for patients receiving thrombolytic therapy.

Nursing implications for patients receiving thrombolytic therapy vary depending on the stage of treatment. Nurses administering thrombolytics must obtain a complete history that identifies any contraindications for the therapy. There is no antidote for thrombolytics once they have been administered. The only treatment is to wait for them to be metabolized and administer blood transfusions as necessary. Vascular access lines, usually more than one, must be established before administration of thrombolytics. After administration, nurses must monitor for complications such as bleeding or dysrhythmias. The nursing diagnosis most applicable for this patient group is high risk for injury related to bleeding or dysrhythmias. Interventions include the administration of antiarrhythmics and preventing trauma or invasive procedures after thrombolytics are administered.

12. Define cardiogenic shock and common causes associated with cardiogenic shock.

Cardiogenic shock occurs when the heart cannot maintain enough cardiac output to meet the body's demands. The most common cause is myocardial infarction, but other cardiac disorders such as end-stage cardiomyopathy, valvular heart disease, cardiopulmonary bypass, and cardiac tamponade may be the precipitating events. Cardiogenic shock has been linked to the destruction of 40% or more of the left ventricle. The incidence of cardiogenic shock following MI is 10% to 15% with a mortality rate of 85% to 100% (Clochesy et al., 1993).

13. What is the prognosis for the patient with cardiogenic shock?

The prognosis is generally poor with cardiogenic shock. Dobutamine, dopamine, and other inotropic agents may be used in an effort to hemodynamically stabilize the patient, or an intraaortic balloon pump (IABP) may be placed. However, the mortality rate is 85% to 100% even with the IABP and medications (Clochesy et al., 1993).

14. Discuss the pathophysiologic process involved in cardiogenic shock.

The pathophysiologic process involved in cardiogenic shock is self-perpetuating. Loss of cardiac muscle leads to decreased pumping ability of the ventricles and reduced stroke volume that causes a decreased cardiac output. The decreased cardiac output perpetuates a decrease in blood pressure and coronary perfusion, which causes progressive myocardial ischemia and cellular dysfunction (Von Rueden & Walleck, 1989).

15. What changes are seen in the hemodynamic parameters in the patient with cardiogenic shock?

Hemodynamic parameters are severely altered in the patient with cardiogenic shock. Cardiac output and cardiac index (CI) are dramatically lowered. Tachycardia occurs as the body attempts to compensate for the drop in systolic blood pressure. The pulmonary artery (Swan-Ganz) catheter readings show an increase in the central venous pressure (CVP), the pulmonary capillary wedge pressure (PCWP), and systemic vascular resistance (SVR), reflecting an increase in preload and afterload (Thompson et al., 1989).

The hemodynamic diagnosis of cardiogenic shock is based on a depression of blood pressure (usually systolic pressure below 80 to 90 mm Hg or a reduction of 70 mm Hg or more), CI of less than 1.8 L/min/m² with elevation of left ventricular filling pressure (PAWP above 16 to 18 mm Hg), and clinical signs of hypoperfusion (e.g., oliguria, mental obtundation, pallor, sweating, and tachycardia) (AHA, 1992, p. 18).

Mrs. Adams showed hemodynamic changes consistent with cardiogenic shock at 2 PM the day of admission. Her systolic blood pressure dropped to 80 mm Hg. Her heart rate increased to 130 bpm, cardiac output dropped from its previous reading of 4 to 2.5 L/min, and CI also dropped from 2 to 1.5 L/min/m². The PCWP increased from 12 to 20 mm Hg, and her SVR increased to 1800 dyne/s/cm^{-5}.

16. Discuss the role of preload and afterload in the management of cardiogenic shock.

Preload is a measurement of the stretch of the ventricles during end of diastole. Because the stretch is difficult to measure, the pressure in the ventricle at the end of diastole is measured. The right ventricle's pressure is reflected in the CVP, whereas the left ventricle's pressure is measured by the PCWP (Hollingsworth, 1992).

The Frank-Starling law states that increased stretch of a muscle causes a more forceful contraction. When a muscle is damaged and less compliant, an increased stretch, using an increased volume, may simply increase pressure without increasing the strength of the contraction. In cardiogenic shock the treatment is aimed at decreasing the preload to relieve pulmonary congestion. However, if the preload is decreased too much, both stroke volume and cardiac output will fall. Some sources recommend a PCWP of 15 mm Hg as the optimum level in cardiogenic shock (Von Rueden & Walleck, 1989).

Afterload is the resistance against which the ventricles eject blood during systole. It is a major determinate of myocardial workload and oxygen consumption. The measurement that reflects afterload for the right ventricle is pulmonary vascular resistance (PVR) and for the left ventricle it is systemic vascular resistance (SVR). The goal in cardiogenic shock is to decrease afterload in an effort to reduce ventricular wall stress, increase ventricular systolic emptying, and lower myocardial oxygen demand (Hollingsworth, 1992).

17. Discuss the role of inotropic agents and vasodilators in cardiogenic shock.

Inotropic agents are a classification of drugs used to increase the contractility of the heart. These include norepinephrine, dopamine, dobutamine, isoproterenol (Isuprel) (rarely used), amrinone (Inocor), milrinone (Primacor), and digitalis (Digoxin). These drugs increase cardiac output and relieve pulmonary congestion (AHA, 1992). Mrs. Adams received dopamine, dobutamine, amrinone, and digoxin.

Dopamine's effects vary depending on the dosage range. At low dosages (1 to 2 µg/kg/min) renal perfusion is increased while heart rate and blood pressure remain unaffected. In midrange dosages (2 to 10 µg/kg/min) dopamine stimulates both β_1- and α-adrenergic receptors, causing an increase in cardiac output resulting from the improved contractility; a mild increase in the SVR and preload often occur. At a dosage range above 10 µg/kg/min, peripheral arterial and venous vasoconstriction occur, causing a marked increase in SVR afterload and preload. Dopamine is usually given when hemodynamically significant hypotension occurs in the absence of hypovolemia. One disadvantage is that dopamine increases cardiac workload without significantly increasing coronary blood flow (AHA, 1992).

Dobutamine has a dosage range of 2.5 to 20 mg/kg/min with usual infusion rates of 5 to 15 µg/kg/min. This drug is a potent inotropic agent that stimulates primarily the β-andrenergic receptors. Dobutamine's primary effect is on the heart, resulting in an increase in contractility and a relatively small increase in heart rate. Dobutamine typically will decrease CVP and PCWP while having little effect on PVR. Like other inotropic agents, dobutamine can increase pulmonary intrapulmonary shunting by augmenting cardiac output, which in turn results in perfusion of poorly ventilated lung regions. In summary, dobutamine when used in patients with congestive heart failure, increases stroke volume and cardiac output while reducing filling pressures in the heart. Dobutamine maintains its hemodynamic effect better than dopamine during continuous infusion, since dopamine depletes myocardial norepinepherine stores (Chernow, 1994).

Digoxin is a cardiac glycoside used to increase myocardial contraction and to control the ventricular response to atrial flutter and fibrillation. Digoxin may be administered both orally and intravenously. When patients begin digoxin treatments they receive loading doses followed by a maintenance dose. Dosages of digoxin should be titrated to the patients cardiac pathology, disease, and age. Digoxin toxicity can occur resulting in numerous arrhythmias, including VT (AHA, 1992; Chernow, 1994).

Vasodilators are agents such as sodium nitroprusside and nitroglycerin. These agents are given to decrease SVR, thereby decreasing afterload and increasing stroke volume. Vasodilators are indicated in hypertensive crisis and in combination with inotropic agents for severe heart failure. Patients must be closely monitored for a decrease in blood pressure (AHA, 1992). Mrs. Adams received only a nitroglycerin patch.

18. Discuss the purpose of volume infusion in cardiogenic shock.

Volume infusion in cardiogenic shock is usually restricted, and diuretics are employed to reduce intravascular volume (Von Rueden & Walleck, 1989). However, when the blood pressure is falling and the PCWP is low, the patient may require volume to increase preload to a therapeutic range. Although Mrs. Adams did not receive volume infusion while in cardiogenic shock, the patient did receive furosemide intravenously to ease pulmonary congestion.

19. What types of mechanical support devices may be used in cardiogenic shock and why?

The patient in cardiogenic shock may require the use of an IABP. The balloon is inserted through the femoral artery and is positioned below the aortic arch and above the renal arteries. The balloon inflates during ventricular diastole to augment diastolic perfusion of the coronary arteries. Deflation occurs during ventricular systole, decreasing afterload (Von Rueden & Walleck, 1989). Mrs. Adams was considered for IABP placement, but this would have necessitated a transfer to another facility. Both the patient and family refused the transfer.

Often patients experiencing cardiogenic shock require mechanical ventilation due to extreme pulmonary edema and weakness. Mrs. Adams and her family stated that under no circumstance were intubation and mechanical ventilation to be initiated.

Other mechanical support devices used include ventricular assist devices (VADs) and extracorporeal membrane oxygenation (ECMO).

Types of VADs include centrifugal, pneumatic, pulsatile, and electrical pulsatile. VADs may be implanted for extended periods of time and are used as a bridge to cardiac transplantation. The mechanical support device, ECMO, is used in children but is poorly tolerated in adults over long periods of time. Major complications occur with VADs and ECMO such as biventricular failure, bleeding, and infection. However, these mechanical devices can be a successful means of supporting patients experiencing cardiac failure who would otherwise die (Clochesy et al., 1993).

20. What are nursing implications for the patient in cardiogenic shock?

Examples of nursing implications for patients in cardiogenic shock are similar to those experiencing AMI. Nursing diagnoses include the following (Von Rueden & Walleck, 1989):

➤ altered cardiac output: decreased related to ventricular mechanical dysfunction
➤ altered renal, cerebral, cardiopulmonary, and peripheral tissue perfusion
➤ impaired gas exchange

Nurses must continually monitor these patients, as they will have pulmonary artery (Swan-Ganz) catheters, arterial lines, numerous vasoactive drips, and possibly mechanical ventilation (IABP, VADs, or ECMO). Careful monitoring of patients is required because medication is based on hemodynamic values. Because patients will require complete bed rest, they will require frequent turning and scrupulous skin care and pulmonary toilet. Cardiac rhythms must be continuously monitored and antiarrhythmic drugs administered as ordered. Kidney function requires close monitoring with measurements of hourly urine outputs. In addition, a close watch must be kept on laboratory values. The patient in cardiogenic shock is critically ill and in need of expert medical and nursing management.

Cardiogenic Shock in Anterior Wall Myocardial Infarction

American Heart Association. (1992). Interim training guidelines for cardiopulmonary resuscitation and emergency cardiac care. *JAMA, 268,* 2171–2302.

Chernow, B. (1994). *Essentials of critical care pharmacology* (2nd ed.). Baltimore: Williams & Wilkins.

Clochesy, J. M., Breu, C., Cardin, S., Rudy, E. B., & Whittaker, A. A. (1993). *Critical care nursing.* Philadelphia: Saunders.

Hanisch, P. J. (1991). Identification and treatment of acute myocardial infarction by electro-cardiographic site classification. *Focus on Critical Care, 18*(6), 481–482.

Hollingsworth, K. W. (1992). Understanding hemodynamic drugs. *Critical Care Choices, 92,* 14–23.

Thompson, J. M., McFarland, G. K., Hirsch, J. E., Tucker, S. M., & Bowers, A. C. (1989). *Mosby's manual of clinical nursing* (2nd ed.). St. Louis: Mosby–Year Book.

Von Rueden, K. T., & Walleck, C. A. (1989). *Advanced critical care nursing: A case study approach.* Rockville, MD: Aspen Publishers.

8

Non-Q-Wave Myocardial Infarction

Sheila Drake Melander, DSN, RN, FCCM

CASE PRESENTATION

Mrs. Jarvis is a 70-year-old, 87.8 kg (194 lb) black woman with a history of insulin-dependent diabetes mellitus, hypertension, atherosclerotic peripheral vascular disease, cancer of the breast and uterus, and congestive heart failure. Mrs. Jarvis presented to an outlying hospital with a complaint of chest pain and shortness of breath. Further questioning revealed that she had been having more frequent episodes of chest pain for the past week accompanied by shortness of breath.

Initial orders

- 2 L oxygen per nasal cannula
- IV line of NSS started at keep open rate
- placed on the cardiac monitor, which showed a normal sinus rhythm without ectopy
- 12-lead electrocardiogram (ECG)
- stat cardiac enzymes to be repeated every 8 hours for 24 hours

Diagnostic data on admission were

BP	190/94	CK	216 U/L
HR	106 bpm	CK-MB	5.6%
Respirations	32/min	LDH	400 U/L
CI	2.2 L/min/m²	AST (SGOT)	25 U/L

ECG ST segment elevation in leads V_2 and V_3

Mrs. Jarvis was given one sublingual nitroglycerin tablets which resolved her pain. She was admitted to the coronary care unit with a diagnosis of "rule out myocardial infarction (MI)."

Her serial cardiac enzymes continued to rise; values from the third set of cardiac enzymes were

CK	350 U/L
CK-MB	5.8%
LDH	680 U/L
AST (SGOT)	52 U/L
CI	1.8 L/min/m^2

Day 2

Mrs. Jarvis had recurrent pain that was not eased with 3 nitroglycerin tablets, diaphoresis, and profound shortness of breath requiring intubation. An ECG demonstrated no change from the previous tracings. Mrs. Jarvis was then taken to the cardiac catheterization laboratory. Cardiac catheterization revealed

- ejection fraction of 35%
- 90% obstruction of the left anterior descending coronary artery (LAD)
- 90% to 95% obstruction of the circumflex artery
- 80% obstruction of the right coronary artery

An intraaortic balloon pump was placed for control of Mrs. Jarvis's refractory chest pain, and a dopamine infusion of 3 µg/kg/min was started. Nitroglycerin at 1.5 µg/ml and heparin at 800 U/h were continued. At this time the patient was transferred to another facility with the diagnosis of non-Q-wave MI and three-vessel disease with the need for emergency bypass surgery. Mrs. Jarvis subsequently underwent bypass surgery on day 3 and has done very well since that time.

Questions

Non-Q-Wave Myocardial Infarction

1. What is the difference between a non-Q-wave MI and a transmural MI?

2. What methods are used in the diagnosis of non-Q-wave MIs?

3. Describe the characteristics of patients diagnosed with a non-Q-wave MI.

4. Which pharmacologic agents may be used in the treatment of a non-Q-wave MI?

5. What are the current recommendations for the use of percutaneous transluminal coronary angioplasty (PTCA) and coronary artery bypass graft (CABG) in the patient with a non-Q-wave MI?

6. Discuss extension of a non-Q-wave MI, including time frame of occurrence and possible outcomes.

7. What are some nursing concerns for the patient with a non-Q-wave MI?

8. What are some nursing actions required for patients taking diltiazem (Cardizem)?

9. What are nursing implications for patients receiving thrombolytic therapy?

QUESTIONS AND ANSWERS

Non-Q-Wave
Myocardial Infarction

1. **What is the difference between a non-Q-wave MI and a transmural MI?**

   The terminology used to classify non-Q-wave and transmural MI has been debated. Several authors have stated that full thickness damage to the myocardium is a transmural MI (Thelan, Davie, Urden, & Lough 1994). ECG changes associated with transmural infarctions involve ST elevations and hyperacute T waves. The hallmark sign associated with transmural MIs is the appearance of a new Q wave. Q waves are deeper (one third to one fourth the height of the R wave) and wider (0.04 seconds or longer in duration) than normal (Boden et al., 1989). Thelan et al. (1994) describe partial thickness damage or nontransmural MIs as either subendocardial, involving the myocardium and endocardium, or as subepicardial, involving the epicardium and the myocardium. Nontransmural MIs typically do not have Q wave changes but do have ST depression.

   Some authors believe this classification is confusing to most and that it does not accurately represent physiological changes to the myocardium. Andre-Fouet et al. (1989) have said that the terminology of Q wave vs. non-Q-wave MI is gaining popularity. It is no longer true that the subendocardium is electrically silent. Older terms such as subendocardial, intramural, and nontransmural are often used interchangeably by cardiologists. Chlochesy, Breu, Cardin, Rudy, and Whittaker (1993) wrote that because of pathology studies we now know that transmural MIs can occur without Q waves and that nontransmural MIs may produce new Q waves. Based on this information MIs should be classified as Q wave or non-Q-wave.

2. **What methods are used in the diagnosis of non-Q-wave MIs?**

   It is estimated that 20% of all MIs have no definable ECG changes (Valle & Lemberg, 1990). Non-Q-wave infarctions generally reveal ST and T wave abnormalities with evolutionary changes. Two dimensional echocardiograms demonstrate regional wall motion abnormalities in 100% of all Q wave infarctions and 86% of non-Q-wave MIs. Diagnostic tools include a daily 12-lead ECG, ECGs with each episode of chest pain, creatine kinase (CK) and CK-MB enzyme measurements for 24 hours, and possibly radionuclear ventriculography to assess wall motion. The ECG should be assessed for nonspecific ST changes such as ST depression or elevation and T wave inversion. CK and CK-MB levels in the non-Q-wave MI patient will be elevated for the first 24 to 36 hours after infarction and then will return to normal (Lewis, 1992).

3. Describe the characteristics of patients diagnosed with a non-Q-wave MI.

Nixon, in a 1994 study found the average age of the non-Q-wave MI patient to be the early 60's; most were women with a history of myocardial infarction who usually presented with a normal ejection fraction. Diagnostic findings of left ventricular hypertrophy and involvement of the anterior wall indicated a poor prognosis. Persistent ST segment depression was associated with high mortality and morbidity. Patients presented with elevated CK and CK-MB values, no Q wave on the ECG, and nonspecific ST and T wave ECG changes. Following are clinical characteristics of the non-Q-wave MI patient (Nixon, 1994):

- lower in-hospital mortality rates
- higher in-hospital reinfarction rates
- postdischarge mortality rates attributed to Q wave MIs
- higher postdischarge rates of reinfarction and recurrence of angina
- higher subsequent mortality and morbidity rates after positive results from a predischarge stress or stress-imaging study
- infarcts smaller in non-Q-wave than in Q wave MIs (therefore better ejection fractions)

4. Which pharmacologic agents may be used in the treatment of a non-Q-wave MI?

Initial care of the MI patient includes the same regimen of care as for the Q wave MI patient: oxygen, cardiac monitoring, cardiac enzyme monitoring, and dysrhythmia management. Thrombolytic therapy for the non-Q-wave MI patient is controversial. The three agents used include streptokinase, tissue plasminogen activator (tPA), and urokinase. Mandelkorn et al. (1983) had positive results with streptokinase with non-Q-wave MI patients, whereas Ambrose et al. (1987) and Nixon (1994) indicated that streptokinase has little effect on the distribution of coronary occlusion after a non-Q-wave MI. For this reason thrombolytic therapy is of little use for the non-Q-wave MI patient. However, emergency room physicians may be unable to predict a Q wave or non-Q-wave MI; therefore thrombolytic therapy at admission is advocated, especially in the presence of ST elevation.

All patients who are at high risk for reinfarction must be referred for cardiac catheterization before discharge to assess the extent of cardiac damage. Patients at low risk and who have normal left ventricular function may be assessed and discharged with a prescribed regimen of diltiazem (Cardizem). Diltiazem is a calcium channel blocker and vasodilator that has been found effective in preventing early reinfarction and severe angina after a non-Q-wave infarction. Diltiazem also was found to have a minor antiplatelet effect (Lewis, 1992; Nixon, 1994). β-Blockers do not reduce in infarct size and have shown little benefit (Gibson et al., 1986). The combination of aspirin and heparin followed by warfarin is the regimen associated with the lowest rate of reinfarction (Cohen et al., 1994). A combination of aspirin and dipyridamole (Persantine, a platelet inhibitor and vasodilator) reduces the incidence of reinfarction in the non-Q-wave MI patient.

5. **What are the current recommendations for the use of percutaneous transluminal coronary angioplasty (PTCA) and coronary artery bypass graft (CABG) in the patient with a non-Q-wave MI?**

According to Nixon (1994) the role of PTCA in the non-Q-wave MI patient is still evolving. Recent studies have shown that PTCA after non-Q-wave MI has been highly successful in improving myocardial function. In the Thrombolysis in Myocardial Infarction (TIMI III) Study conducted by Braunwald, McCabe, Cannon, and Muller (1994), patients were randomized into groups, and the patients who chose the PTCA experienced improvement in their condition. CABG surgery was performed on one fourth of the patients. Outcomes for the PTCA and CABG groups did not differ with respect to MI or death unless categorized by age groups. Holt, Gersh, and Holmes (1988) found in a post-MI study that reinfarction rates and mortality were lower in non-Q-wave MI patients who had PTCA than in those who had CABG. More studies are needed to compare the results from PTCA and CABG revascularization in the non-Q-wave MI patient.

6. **Discuss extension of a non-Q-wave MI, including time frame of occurrence and possible outcomes.**

Historically, non-Q-wave MIs were thought to be benign in most patients; however, current studies have yielded different results. In one study, Lewis (1992) reported that 43% of patients with non-Q-wave MI extended their MIs as compared to only 9% of the patients who presented with Q wave MI. In another study, Berger, Murabito, Evans,

Anderson, and Levy (1992) reported that patients with a history of hypertension before an initial MI were at particular risk for reinfarction or extension of the infarct. Extension generally occurs between the sixth and fourteenth days after the acute event. Lewis stated that reinfarction is thought to be related to spontaneous reperfusion, which renders the viable tissue in the area of the non-Q-wave MI vulnerable. Nixon (1994) reported the average time for reinfarction to be 10 days after a non-Q-wave MI. After reinfarction the mortality for the patients in the study was similar to that for inpatient Q wave MI patients. Further findings revealed that the incidence of congestive heart failure and ventricular arrhythmias increased after reinfarction.

7. **What are some nursing concerns for the patient with a non-Q-wave MI?**

   - Patients must continually be assessed for any signs of chest pain or chest tightness, which could signal reinfarction or the development of unstable angina.
   - Cardiac enzymes must be closely monitored and changes reported to the physician immediately.
   - All regimens of care such as thrombolytic therapy and antithrombolytic medications should be explained to the patient.
   - Before the patient is discharged with any prescribed medications, all possible side effects should be thoroughly explained to the patient.
   - Cardiac rehabilitation should begin while the patient is still in the cardiac intensive care unit (Lewis, 1992).

8. **What are some nursing actions required for patients taking diltiazem (Cardizem)?**

   - Administer oral dose on an empty stomach to promote rapid absorption.
   - Take pulse before each dose. If the pulse is below 50 bpm, withhold the dose and notify the physician.
   - Instruct the patient to slowly change from a sitting or lying position to a standing position to avoid orthostatic hypotension.
   - Instruct patients that if they forget to take a dose of medication, they should take it as soon as they remember it unless it is almost time for the next dose, in which case they should omit the missed dose.
   - To help prevent dizziness and hypotension, instruct the patient to avoid alcohol.
   - Instruct the patient to use good oral hygiene techniques and to schedule regular dental checkups to help reduce the incidence or severity of gingivitis and gingival hyperplasia (McKenry & Salerno, 1992).

9. **What are the nursing implications for patients receiving thrombolytic therapy?**

- Thoroughly assess patient for potential bleeding risks before initiation of thrombolytic therapy.
- Inform the patient and the patient's family of the risk of bleeding after therapy and that any posttherapy bleeding no matter now minor must be reported.
- Explain to the patient the ramifications of the reperfusion phenomenon, which includes pain, dysrhythmias, ECG changes, and CK release.
- Monitor patients for bleeding every 15 minutes for the first hour after therapy is begun, then every 30 minutes for the next 8 hours, and every 4 hours until the therapy is discontinued.
- Monitor vital signs frequently.
- Monitor patients for any signs of internal bleeding, such as bloody sputum, hematuria, hematemesis, dark stools, and flank or abdominal pain.
- Observe and palpate pulses of affected extremities frequently.
- Monitor for dysrhythmias.
- Watch patients at initiation of therapy for an allergic reaction such as bronchospasm or skin rash. If a reaction does occur, discontinue the infusion and treat with epinephrine, bronchodilators, or corticosteroids.
- To prevent bruising, avoid unnecessary handling the patients and keep the side rails padded.
- If bleeding occurs, maintain pressure at the site for at least 30 minutes and check frequently for signs of further bleeding.
- Avoid intramuscular injections because of the danger of a hematoma or bleeding.

Non-Q-Wave Myocardial Infarction

Ambrose, J. A., Monsen, C. H., Borrico, S., Cohen, M., Gorlin, R., & Fuster, V. (1987). Quantitative and qualitative effects of intracoronary streptokinase in unstable angina and non-Q-wave infarction. *Journal of the American College of Cardiology, 9*(5), 1156–1164.

Andre-Fouet, X., Pillot, M., Leizorovicz, A., Finet, G., Gayet, C., & Milon, H. (1989). "Non Q-wave," alias "nontransmural," myocardial infarction: A specific entity. *American Heart Journal, 117*(4), 892–901.

Berger, C., Murabito, J., Evans, J., Anderson, S., & Levy, D. (1992). Prognosis after first myocardial infarction: Comparison of Q-wave myocardial infarction in the Framingham heart study. *JAMA, 268*(12), 1545–1551.

Boden, W., Gibson, R., Schechtmen, K., Kleiger, R., Schwartz, D., Capone, R., & Roberts, R. (1989). ST segment shifts are poor predictors of subsequent Q wave evolution in acute myocardial infarction. *Circulation, 79*(3), 537–547.

Braunwald, E., McCabe, C., Cannon, C., & Muller, J. (1994). Effects of tissue plasminogen activator and a comparison of early invasive conservative strategies in unstable angina and non Q-wave myocardial infarction: Results of the TIMI IIIB trial. *Circulation, 89*(4), 1545–1554.

Clochesy, J., Breu, C., Cardin, S., Rudy, E., & Whittaker, A. (1993). *Critical care nursing.* Philadelphia: Saunders.

Cohen, M., Adams, P., Parry, G., Xiong, J., Chamberlain, D., Wieczorek, I., Fox, A., Chesebro, J., Strain, J., Keller, A., Lancaster, G., Ali, J., Kronmal, R., & Fuster, V. (1994). Combination antithrombotic therapy in unstable rest angina and non Q-wave infarction in nonprior aspirin users. *Circulation, 89*(1), 81–88.

Gibson, R., Boden, W., Theroux, P., Strauss, H., Pratt, C., Gheorghiade, M., Capone, R., Crawford, M., Schlant, R., Kleiger, R., Young, P., Schechtman, K., Perryman, M., & Roberts, R. (1986). Diltiazem and reinfarction in patients with non Q-wave myocardial infarction. *New England Journal of Medicine, 315*(7), 423–428.

Holt, G., Gersh, B., & Holmes, D. (1988). Results of percutaneous transluminal coronary angioplasty for angina pectoris after non Q-wave myocardial infarction. *American Journal of Cardiology, 61*(15), 1238–1242.

Lewis, P. (1992). Clinical implications of non Q-wave (subendocardial) myocardial infarctions. *Focus on Critical Care, 19*(1), 29–33.

Mandelkorn, J., Wolf, N., Singh, S., Shecter, J., Kersh, R., Rodgers, D., Workman, M., Bentivoglio, L., LaPorte, S., & Meister, S. (1983). Intracoronary thrombus in nontransmural myocardial infarction and in unstable angina. *American Journal of Cardiology, 52*(1), 1–6.

McKenry, L., & Salerno, E. (1992). *Pharmacology in nursing.* St. Louis: Mosby–Year Book.

Nixon, J. (1994). Non Q-wave myocardial infarction. *Postgraduate Medicine, 95*(5), 211–223.

Thelan, L., Davie, J., Urden, L., & Lough, M. (1994). *Textbook of critical care nursing.* St. Louis: Mosby–Year Book.

Valle, B., & Lemberg, L. (1990). Non Q-wave versus nontransmural infarction. *Heart and Lung, 19*(2), 208–211.

9

Congestive Heart Failure

Kelly A. Hertel, BSN, RNC, CCRN, CEN

CASE PRESENTATION

John Arnold, age 80 years, was admitted to the hospital after visiting his primary physician with complaints of having experienced general malaise for 3 to 4 days, shortness of breath, and abdominal pain. Initial assessment revealed bibasilar crackles, an audible S_3, and tachycardia. Mr. Arnold also informed the nurse of occasional epigastric pain, which he attributed to his "ulcer acting up."

Mr. Arnold's history includes diabetes for more than 30 years, peptic ulcer, and hypertension and coronary artery disease (past examinations indicated an 80% blockage of the left carotid artery and 60% blockage of the right carotid artery). Following are admission diagnostic data:

BP	150/72		
HR	102–123 bpm and irregular		
Respirations	24–32/min		
Temperature	37.3° C (99.2° F) (Tympanic)		
Height	175 cm (5'10")		
Weight	79 kg (175 lb) Patient stated his weight had increased approximately 3 kg (6 lb) during the last 3 days.		
Urine	yellow and cloudy		
Na+	140 mmol/L	BUN	17 mg/dl
K+	4.2 mmol/L	Glucose	332 mg/dl
Hgb	11.8 g/dl	Creatinine	1.2 mg/dl
Hct	36.2%	LDH	705 U/L
AST (SGOT)	134 U/L	CK	587 U/L
Cl–	102 mmol/L		

CXR	Mild congestive heart failure (CHF) superimposed on chronic obstructive pulmonary disease (COPD) and chronic pulmonary parenchymal changes
ECG	Sinus rhythm with a left bundle branch block, long QT interval

Shortly after admission, Mr. Arnold became cold and clammy. Respirations were labored, and he complained of epigastric pain. Physical examination found the patient diaphoretic, gasping for air, with jugular venous distension. Bilateral crackles were present with an expiratory wheeze. Audible crackles were also heard with respirations. The patient was placed in a high-Fowler position, and oxygen therapy of 4 L/min was initiated. It was noted that urinary output had been scant since admission.

Status progressed to critical within 30 minutes. With a diagnosis of pulmonary edema, Mr. Arnold was transferred to the cardiac care unit (CCU) for aggressive diuretic therapy. CK-MB was confirmed at this time to be 7.5%.

Routine CCU orders were initiated, and the plan of care was briefly explained to the patient. The patient's heart monitor showed atrioventricular dissociation with periods of ventricular standstill. Furosemide (Lasix) 100 mg IV, atropine sulfate 0.5 mg IV, and dobutamine (Dobutrex) 1 g/250 NS at 5 µg/kg/min were begun. Overall status continued to deteriorate, and a cardiac consult was requested. The patient was prepared for the placement of a temporary 7.5 transvenous pacing catheter in the right subclavian vein. Initial settings were MA 15, rate 80, and full demand. The heart monitor then showed a paced rhythm with a rate of 80 bpm. Additional diagnostic data were

BP	190/100	CO	4.64 L/min	pH	7.46*
HR	123 bpm	CVP	19 cm H_2O	$PaCO_2$	31 mm Hg
Respirations	42/min	SVR	1810 dyne/s/cm^{-5}	PaO_2	80 mm Hg
PAP	50/22 mm Hg	CI	2.34 L/min/m^2	SaO_2	96%
PCWP	24 mm Hg			HCO_3^-	24 mmol/L

*On 4 L oxygen by nasal cannula.

At this point the patient's dobutamine drip was increased to 10 µg/kg/min. Nitroglycerin (Tridil) 50 mg/250 ml NS was initiated and titrated to 50 µg/kg/min. A dopamine drip was ordered to be on standby. An additional 200 mg of furosemide (Lasix) was administered IV, and a marked improvement in urinary output was obtained.

Within a short time the patient said that he found it "easier to breathe." Hemodynamic and laboratory results are as follows:

BP	140/90	CO	5.5 L/min	pH	7.43*
HR	109 bpm	CVP	8 cm H_2O	$PaCO_2$	36 mm Hg
Respirations	24/min	SVR	1340 dyne/s/cm^{-5}	PaO_2	89 mm Hg
PAP	30/10 mm Hg	CI	2.8 L/min/m^2	SaO_2	98%
PAWP	12 mm Hg			HCO_3^-	25 mmol/L

*On 2 L oxygen by nasal cannula.

Over the next 4 days, several attempts were made to wean the patient from the IV drips. Eventually all drips, temporary pacing catheter, and Foley catheter were removed. The heart monitor showed a slightly irregular sinus rhythm. The patient was transferred to the medical-surgical floor. Treatment included digoxin (Lanoxin) 0.125 mg daily, furosemide (Lasix) 160 mg PO b.i.d., captopril (Capoten) 25 mg q6h, sucralfate (Carafate) 1 g ac and hs, nitroglycerin ointment 5 cm (2 in.) q6h and a K^+ supplement q6h. The appropriate departments were notified to assist Mr. Arnold in planning his home management.

QUESTIONS

Congestive Heart Failure

1. Discuss the pathophysiology of CHF.

2. Discuss Mr. Arnold's signs and symptoms that were consistent with CHF.

3. Compare the characteristics of right- and left-sided heart failure.

4. Describe the predisposing factors that placed Mr. Arnold at risk for CHF.

5. List the nursing diagnoses appropriate to Mr. Arnold's care.

6. Briefly define the following terms: cardiac output, preload, afterload, contractility, and stroke volume.

7. Describe the benefits of using a pulmonary artery catheter during CHF.

8. Briefly describe the pathophysiology of pulmonary edema.

9. List the pharmacologic agents used in Mr. Arnold's care and explain their importance to his treatment.

10. Discuss homecare management of an individual with a history of CHF.

11. The number of hearts available for transplantation does not meet demand. What other treatment options do individuals with CHF have?

QUESTIONS AND ANSWERS

Congestive Heart Failure

1. **Discuss the pathophysiology of CHF.**

Cross (1993, p. 589) described CHF as a "condition in which the ventricles fail to pump adequately." One can view heart failure as a series of events that occurs throughout the heart. Tracing the flow of the heart in reverse, starting in the left ventricle, the series begins with failure of the left ventricle to adequately empty during contraction. The left ventricle often fails because of ischemia. As blood begins to accumulate in the ventricle, elevated pressures are reflected in the left atrium and pulmonary veins. If the condition is allowed to progress, eventually elevated pressures will be noted in the right ventricle and atrium. Right-sided heart failure is most commonly caused by left-sided heart failure (Hartshorn, Lamborn, & Noll, 1993).

Several parameters are affected by heart failure. For instance, failure of the left ventricle decreases cardiac output, thereby reducing the amount of oxygenated blood available for distribution throughout the body. As a result of elevated pressures and fluid accumulation within the lungs, gas exchange may be affected. To rid the body of excess carbon dioxide, the respiratory rate increases, simultaneously increasing the heart rate. This increased heart rate decreases emptying time for the ventricles, worsening the CHF. If pressures continue to increase and right-sided failure occurs, venous return to the heart will also be reduced (Hartshorn et al., 1993).

2. **Discuss Mr. Arnold's signs and symptoms that were consistent with CHF.**

On initial assessment, Mr. Arnold complained of fatigue and shortness of breath. Physical findings revealed bibasilar crackles, an audible S_3, tachycardia, and recent weight gain. As Mr. Arnold's condition worsened, he became diaphoretic. He developed dysrhythmias, and his filling pressures were elevated with a decrease in cardiac output.

3. **Compare the characteristics of right- and left-sided heart failure.**

The findings listed in the answer to question 2 represent Mr. Arnold's signs and symptoms indicative of heart failure. Signs and symptoms can often be associated with either left- or right-sided failure. In Table 9–1 are the characteristics listed by Alspach (1991, p. 243).

4. **Describe the predisposing factors that placed Mr. Arnold at risk for CHF.**

Bridges and Strong (1993, p. 17) wrote that "Congestive heart failure is the most common medical diagnosis among individuals 65 years and older." Mr. Arnold was 80 years old at the time of this incident. Gupta (1991, p. 83) stated that the incidence of CHF "doubles for each decade of life from the age of 45–75." Mr. Arnold's history was also positive for diabetes and hypertension. Both factors contribute to the occurrence of CHF.

5. **List the nursing diagnoses appropriate to Mr. Arnold's care.**

According to Hartshorn et al. (1993), the following are appropriate nursing diagnoses for the patient diagnosed with CHF:

Table 9–1   Signs and Symptoms of Left- and Right-sided Heart Failure

Left-sided Heart Failure	Right-sided Heart Failure
Anxiety	Hepatomegaly
Orthopnea	Splenomegaly
Dyspnea, dyspnea on exertion, nocturnal dyspnea	Dependent pitting edema
Cough with frothy sputum	Venous distension
Tachypnea	Hepatojugular reflux
Diaphoresis	Bounding pulses
Basilar crackles, rhonchi	Oliguria
Cyanosis	Dysrhythmias
Hypoxia, respiratory acidosis	Elevated central venous, right atrial, and right ventricular pressures
Elevated pulmonary artery diastolic pressure and pulmonary capillary wedge pressure	Kussmaul's sign
Nocturia	Murmur of tricuspid insufficiency
Mental confusion	Audible S_3 and S_4 heart sounds
Audible S_3 and S_4 heart sounds	Fatigue, weakness
Fatigue, weakness, lethargy	Abdominal pain
Murmur of mitral insufficiency	Anorexia
CXR shows enlarged left ventricle and left atrium, pleural effusion	CXR shows enlarged right atrium and right ventricle
Pulsus alternans	Weight gain

➤ alteration in cardiac output: decreased, related to decreased myocardial contractility

➤ alteration in cardiac output: decreased, related to increased afterload

➤ impaired gas exchange related to ventilation-perfusion imbalance

➤ high risk for fluid volume deficit related to excessive diuresis

➤ high risk for injury: dysrhythmias related to electrolyte imbalance.

➤ activity intolerance related to generalized weakness and imbalance between oxygen supply and demand

➤ alteration in tissue perfusion: decreased related to decreased cardiac output

6. **Briefly define the following terms: cardiac output, preload, afterload, contractility and stroke volume.**

Cardiac output: The amount of blood ejected from the heart per minute.

Preload: The stretch of the ventricular myocardium before contraction. This stretch is determined by the amount of blood within the ventricles. It is important to remember that fibers can stretch beyond a point where they no longer enhance contraction (Alspach, 1991).

Afterload: The amount of resistance the ventricles must pump against to circulate blood through the body (Alspach, 1991).

Contractility: The property of the ventricles that contracts and assists in emptying the heart's contents.

Stroke volume: The amount of blood ejected by left ventricular contraction during each systole (Alspach, 1991).

7. **Describe the benefits of using a pulmonary artery catheter during CHF.**

Pulmonary artery catheters allow a more accurate picture of a patient's fluid balance and hemodynamic status. The following readings may be obtained through the use of the catheter.

Central Venous Pressure (CVP)

CVP provides information concerning right ventricular pressure. For example, a patient experiencing hypovolemia will have a low CVP reading. In right-sided heart failure, readings will be higher than normal. Normal CVP readings are 0 to 12 cm H_2O or 0 to 4 mm Hg (Hartshorn et al., 1993).

Pulmonary Artery Pressure (PAP)

PAP measurements contain both a systolic and diastolic reading. Alspach (1991, p. 196) stated that "PA systolic pressure represents pressure produced by RV and PA diastolic pressure reflects LVEDP and is used as a measure of LV function and diastolic filling pressures." Normal PA systolic pressures are 20 to 30 mm Hg. PA diastolic pressures are normally less than 10 to 20 mm Hg (Alspach, 1991).

Pulmonary Capillary Wedge Pressure (PCWP)

"PCWP is a reflection of LA pressure and is used to assess LV filling pressures (LVEDP)" (Alspach, 1991, p. 197). Normal PCWP pressures should measure 4 to 12 mm Hg (Alspach, 1991).

Systemic Vascular Resistance (SVR)

Systemic or arterial afterload is measured by the systemic vascular resistance. Normal SVR is 800 to 1200 dyne/s/cm^{-5} (Thelan, Davie, Urden, & Lough, 1994).

Mr. Arnold also required temporary pacing because of AV dissociation. Certain pulmonary catheters are designed with this pacing feature.

8. **Briefly describe the pathophysiology of pulmonary edema.**

Because of increased pressures within the left atrium and ventricle, fluid accumulates in the pulmonary vascular system. As this system becomes saturated, gas exchange at the alveoli is inhibited. This decrease in gas exchange produces hypoxemia and leaves the patient short of breath and anxious (Thelan et al., 1994).

9. **List the pharmacologic agents used in Mr. Arnold's care and explain their importance to his treatment.**

Furosemide (Lasix)

Often patients diagnosed with CHF present with edema, pulmonary congestion, or both. Edema is apparent in right-sided heart failure because of the increase in fluid within the venous system. Pulmonary congestion can be detected on ausculation when the left ventricle fails to empty during contraction, leading to increased pressure within the lungs. Diuretics facilitate not only the elimination of sodium and water but also prevention of the reabsorption of these materials, thereby reducing preload (Cuny & Enger, 1993). Furosemide acts on the loop of Henle. Diuresis is usually quite rapid, with a relief in symptoms noted before actual urinary output increases. Whalen and Izzi (1993, p. 262) stated that "loop diuretics, such as furosemide, are employed in acute management because they maintain their effectiveness even in the presence of the reduced renal perfusion and glomerular filtration seen in acute CHF." Because of the rapid action of these diuretics, electrolyte levels, such as potassium and magnesium, should be monitored closely.

Dopamine (Intropin)

Although dopamine was not used in Mr. Arnold's case, it is important to discuss its use and dose-related effects. At a low dosage of 0.5 to 2 µg/kg/min, this inotropic agent increases renal perfusion, which aids in fluid elimination and preload reduction. At a dosage of 2 to 10 µg/kg/min, β-adrenergic receptors are stimulated, increasing contractility, stroke volume, and heart rate. Dosages over 10 µg/kg/min produce alpha effects resulting in vasoconstriction, which increases blood pressure. At high dosage levels, however, this vasoconstriction leads to decreased renal perfusion (Brown, 1993).

Dobutamine (Dobutrex)

Dobutamine is a sympathomimetic that stimulates both β- and α-adrenergic receptors. However, dobutamine is more specific to β_1-adrenergic receptors (myocardium) than β_2-adrenergic receptors (peripheral vessels and bronchioles). At a dosage of 2.5 to 10 µg/kg/min, dobutamine increases contractility, stroke volume, and cardiac output (Cross, 1993). At dosages over 10 µg/kg/min, β_2-adrenergic receptors are stimulated but not to the degree that β_1-adrenergic receptors are stimulated (Brown, 1993).

Vasodilators (Nipride)

Vasodilators are used to reduce preload and afterload. Arteriolar vasodilation assists in increasing cardiac output by decreasing systemic vascular resistance. Vasodilation of the venous system decreases the amount of blood used during preload. Vasodilators also assist in decreasing the myocardial oxygen consumption, which helps to relieve myocardial ischemia (Hartshorn et al., 1993).

Digitalis (Digoxin)

Digitalis is a cardiac glycoside that works by inhibiting the sodium-potassium pump. As a result, increased intracellular sodium is exchanged for extracellular calcium. Higher levels of intracellular calcium now assist in increasing the force of the heart's contraction. Digitalis also possesses a negative chronotropic effect. This slower conduction through the heart allows for a longer diastolic filling time, which in turn improves stroke volume and cardiac output (Cross, 1993).

Captopril (Capoten)

Angiotensin II is a potent vasoconstrictor that strengthens vascular resistance and increases sodium and water retention through the release of aldosterone from the adrenal cortex. Captopril blocks the enzyme that converts angiotensin I to angiotensin II. This helps to reduce both preload and afterload by attenuating vasoconstriction and decreasing sodium and water retention (Khosla & Somberg, 1993).

10. **Discuss homecare management of an individual with a history of CHF.**

Alspach (1991) listed several steps that should be considered in the evaluation or discharge phase of patient teaching. First, information concerning the patient's dietary needs and restrictions should be discussed. Meals should be low in sodium because of the potential for fluid accumulation. Before discharge, foods high in sodium should be reviewed with the patient or the individual responsible for food preparation. Second, patients with a history of CHF usually require a daily diuretic, which decreases potassium levels. Therefore, consumption of foods high in potassium should be discussed to prevent low potassium levels. Third, since digoxin has been prescribed for Mr. Arnold, he requires instruction in the proper technique for monitoring his pulse and should adequately demonstrate the technique. Digoxin normally is reserved for a heart rate less than 60 bpm.

As patients are discharged from the hospital, many ask, When should I become concerned? or When should I call the doctor? A basic review of symptoms such as weight gain, difficulty breathing, or fatigue should be discussed with the patient along with any possible side effects of medications. Recording a daily weight may be an excellent way to detect heart failure before actual symptoms appear (Cuny & Enger, 1993). Finally, the medications that will be sent home should be reviewed with the patient and significant others. The importance of each medication and possible side effects should be discussed. The patient should be instructed not to discontinue medications without consulting his physician (Alspach, 1991).

11. **The number of hearts available for transplantation does not meet demand. What other treatment options do individuals with CHF have?**

Following are three options for treatment of CHF cited in the September issue of *Nursing 93* (p. 32F):

Dynamic Cardiomyoplasty

The patient's skeletal muscle is used to reinforce the heart. This new muscle learns to contract simultaneously with each cardiac cycle.

Assisting the Ventricle

This approach is slightly more complicated than dynamic cardiomyoplasty. A pouch made from skeletal muscle is attached to the aorta, where excess blood is deposited. While the heart is in diastole, a pace-maker stimulates the pouch to contract. This contraction empties the contents of the pouch into the circulatory system.

Continuous Ambulatory Peritoneal Dialysis (CAPD)

This procedure helps to rid the body of excess fluid while maintaining an adequate electrolyte balance.

REFERENCES

Congestive Heart Failure

Alspach, J. (1991). *Core curriculum for critical care nursing* (4th ed.). Philadelphia: Saunders.

Bridges, J., & Strong, A. (1993). Angiotensin converting enzyme inhibition: Pharmacologic management to minimize postinfarction heart failure. *Critical Care Nursing Quarterly, 16*(2), 17–26.

Brown, K. (1993, April). Boosting the failing heart with inotropic drugs. *Nursing 93*, pp. 34–44.

Cross, J. (1993). Pharmacologic management of heart failure: Positive inotropic agents. *Nursing Clinics of North America, 5*(4), 589–596.

Cuny, J., & Enger, E. (1993). Medical management of chronic heart failure: Direct-acting vasodilators and diuretic agents. *Nursing Clinics of North America, 5*(4), 575–587.

Gupta, S. (1991). Congestive heart failure in the elderly. *Postgraduate Medicine, 90*(7), 83–87.

Hartshorn, J., Lamborn, M., & Noll, M. (1993). *Introduction to critical care nursing.* Philadelphia: Saunders.

Khosla, S., & Somberg, J. (1993). Mild heart failure: Why the switch to ACE inhibitors? *Geriatrics, 48*(11), 47–54.

Reviewing new treatments for congestive heart failure. (1993, September). *Nursing 93, 23,* 32F.

Thelan, L., Davie, J., Urden, L., & Lough, M. (1994). *Critical care nursing* (2nd ed.). St. Louis: Mosby–Year Book.

Whalen, D., & Izzi, G. (1993). Pharmacologic treatment of acute congestive heart failure resulting from left ventricular systolic or diastolic dysfunction. *Nursing Clinics of North America, 5*(4), 261–269.

10

Carotid Endarterectomy

Pam B. Koob, MA, MSN, RN, CCRN

CASE PRESENTATION

Maxine Hamilton, age 62 years, has a history of coronary artery disease (CAD) and a four-vessel coronary artery bypass graft (CABG) completed 4 years ago. Two years before her cardiac surgery, she had a silent inferior myocardial infarction (MI). This MI was not discovered until she was seen in her physician's office for her usual physical examination, which included an electrocardiogram (ECG) and cardiac enzyme determination. She did not remember having any unusual episodes of chest pain before the discovery of the MI, other than her usual "indigestion." She had been doing well since her CABG, but during the past 6 months, Mrs. Hamilton has had at least three transient ischemic attacks (TIAs).

The first TIA involved numbness of her left arm and leg, dizziness, and a headache. The second TIA was identical. The third TIA did not include a headache, but she did again have numbness of her left arm and leg and dizziness. Each episode lasted approximately 15 minutes.

After the first TIA, Dr. Allen found bruits over the carotid arteries bilaterally and bright yellow plaques of cholesterol (Hollenhorst plaques) on retinal examination. After obtaining these findings, he performed a Doppler ultrasound of the carotid arteries and a head computed tomography (CT) scan to assist in determining the cause of the TIAs.

The results of the Doppler ultrasound and the CT scan indicated stenosis of both carotid arteries, more severe on the right side. After options were discussed with Mrs. Hamilton, a conservative medical approach was agreed on. Dr. Allen ordered aspirin (Bayer) 325 mg/d.

After the second TIA, Dr. Allen encouraged Mrs. Hamilton to consider surgery, but she declined. After the third TIA, Mrs. Hamilton agreed to have a cardiac catheterization and an arch angiography. Her precath ECG revealed an old MI, with Q waves in leads II, III, and aVF.

Results of the cardiac catheterization revealed minimal (25%) occlusion of the right coronary artery. The remaining coronary vessels were 10% occluded. The two-vessel arteriography report revealed bilateral carotid disease with 95% stenosis of the right internal carotid artery and 80% occlusion of the left internal carotid artery.

Intensive Care Admission

After undergoing a right carotid endarterectomy (RCEA), Mrs. Hamilton was admitted directly to the ICU at 11:45 AM. Initial postoperative vital signs and assessment revealed:

Height   162.5 cm (5'5")
Weight   63 kg (140 lb)
BP   124/78
HR   80 bpm
Respirations 24/min
Temperature   36.8° C (98.2 F) (oral)

A clean dry dressing was placed over the right carotid area with a Jackson-Pratt drain in place. Her right neck area was slightly swollen. Physician's orders were as follows:

- cardiac monitor
- continuous pulse oximetry
- arterial line (A-line) for direct BP measurement
- oxygen at 2 L/min by nasal cannula
- D5 in 0.25 NSS with 20 mEq KCl at 75 ml/h
- nitroprusside (Nipride) to keep BP < 140 (currently 10 ml/h [33 µg/min] mixed as nitroprusside 50 mg in 250 ml D_5W).
- CBC, BUN, K^+, ECG, and CXR in AM
- meperidine hydrochloride (Demerol) 25 mg IM q3–4h prn
- elevate head of bed 30 degrees
- neuro checks q15min for 2 hours, q1h for 4 hours, q2h for 6 hours, then q4h

At 12 noon, 15 minutes after the initial assessment, the following data were obtained:

BP   172/92 (cuff); 180/98 (arterial line)
HR   98 bpm
Respirations 26/min
Temperature   37.2° C (98.9° F) (oral)

Breath sounds were clear, with a pulse oximetry reading of 96%. The trachea was midline with airflow auscultated over the trachea. ECG monitor revealed normal sinus rhythm at 98 bpm. The patient was easily aroused and oriented to person, place, and time. Hand grips were strong bilaterally with equal strength. Plantar flexion and dorsiflexion were intact. Mrs. Hamilton's speech was clear. Pupils were equal, round, and reacted to light. Cranial nerves were intact.

Glucose	80 mg/dl
BUN	11 mg/dl
Creatinine	0.9 mg/dl
Na$^+$	139 mmol/L
K$^+$	3.9 mmol/L
Cl$^-$	106 mmol/L
Hgb	12.3 g/dl
Hct	39.3%

Nitroprusside (Nipride) is now infusing at 15 ml/h (50 µg/min).

QUESTIONS

Carotid Endarterectomy

1. Briefly describe the anatomy of the cerebral circulation and the pathophysiology of the carotid circulation that can require surgical intervention. What are the causative factors leading to stroke?

2. Define carotid endarterectomy.

3. What are the purpose and goal of carotid endarterectomy? Why was this procedure the best option for Mrs. Hamilton?

4. Mrs. Hamilton underwent the two most common diagnostic studies to determine blood flow and specific occlusion. Describe these studies and their typical findings. What are the risks and benefits of these studies?

5. Which study demonstrates when carotid endarterectomy should be selected over medical treatment? What criterion is used?

6. What are the clinical manifestations of atherosclerotic carotid artery disease? What are the three categories of patients with the disease?

7. Define TIA, amaurosis fugax, and RIND. What signs and symptoms did Mrs. Hamilton exhibit?

8. Describe the effect Mrs. Hamilton's hypertension could have postoperatively. What goals and treatment modalities would be expected?

9. Why do some patients develop postoperative hypotension? What are the nurse's responsibilities?

10. What should be included in Mrs. Hamilton's neurologic assessment?

11. Discuss how carotid endarterectomy can damage certain cranial nerves. What are the clinical manifestations of specific nerve damage? What precautions should be taken to prevent cranial nerve damage?

12. What are the signs of decreased cerebral functioning related to decreased cerebral blood flow that should be assessed in Mrs. Hamilton and immediately reported to the physician?

13. Twelve hours after surgery the nurse notices a hematoma around Mrs. Hamilton's incision site. What causes a hematoma following a carotid endarterectomy? Discuss the danger posed by this finding.

14. What are other potential complications to keep in mind for Mrs. Hamilton?

15. What instructions should Mrs. Hamilton receive regarding restriction of neck movement immediately after surgery?

16. After surgery, Mrs. Hamilton made good progress and was discharged home on the third postoperative day. Discharge medications included nifedipine (Procardia) 20 mg PO q8h and dipyridamole (Persantine) 50 mg b.i.d. Describe the pharmacodynamics and clinical effects of these drugs. What instructions regarding her medications should be given to Mrs. Hamilton before her discharge?

QUESTIONS AND ANSWERS

Carotid Endarterectomy

1. **Briefly describe the anatomy of the cerebral circulation and the pathophysiology of the carotid circulation that can require surgical intervention. What are the causative factors leading to stroke?**

The brain receives 85% of its blood supply from the anterior circulation (bilateral carotid arteries) and 15% of its posterior blood supply from the posterior circulation (bilateral vertebral arteries). The common carotid arteries bifurcate extracranially into external and internal branches, with the external carotid artery carrying blood to the face and scalp and the internal carotid artery sending blood to the cerebral hemispheres. The internal carotid artery has four major intracranial branches: anterior cerebral artery, middle cerebral artery, ophthalmic artery, and posterior communicating artery (Clochesy, Breu, Cardin, Rudy, & Whittaker, 1993; Fode, 1990; Sanchez, 1988).

Patients with carotid artery stenosis who require a carotid endarterectomy have developed an obstruction of the blood flow to the brain. The obstruction usually occurs at the bifurcation of the common carotid artery and is typically a result of atherosclerosis. When fatty deposits are coated by fibrous tissue, a plaque develops, leading to stenosis. As this plaque increases in size, cerebral blood flow decreases. When the intimal lining of the artery is no longer intact, the plaque may become ulcerated and expose the roughened area. This, in turn, attracts more debris and can eventually lead to embolization. Cerebral blood flow decreases because of the narrowed vessel, and release of microemboli from the atheroma occurs. If the emboli are of platelet origin, vasospasm and additional obstruction can occur as a result of the release of vasoactive substances such as thromboxane A_2 and create even further vasoconstriction. This further compromise to cerebral tissue leads to cerebral ischemia and infarction (Clochesy et al., 1993; Johnson & Anderson, 1991; Kane & Wilson, 1993).

Causative factors include atherosclerosis, fibromuscular dysplasia, aneurysms, trauma, Takayasu's arteritis, and spontaneous dissection (Clochesy et al., 1993; Johnson & Anderson, 1991).

2. Define carotid endarterectomy.

A carotid endarterectomy is the surgical removal of an atheroma (fatty plaque) at the carotid bifurcation in an attempt to prevent stroke (Kane & Wilson, 1993).

3. What are the purpose and goal of carotid endarterectomy? Why was this procedure the best option for Mrs. Hamilton?

Carotid endarterectomy is the therapy of choice in symptomatic patients with high-grade internal carotid artery stenosis (Feussner, 1993; O'Brien & Ricotta, 1994). The goal is removal of the atherosclerotic plaque formation in an effort to prevent stroke (Johnson & Anderson, 1991). Because of Mrs. Hamilton's high-grade stenosis and history of TIAs, the surgical procedure is indicated as the best option for preventing stroke or cerebrovascular accident (CVA).

4. Mrs. Hamilton underwent the two most common diagnostic studies to determine blood flow and specific occlusion. Describe these studies and their typical findings. What are the risks and benefits of these studies?

The most common studies include a Doppler ultrasound of the carotid arteries and a cerebral angiography. The Doppler ultrasound assesses peripheral arterial or cerebrovascular blood flow and velocity by picking up sound generated by blood moving through the underlying vessels. Vessels that are totally occluded do not transmit sound. No particular risk is associated with this study.

A cerebral angiography is performed by injecting a contrast material into one or more arteries to obtain radiographic visualization of the targeted circulation. Preprocedure care involves premedication and signing of an informed consent. Postprocedure care involves checking the site for bleeding or hematoma formation. A major complication of this procedure can be a stroke caused by accidental dislodging of an atherosclerotic plaque from the artery wall or a clot that formed at the end of the catheter or needle (Alspach, 1991).

5. Which study demonstrates when carotid endarterectomy should be selected over medical treatment? What criterion is used?

The North American Symptomatic Carotid Endarterectomy Trial (NASCET) has demonstrated that in patients with over 75% occlusion of the internal carotid artery, carotid endarterectomy offers a clear benefit to the patient (O'Brien & Ricotta, 1994).

6. **What are the clinical manifestations of atherosclerotic carotid artery disease? What are the three categories of patients with the disease?**

According to Johnson and Anderson (1991), patients with atherosclerotic carotid artery disease may present with stroke or TIA or be asymptomatic. Three categories of patients have been identified by Moore and Quinones-Baldrich (1991): (1) patients with no symptoms but with a documented significant lesion or nonocclusive ulceration and no permanent neurologic deficits, (2) patients with TIAs, the most frequent sign of carotid artery disease and (3) patients with completed cerebral infarction.

7. **Define TIA, amaurosis fugax, and RIND. What signs and symptoms did Mrs. Hamilton exhibit?**

A TIA is a temporary focal episode of neurologic dysfunction of vascular origin that may last from a few minutes up to 24 hours (Fode, 1990).

By definition, neurologic examination must be normal or baseline within 24 hours. Typically, the neurologic deficit lasts 10 to 20 minutes and consists of hemiparesis with or without dysarthria, hemisensory loss, hemianopia, dysphasia, or monocular visual loss (Bruno, 1993, p. 26).

Permanent damage is rarely associated with a TIA. When the symptoms are the same for each attack, the cause is usually the extracranial circulation. Patients with cardiac emboli tend to have variable symptoms.

The most common symptoms are contralateral hemiparesis and/or hemiparesthesia, visual changes, receptive and/or expressive aphasia, vertigo, syncope, headaches, and ataxia. A classic symptom of carotid TIAs is transient spells of ipsilateral monocular blurring or blindness commonly called amaurosis fugax (Johnson & Anderson, 1991, p. 501).

A minor stroke lasts more than 24 hours but usually resolves (Kane & Wilson, 1993).

Amaurosis fugax, a transient spell of monocular blindness, is commonly referred to as a retinal TIA. "The onset is rapid and the patient often describes the event as a shade coming down slowly over one eye. Patients may not be able to determine which eye is affected" (Fode, 1990, p. 26).

"A reversible ischemic neurologic deficit (RIND) is neurologic dysfunction which persists beyond the 24 hour period of a TIA but eventually resolves." By definition, the deficit resolves "within 1 week" (Fode, 1990, p. 26).

Mrs. Hamilton's symptoms accompanying her TIAs included dizziness, numbness of her left arm and leg, and a headache.

8. **Describe the effect Mrs. Hamilton's hypertension could have postoperatively. What goals and treatment modalities would be expected?**

Frequent changes in blood pressure often occur during the immediate postoperative period. Baroreceptors located in the carotid sinus may have been disturbed during the surgical procedure, resulting in hypertension (Kane & Wilson, 1993). "Significant hypertension has been reported in 19% to 25% of patients" (O'Brien & Ricotta, 1994, p. 2). Research indicates that hypertension usually occurs during the early postoperative period and generally lasts an average of 5 to 6 hours after surgery (Hartshorn, Lamborn, & Noll, 1993; O'Brien & Ricotta, 1994).

One danger of hypertension includes rupture of the operative vessels. In addition, sustained hypertension puts the patient at risk for an intracerebral hemorrhage, edema, and stroke (Kane & Wilson, 1993).

Sodium nitroprusside or nitroglycerin are vasodilators that are frequently used to maintain the patient's blood pressure within a range of 1 to 20 mm Hg of the patient's preoperative baseline.

9. Why do some patients develop postoperative hypotension? What are the nurse's responsibilities?

Patients with chronic hypertension may develop reflex hypotension and bradycardia, which could require vigorous treatment with vasopressors. "Hypotension places the patient at risk for decreased cerebral blood flow and perfusion, causing changes in mentation and increasing the chances for neurologic deficits" (Johnson & Anderson, 1991, p. 504). The nurse must carefully titrate vasoactive drugs such as nitroprusside (Nipride) or nitroglycerin to avoid hypotension (Kane & Wilson, 1993). In the event that hypotension does occur and reduction in the rate of the vasodilating drug being used is not effective, vasoactive drugs such as dobutamine or dopamine may be required.

10. What should be included in Mrs. Hamilton's neurologic assessment?

a. Level of consciousness and orientation
b. Ability to follow commands
c. Speech
d. Extremity movement and strength
e. Pupil size and reaction to light; visual field acuity
f. Cranial nerves
   (1) ability to position the tongue midline (hypoglossal)
   (2) ability to smile (facial)
   (3) ability to speak (vagus)
   (4) ability to raise arms and sustain for 3 seconds (spinal accessory)
     (Kane & Wilson, 1993)

11. Discuss how carotid endarterectomy can damage certain cranial nerves. What are the clinical manifestations of specific nerve dam-

age? What precautions should be taken to prevent cranial nerve damage?

Injuries to cranial nerves can occur from intraoperative trauma (such as inadvertent transection or retractor injuries) and edema, resulting in nerve compression. According to O'Brien and Ricotta (1994), cranial nerve damage occurs in 16% of patients undergoing carotid endarterectomy. These injuries usually resolve; however, 1% to 4% do not resolve. The following cranial injuries may occur:

- XII, hypoglossal (located under the carotid artery): inability to position the tongue midline
- X, vagus (laryngeal branch): hoarseness, loss of cough mechanism
- VII, facial (marginal mandibular branch): drooping of the lip ipsilateral to the surgery site
- XI, spinal accessory: inability to shrug shoulders (Johnson & Anderson, 1991; Kane & Wilson, 1993; O'Brien & Ricotta, 1994).

The presence of cranial nerve deficits should be determined before giving the patient any ice chips, water, or food. Once the gag reflex has returned, the patient should be given liquids only initially and cautiously when awake. The head of the bed should be elevated at all times. Suctioning equipment should be available and ready for use. In addition, the patient should be closely observed for respiratory difficulties or other signs of hypoxemia.

12. **What are the signs of decreased cerebral functioning related to decreased cerebral blood flow that should be assessed in Mrs. Hamilton and immediately reported to the physician?**

- ipsilateral vascular-type headaches
- decreased level of consciousness
- unequal, dilated, or sluggish pupils
- motor weakness or hemiplegia
- visual disturbances
- respiratory or breathing pattern changes
- dysphasia
- seizures
- Widening pulse pressure (late and ominous sign) (Johnson & Anderson, 1991, p. 504)

13. **Twelve hours after surgery the nurse notices a hematoma around Mrs. Hamilton's incision site. What causes a hematoma following a carotid endarterectomy? Discuss the danger posed by this finding.**

Development of a hematoma is a serious, potentially life-threatening complication. A hematoma in the neck area can contribute to airway occlusion, tracheal deviation, or rupture of the operative vessel. The patient should be monitored for bleeding and the following reported to the physician: edema, bright red drainage from the incision site, decreased hematocrit, and hypotension. In some cases the patient may be required to return to surgery for reexploration and evacuation of the hematoma (Johnson & Anderson, 1991; Kane & Wilson, 1993).

14. What are other potential complications to keep in mind for Mrs. Hamilton?

Stroke due to embolization, thrombosis, or hemorrhage can occur. Also, postoperative MI is a major complication of carotid endarterectomy. Mrs. Hamilton is a potential candidate for an MI because of her history of preexisting cardiovascular disease (Kane & Wilson, 1993). MI occurs infrequently but is the most common cause of death following carotid endarterectomy (0.8% to 3%); the risk of MI is increased in patients with a history of angina (13%) (O'Brien & Ricotta, 1994).

15. What instructions should Mrs. Hamilton receive regarding restriction of neck movement immediately after surgery?

The patient should avoid any sharp turns of the neck. Nothing should be placed on the site that might cause injury or damage. The head should be supported at all times (Hartshorn et al., 1993).

16. After surgery, Mrs. Hamilton made good progress and was discharged home on the third postoperative day. Discharge medications included nifedipine (Procardia) 20 mg PO q8h and dipyridamole (Persantine) 50 mg b.i.d. Describe the pharmacodynamics and clinical effects of these drugs. What instructions regarding her medications should be given to Mrs Hamilton before her discharge?

According to Katsung (1992), calcium channel blockers, such as nifedipine, relax vascular smooth muscle, specifically arterioles and veins, without causing orthostatic hypotension, thus reducing blood pressure. Peripheral vascular resistance is reduced, especially with nifedipine. Calcium channel blockers also reduce cardiac contractility and cardiac output in a dose-dependent fashion. Some research has indicated that calcium channel blockers may interfere with the development of atheromatous lesions. The most important adverse side effect is cardiac depression, including cardiac arrest, bradycardia, atrioventricular block, and congestive heart failure. Minor toxicity caused by calcium channel blockers includes flushing, edema, dizziness, nausea, and constipation. Mrs. Hamilton should be taught how to take her pulse before taking this drug and to report a pulse of less than 50 bpm to her physician, as well as the side effects addressed above.

Dipyridamole (Persantine) is a platelet adhesion inhibitor. Its mechanism of action is not yet fully understood. Adverse reactions with therapeutic doses are usually minimal and transient. Transient dizziness, abdominal discomfort, and rash have been reported in the literature (Katsung, 1992). Mrs. Hamilton should be instructed to report persistent symptoms to her doctor.

Carotid Endarterectomy

Alspach, J. G. (Ed.). (1991). *Core curriculum for critical care nursing.* Philadelphia: Saunders.

Bruno, A. (1993). Ischemic stroke, part 1: Early, accurate diagnosis. *Geriatrics, 48*(3), 26–34.

Clochesy, J. M., Breu, C., Cardin, S., Rudy, E. B., & Whittaker, A. A. (1993). *Critical care nursing.* Philadelphia: Saunders.

Feussner, J. R. (1993). Indications for endarterectomy and for nonsurgical treatment. *Consultant, 33*(2), 35–37.

Fode, N. C. (1990). Carotid endarterectomy: Nursing care and controversies. *Journal of Neuroscience Nursing, 22*(1), 25–31.

Hartshorn, J., Lamborn, M., & Noll, M. L. (1993). *Introduction to critical care nursing.* Philadelphia: Saunders.

Johnson, S. M., & Anderson, B. (1991). Carotid endarterectomy: A review. *Critical Care Clinics of North America, 3*(3), 499–506.

Kane, H. L., & Wilson, L. B. (1993). Practical points in the care of the post-carotid endarterectomy. *Journal of Post Anesthesia Nursing, 8*(6), 403–405.

Katsung, B. G. (Ed.). (1992). *Basic and clinical pharmacology.* Norwalk, CT: Appleton & Lange.

Moore, W., & Quinones-Baldrich, W. (1991). External cerebral vascular disease: The carotid artery. In Moore, W. (Ed.). *Vascular surgery: A comprehensive review* (pp. 434–472). Philadelphia: Saunders.

O'Brien, M. S., & Ricotta, J. J. (1994). Postoperative treatment of patients undergoing carotid endarterectomy. *Journal of Vascular Nursing, 12*(1), 1–5.

Sanchez, F. (1988). Carotid endarterectomy: A comprehensive approach to care. *Journal of Post Anesthesia Nursing, 1*(2), 97–106.

11

Acute Renal Failure

Sheila Drake Melander, DSN, RN, FCCM

CASE PRESENTATION

Sarah Banks, age 68 years, initially was admitted to the hospital for elective surgical repair of an abdominal aortic aneurysm. Her surgery was documented as uneventful. However, her postoperative period was complicated as a result of a small bowel perforation that developed during her fifth postoperative day.

Postoperative Day 5

Current vital signs and laboratory results are as follows:

BP	170/94
HR	110 bpm
Respirations	30/min
Temperature	38.6° C (101.4° F) (Rectal)
Hgb	10.1 g/dl
Hct	30%
RBCs	3.5 x 10^6/mm^3
WBCs	20,000/mm^3

Urine

Creatinine	0.6 g/24 h	Na^+	45 mmol/d
Osmolality	460 mOsm/kg	K^+	15 mmol/d
Specific gravity	1.01	Cl^-	48 mmol/d
pH	9.0		

Serum

Na$^+$	135 mmol/L	Creatinine	1.4 mg/dl
K$^+$	4.8 mmol/L	Uric acid	9 mg/dl
Cl$^-$	88 mmol/L	Phosphorus	5.2 mg/dl
Ca	6 mg/dl	Alkaline phosphatase	14.8 King-Armstrong U/dl
BUN	27 mg/dl		

Laboratory results and vital signs were telephoned to her physician. Her physician's orders included the following:

- hydralazine (Apresoline) at 10 mg q.i.d.
- gentamicin sulfate (Garamycin) IV at 5 mg/kg t.i.d. in divided doses
- piperacillin sodium (Pipracil) 3 g q12h

Gastrointestinal Fistula Repair

As a result of an abnormal abdominal x-ray, Mrs. Banks was returned to surgery for repair of a small bowel perforation. Four days after Mrs. Banks' bowel surgery, she developed a gastrointestinal fistula. She was again taken to surgery for repair of the fistula. Postoperatively, her blood pressure dropped to 80/52 and her urine output was 20 ml/h, requiring invasive monitoring. Mrs. Banks' oxygen saturations and arterial blood gases dropped significantly. She required intubation and was transferred to the intensive care unit (ICU).

Intensive Care Admission

After Mrs Banks' admission to the ICU, the staff took a complete history that revealed her history of congestive heart failure. Mrs. Banks weighed 76.5 kg (170 lb) (preoperative weight was 71 kg [158 lb]) and evidenced 2+ pitting edema in her lower extremities. Her skin was pale, shiny, and dry. She complained of nausea and stated that she "felt as if she had no energy left." The past 24 hours' intake was 1400 ml, while her output was 510 ml. Jugular vein distension was noted, and crackles were auscultated bilaterally in the lung bases. The initial cardiac rhythm was tachycardia with a rate of 110 bpm, a PR interval of 0.18 seconds, QRS of 0.14 seconds, and peaked T waves.

A fluid challenge was administered unsuccessfully. Despite volume replacement and diuretics, Mrs. Banks' renal status deteriorated further, and she was diagnosed with acute renal failure (ARF). Dopamine (Intropin) was started at 2 μg/kg/min and dobutamine (Dobutrex) at 3 μg/kg/min, and continuous arteriovenous hemofiltration dialysis (CAVHD) was begun. Diagnostic data at this time were:

Weight	82 kg (182 lb)	PAP	36/16
HR	124 bpm	PAWP	15 mm Hg
BP	90–100 mm Hg systolic		
Urine output	15 ml/h		

Na⁺ 146 mmol/L	Ca	7 mg/dl

Na⁺ 146 mmol/L   Ca   7 mg/dl
K⁺ 5.8 mmol/L   BUN   36 mg/dl
Cl⁻ 98 mmol/L   Creatinine 3.9 mg/dl

After 4 days of CAVHD, BUN and creatinine levels began falling and blood pressure stabilized with a decrease in weight and edema. Electrolyte and laboratory values returned to normal limits. Mrs. Banks was started on total parenteral nutrition (TPN), and renal function continued to improve until CAVHD was discontinued 5 days later.

Acute Renal Failure

1. Discuss the pathophysiology involved in ARF.

2. Describe the four phases in the clinical course of ARF.

3. Compare and contrast oliguric and nonoliguric renal failure.

4. What clinical assessment data support the diagnosis of ARF for Mrs. Banks? What other diagnostic information may be useful in the diagnosis of ARF?

5. What is the significance of the use of gentamicin sulfate (Garamycin) and piperacillin sodium (Pipracil) in Mrs. Banks' treatment regimen?

6. Discuss the major nephrotoxic drug classifications, including risk factors and prevention of nephrotoxicity.

7. What is the rationale for including dopamine (Intropin) in Mrs. Banks' treatment plan?

8. Identify other pharmacologic agents used in the treatment of ARF and the rationale for their use.

9. Discuss the dietary management of the patient in ARF.

10. Discuss the three different forms of dialysis used in the treatment of ARF including the indications and contraindications for each. Why was CAVHD indicated in Mrs. Banks' case?

11. List nursing diagnoses appropriate for care of the patient with ARF.

12. What are the nursing responsibilities and potential complications related to CRRT?

QUESTIONS AND ANSWERS

Acute Renal Failure

1. **Discuss the pathophysiology involved in ARF.**

Definition

Baer and Lancaster (1992) defined ARF as "the abrupt cessation of renal function." A more relevant definition of ARF involves an understanding of the onset, duration, and prognosis of the disease as it relates to individual patients. The onset of ARF generally is sudden and characterized by either anuria (<100 ml/24 h), oliguria (100–400 ml/24 h), or polyuria (>400 ml/24 h). Oliguria is the most common urine volume seen in ARF, whereas anuria is seen least frequently (Baer & Lancaster, 1992). The duration of ARF is typically 10 to 25 days and involves different phases according to time span, renal flow, oxygen consumption, and urine volume and filtration (Baer & Lancaster, 1992). The prognosis for ARF is good in that in 50% to 60% of the patient population kidney function returns to normal. Of the remaining patients, 25% to 30% develop chronic renal failure, and a mortality rate of 15% to 20% exists as a result of systemic effects (Baer & Lancaster, 1992).

Etiology

ARF can be classified as having prerenal, postrenal, or intrarenal, (parenchymal) causes (Clochesy, Breu, Cardin, Rudy, & Whittaker, 1993). Prerenal causes are the result of decreased renal perfusion due to hemorrhage, dehydration, decreased cardiac output, or fluid shifts. Postrenal causes are due to an obstruction in the flow of urine from such conditions as benign prostatic hypertrophy, tumor, and bladder, renal, or ureteral calculi. Parenchymal causes involve a direct insult to kidney tissue, such as occurs in acute tubular necrosis (ATN), glomerulonephritis, renal vascular disease, and interstitial nephritis (Chambers, 1987).

According to Alspach (1991) the most common form of ARF in the critically ill patient is ATN resulting from ischemic or toxic damage to the nephrons. Individuals at risk for developing ATN include those who have suffered a decrease in blood pressure as a result of hypovolemia or sepsis. Also at risk are those patients exposed to nephrotoxic drugs, heavy metals, pigments such as myoglobin released during trauma, and hemoglobin from mismatched transfusions (Norris, 1989). Endogenous toxins produced from septicemia or multiple organ failure are also causative agents.

Pathophysiology

The pathophysiology of ATN involves changes in renal hemodynamics, cellular metabolism, and nephron structure and function. A decrease in the mean arterial pressure (MAP) leads to decreased renal blood flow and perfusion pressure. As stated by Ulrich (1989), the kidney receives approximately 25% of the cardiac output, or 1200 ml/min. As a result of a decreased blood flow, ischemia may lead to a release of renin, activating the renin-angiotensin-aldosterone system. Once activated, this system causes the renal afferent arterioles to constrict and the glomerular blood flow, hydrostatic pressure, and filtration rate to decrease, which leads to tubular dysfunction and oliguria. Other changes contributing to renal vasoconstriction and tubular cellular injury include the production of adenosine, the decrease in prostaglandin synthesis, and blood flow redistribution from the outer to the inner cortex (Baer & Lancaster, 1992; Clochesy et al., 1993).

The amount of renal cell damage depends on the ischemic time period (Baer & Lancaster, 1992). Ischemia leads to anaerobic metabolism resulting in a decreased production of adenosine triphosphate (ATP). A lack of ATP causes an alteration in the sodium-potassium pump and sodium-calcium exchange. An increased intracellular sodium content leads to cellular swelling and cell death, which raises tissue pressures and further impedes arteriole blood flow (Baer, 1990). As a result of tubular cell swelling and necrosis, tubular obstruction occurs from an accumulation of cellular debris. The tubular obstruction leads to an increased hydrostatic pressure in the Bowman's capsule, resulting in a decreased glomerular filtration rate. The damaged tubular membrane increases tubular permeability, which allows a back leak of tubular filtrate into the plasma, further decreasing the amount of tubular filtrate present (Baer & Lancaster, 1992; Ulrich, 1989).

In toxic ATN, toxins cause initial injury to the tubular cells. After this initial injury, the pathophysiology of toxic and ischemic ATN are similar. However, the tubular basement membrane may not be damaged in toxic ATN, resulting in a faster healing process and presence of nonoliguric rather than oliguric ARF (Baer & Lancaster, 1992).

2. Describe the four phases in the clinical course of ARF.

The four phases of ARF include the (1) onset phase, (2) oliguric-anuric phase, (3) diuretic phase, and (4) convalescent or recovery phase.

Onset Phase

The onset phase can last up to 2 days and is characterized by renal blood flow and oxygen consumption at 25% of normal, urine volume at 20% of normal, and filtration clearance at 10% of normal (Baer & Lancaster, 1992). The most important factor affecting this phase is the alteration in systemic hemodynamics as evidenced by decreased cardiac output (Alspach, 1991).

Oliguric-Anuric Phase

The oliguric-anuric phase lasts about 8 to 14 days and is characterized by a further decrease in urine volume to 5% of normal. The oliguric phase occurs as a result of obstruction of the tubules, total reabsorption of urine filtration, tubular cell damage, and renal vasoconstriction (Alspach, 1991). The longer the patient remains in this phase, the poorer the prognosis. As reported by Alspach (1991), the nonoliguric phase is reflective of decreased tubular damage. Duration of this phase is generally short, with the patient reaching the recovery phase in 5 to 8 days.

Diuretic Phase

The diuretic phase lasts about 10 days and is made up of two phases. Early diuresis is characterized by a renal blood flow and oxygen consumption increase to 30% of normal, a urine volume to 150% of normal, and stabilization of laboratory values. Late diuresis is said to have begun once the BUN and creatinine levels begin to fall. In this stage, renal blood flow increases to 50% of normal, urine volume increases to 200% of normal, and filtration clearance increases to 50% of normal (Baer & Lancaster, 1992). This stage is complete when the laboratory values stabilize and return to normal limits (Ulrich, 1989).

Convalescent or Recovery Phase

The convalescent or recovery phase begins with the stabilization of laboratory values and can range from 3 to 12 months. Kidney function must be monitored very closely during the recovery phase. Patient education must include the fact that the recovery phase may conclude with residual impairment of kidney function (Alspach, 1991).

3. **Compare and contrast oliguric and nonoliguric renal failure.**

Oliguric ATN

Oliguric ATN involves tubular damage resulting in a tubular backleak of filtrate and tubular obstruction. During oliguria, the kidney is unable to concentrate urine, resulting in excretion of urine that is rich in sodium but lacking in excess volume, electrolytes, and waste (Stark, 1992b). The patient exhibits fluid, electrolyte, and acid-base imbalances, requiring frequent dialysis, resulting in a poorer prognosis.

Nonoliguric ATN

In contrast, tubular damage in the nonoliguric kidney is less severe, resulting in a concentrating defect vs. an impairment of urinary flow with tubular backleak and obstruction. The nonoliguric kidney has normal to excess output, requiring less frequent dialysis. Nonoliguric ATN is demonstrated as a shortened course with a 50% reduction in mortality (Stark, 1992a). Therefore, when prevention of ATN in the critically ill patient is not possible, creation of a nonoliguric ATN by improving renal blood flow may help decrease the amount of tubular damage. Protective agents that can accomplish this include volume expanders such as mannitol (Osmitrol), furosemide (Lasix), and dopamine (Intropin). Prostaglandins, even though experimental, may also be used for their vasodilating benefits (Stark, 1992a).

4. **What clinical assessment data support the diagnosis of ARF for Mrs. Banks? What other diagnostic information may be useful in the diagnosis of ARF?**

Assessment Data

Mrs. Banks' assessment information included jugular vein distension, pulmonary congestion, tachypnea, tachycardia, and intake and output imbalances. The cardiac monitor revealed peaked T waves and widened QRS complexes. Mrs. Banks also complained of lethargy and nausea and vomiting (Clochesy et al., 1993). Mrs. Banks' assessment data are supportive of the diagnosis of ARF (Clochesy et al., 1993).

Client History

Aspects of the patient's history that are important in diagnosing ARF include renal symptoms, systemic diseases, laboratory results, and medication history. Mrs. Banks had a positive history for cardiovascular disease and experienced a hypotensive episode postoperatively along with sepsis. These findings in addition to other system diseases, such as hematopoietic or immunologic diseases, have a direct impact on the renal system. Also, Mrs. Banks is being treated with two nephrotoxic agents, gentamicin sulfate (Garamycin) and piperacillin sodium (Pipracil).

Laboratory Data

The best measure to assess renal function is urinary creatinine clearance (Hartshorn, Lamborn, & Noll, 1993). If this is not readily available, serum creatinine and BUN levels should be monitored daily for evaluations. Mrs. Banks' creatinine and BUN levels were both elevated. BUN levels are the least helpful of the two measures, as the BUN is often influenced by bleeding, volume depletion, and catabolism. Mrs. Banks was in an oliguric state; however, urine volume is not always a good measure of renal function, since some patients may exhibit oliguric or polyuric renal failure. Patterns of urine output must be monitored to identify renal perfusion status. Mrs. Banks demonstrated elevations in sodium, potassium, chloride, phosphorus, uric acid, and alkaline phosphatase levels that support the diagnosis of ARF. A decreased calcium level and a high normal magnesium level may also be evident in ARF (Baer & Lancaster, 1992).

Urine laboratory values supporting ARF include the following:

- a decrease in creatinine, osmolality, sodium, potassium, chloride, calcium, and phosphorus levels
- increased pH
- fixed specific gravity and normal glucose and protein levels. It should be noted, however, that urinary laboratory values vary depending on the pathophysiology involved. For example, in ATN the urinary sodium is usually elevated (Norris, 1989).

Diagnostic Information

Noninvasive diagnostic procedures that should be evaluated in Mrs. Banks and other patients with ARF include intake and output, daily weights, and the kidney, ureters, and bladder (KUB) x-ray. Invasive procedures that may be used include IV pyelography, computed tomography (CT), renal angiography, renal scan, nephrosonography, and renal biopsy (Hartshorn et al., 1993).

5. **What is the significance of the use of gentamicin sulfate (Garamycin) and piperacillin sodium (Pipracil) in Mrs. Banks' treatment regimen?**

Gentamicin and piperacillin are both nephrotoxic agents. Piperacillin sodium (Pipracil), a penicillin, may lead to interstitial nephritis with ARF due to a hypersensitive reaction. Gentamicin sulfate (Garamycin), an aminoglycoside, may lead to renal dysfunction with ATN. Aminoglycosides primarily affect the proximal tubule. Toxicity is evident in 10% to 25% of patients receiving the drug (Garfinkel, Porter, & Whelth, 1988).

6. **Discuss the major nephrotoxic drug classifications, including risk factors and prevention of nephrotoxicity.**

Nephrotoxic Drug Classifications

Ninety-five percent of drug-related renal failure may be attributed to use of antibiotics, nonsteroidal antiinflammatory agents (NSAIDs), and radiographic contrast media. Antibiotics may lead to interstitial nephritis and tubular dysfunction. NSAIDs alter renal blood flow and glomerular filtration. Radiographic contrast material may alter intrarenal blood flow and cause obstruction (Clochesy et al., 1993; Garfinkle et al., 1988). Patients at risk for drug-induced renal disease include those characterized by the following: (1) significant volume dysfunction, such as those individuals with liver or cardiac disease; (2) preexisting renal insufficiency; (3) administration of more than one nephrotoxic agent; and (4) age over 60 years (Garfinkle et al., 1988).

Prevention of Nephrotoxicity

Nephrotoxicity may be prevented by identifying risk factors, providing correct drug dosages, and monitoring serum drug levels. Serum creatinine and creatinine clearance levels should be monitored while a patient receives nephrotoxic agents. Alternate diagnostic measures should be considered before a contrast medium is administered to individuals at risk for renal dysfunction. Prehydration and the use of mannitol or furosemide (Lasix) may also decrease nephrotoxic effects. The simultaneous use of more than one nephrotoxic agent should be avoided (Garfinkle et al., 1988).

7. **What is the rationale for including dopamine (Intropin) in Mrs. Banks' treatment plan?**

Dopamine (Intropin), a vasopressor, will lead to an improvement in cardiac output and renal perfusion by causing vasodilation of the renal vasculature. The vasodilating effect is most evident with lower doses of the drug between 0.5 and 3 $\mu g/kg/min$. With higher doses the vasoconstrictive properties of dopamine are more evident, thus decreasing urinary output (Dolleris, 1992).

8. **Identify other pharmacologic agents used in the treatment of ARF and the rationale for their use.**

Pharmacologic Management

In addition to dopamine (Intropin), loop diuretics such as furosemide (Lasix) and osmotic diuretics such as mannitol are used in the treatment of ARF. Diuretics are used in ARF to increase urinary flow with the intent of flushing out the cellular debris causing tubular obstruction and possibly creating a nonoliguric ATN. Osmotic diuretics and loop diuretics have been found to dilate renal arteries by increasing the synthesis of prostaglandins, resulting in restoration of renal blood flow (Dolleris, 1992). Since the decrease in renal perfusion has its greatest impact in the initial stages of ARF, it is crucial to use diuretics as an early intervention. It is recommended that mannitol be used in hypovolemic or normovolemic patients, whereas loop diuretics such as furosemide should be used in volume-overloaded patients (Dolleris, 1992). Larger dosages may be required, as the secretion of these agents into the proximal tubules may be limited by the presence of uremic toxins (Dolleris, 1992).

9. **Discuss the dietary management of the patient in ARF.**

According to Baer and Lancaster (1992), the goals of dietary management are to minimize uremic toxicity, minimize fluid and electrolyte
imbalances, and maintain an anabolic state. Tissue catabolism develops
frequently in ARF, which in turn leads to increases in BUN levels,
metabolic acidosis, and hyperkalemia. The patient requires a high-calorie, low-protein diet. The protein must have a high biologic value
(HBV), since these protein foods contain all the essential amino acids
and reduce the urea nitrogen produced during metabolism. Examples
of such foods include meat, poultry, eggs, and milk. The daily HBV
protein intake should be 1 g/kg of body weight for dialysis patients and
40 g/d in nondialyzed patients (Baer & Lancaster, 1992). ARF patients
usually require diets restricted in sodium and potassium. Fluids typically
are restricted to 600 to 1000 ml/d plus the amount of urine excreted
per day (Baer & Lancaster, 1992). The dialysis patient requires supplements of vitamin B, vitamin C, and folic acid. For patients who are unable to eat, TPN is indicated. A TPN calorie-to-nutrient ratio of greater
than 450:1 is recommended to prevent protein catabolism and BUN
level elevations (Baer & Lancaster, 1992).

10. **Discuss the three different forms of dialysis used in the treatment
of ARF, including the indications and contraindications for each.
Why was CAVHD indicated in Mrs. Banks' case?**

The three dialysis options in the critically ill patient include hemodialysis, peritoneal dialysis, and continuous renal replacement therapy (CRRT) (Stark, 1992b).

Hemodialysis

Hemodialysis provides ultrafiltration for rapid water removal and diffusion for solute removal. It is indicated for uremia, electrolyte imbalances, fluid overload, and severe metabolic acidosis. Contraindications
include hemodynamic instability, lack of access, and decreased clotting
ability.

Peritoneal Dialysis

Peritoneal dialysis is a slow, efficient form of dialysis that involves an exchange of fluid and solutes between the peritoneal cavity and peritoneal
capillaries. Peritoneal dialysis is indicated for uremia, fluid and electrolyte imbalances, and hemodynamic instability. However, it is contraindicated in emergency situations unless all other forms of dialysis are
unavailable or contraindicated. It is also contraindicated in abdominal
conditions or sepsis (Stark, 1992b).

Continuous Renal Replacement Therapy

Three forms of CRRT include slow continuous ultrafiltration (SCUF), continuous arteriovenous hemofiltration (CAVH), and continuous arteriovenous hemofiltration dialysis (CAVHD). CRRT is an ongoing therapy that may be used for days or months by allowing slow volume removal while maintaining hemodynamic stability (Bosworth, 1992; Clochesy et al., 1993). SCUF employs principles of ultrafiltration for fluid removal, whereas CAVH is used for both solute and fluid removal. In addition to ultrafiltration, CAVHD allows for removal of solutes via passive diffusion (Stark, 1992b). CRRT is indicated for hypervolemic patients unresponsive to diuretics, hemodynamically unstable patients, oliguric patients requiring large amounts of volume replacement, and patients without adequate anticoagulation (Lawyer & Velasco, 1989; Stark, 1992b). Disadvantages of CRRT include the need for arterial access, restrictions on the patient's activity level, and lack of dramatic reduction in urea due to the absence of a circuit blood pump (Bosworth, 1992). In CRRT, a blood pump is not necessary, as a pressure gradient is formed with blood flow from an artery to a vein. Hydrostatic pressure is exerted by the MAP, and negative pressure is created by the level of the drainage bag (Bosworth, 1992).

CRRT was an appropriate dialysis option for Mrs. Banks, since she was hemodynamically unstable. Mrs. Banks may not have tolerated traditional hemodialysis because of her hemodynamic instability and hypotension. Mrs. Banks also had a large daily fluid requirement that included TPN. Mrs. Banks' unresponsiveness to diuretic therapy also supports the need for CRRT.

11. **List nursing diagnoses appropriate for care of the patient with ARF.**

As cited by Hartshorn et al. (1993), the following nursing diagnoses should be considered in the care of the patient with ARF.

- ➤ alteration in fluid and electrolyte and acid-base balance
- ➤ alteration in cardiac output
- ➤ high risk for infection
- ➤ alteration in coagulation
- ➤ alteration in breathing patterns
- ➤ alteration in nutrition
- ➤ alteration in bowel elimination
- ➤ impaired physical mobility
- ➤ high risk for injury
- ➤ sensory-perceptual alterations
- ➤ alteration in thought processes

➤ high risk for impaired skin integrity
➤ alteration in oral mucous membranes
➤ knowledge deficit
➤ alteration in urinary elimination

12. What are the nursing responsibilities and potential complications related to CRRT?

Nursing Responsibilities

Before CRRT is begun, patient and family teaching concerning the procedure should be completed. Once the therapy has started, it is crucial to monitor the patient's hemodynamic status frequently to observe the patient's response to fluid removal. Any changes in heart rate, blood pressure, central venous pressure, and pulmonary capillary wedge pressure may indicate hypovolemia, requiring the need for a crystalloid infusion and adjustment of the ultrafiltration rate (Bosworth, 1992). The nurse should also monitor the partial thromboplastin times and observe the patient for any signs of bleeding. Electrolyte loss in ultrafiltration can be significant, indicating the need for close monitoring of electrolyte imbalances. Patients receiving CRRT therapy are at risk for hyponatremia, hypokalemia, and hypocalcemia. The patient should also be monitored for acid-base imbalances, as bicarbonate is easily removed with CRRT. Replacement fluids usually have a bicarbonate base. If metabolic alkalosis occurs during therapy, replacement solutions may be changed to normal saline until the pH and bicarbonate levels are normal (Bosworth, 1992). Drug levels also must be monitored closely, as CRRT may remove many of the drugs that are typically used in critical care patients (Bosworth, 1992).

The position and patency of the hemofilter and arteriovenous system must be checked frequently. When using a femoral catheter, the patient's legs must be positioned straight to avoid kinking of the catheter (Lievaart & Voerman, 1991). Access sites must be inspected frequently for signs of infection or bleeding. A transparent permeable dressing should be applied and changed every 3 to 5 days. Fluid balance should be calculated every 4 to 6 hours and the amount of ultrafiltration noted every 30 minutes to monitor for a hypovolemic or hypervolemic episode (Lievaart & Voerman, 1991).

Prevention of Complications

Prevention of complications related to CRRT requires early intervention by the nursing staff. Restrictions on patient activity may lead to complications related to skin integrity, requiring a turning schedule via "log rolling." Dislodgment of the arterial catheter may lead to hemorrhage. Therefore, patients receiving CRRT therapy may require restraints or sedation (Bosworth, 1992). Sutures around the catheter and connection ports must be inspected frequently for patency. Thrombosis is another potential complication that requires close monitoring of distal extremity pulses and perfusion. Infection may be prevented by changing the occlusive dressing at the catheter site every 5 days. The site should be observed for signs of infection, and any lines and solutions should be changed according to hospital policy (Bosworth, 1992).

REFERENCES

Acute Renal Failure

Alspach, J. G. (1991). *Core curriculum for critical care nursing*. Philadelphia: Saunders.

Baer, C. L. (1990). Acute renal failure: Recognizing and reversing its deadly course. *Nursing, 6,* 34–39.

Baer, C. L., & Lancaster, L. E. (1992). Acute renal failure. *Critical Care Nursing Quarterly, 14*(4), 1–21.

Bosworth, G. (1992). SCUF/CAVH/CAVHD: Critical differences. *Critical Care Nursing Quarterly, 14*(4), 45–55.

Chambers, J. K. (1987). Fluid and electrolyte problems in renal and urologic disorders. *Nursing Clinics of North America, 22*(4), 815–826.

Clochesy, J. M., Breu, C., Cardin, S., Rudy, E. B., & Whittaker, A. A. (1993). *Critical care nursing*. Philadelphia: Saunders.

Dolleris, P. M. (1992). Diuretic and vasopressor usage in acute renal failure: A synopsis. *Critical Care Nursing Quarterly, 14*(4), 28–31.

Garfinkel, H., Porter, G. A., & Whelth, A. (1988). Renal failure: Are drugs the cause? *Patient Care, 9/15,* 71–87.

Hartshorn, J., Lamborn, M., & Noll, M. L. (1993). *Introduction to critical care nursing*. Philadelphia: Saunders.

Lawyer, L. A., & Velasco, A. (1989). Continuous arteriovenous hemodialysis in the ICU. *Critical Care Nursing Quarterly, 14*(4), 72–77.

Lievaart, A., & Voerman, H. J. (1991). Nursing management of continuous arteriovenous hemodialysis. *Heart and Lung, 20*(2), 152–158.

Norris, M. K. (1989). Acute tubular necrosis: Preventing complications. *Dimensions of Critical Care Nursing, 8*(1), 16–25.

Stark, J. (1992a). Acute tubular necrosis: Differences between oliguria and nonoliguria. *Critical Care Nursing Quarterly, 14*(4), 22–27.

Stark, J. (1992b). Dialysis options in the critically ill patient: Hemodialysis, peritoneal dialysis and continuous renal replacement therapy. *Critical Care Nursing Quarterly, 14*(4), 40–44.

Ulrich, B. T. (1989). *Nephrology nursing*. Philadelphia: Saunders.

Chronic Renal Failure and Renal Transplantation

Gail Stamper Franks, MSN, RN

CASE PRESENTATION

Richard Morgan, age 67 years, was diagnosed with end-stage renal disease (ESRD) secondary to chronic pyelonephritis. He received hemodialysis at an outpatient clinic three times per week. He traveled with his wife approximately 75 miles to reach the clinic. A short experience with home dialysis was unsuccessful, and Mr. Morgan had begun to miss one and sometimes two clinic appointments each week. Mr. Morgan had no active malignancy or infectious process. He had a strong support system with siblings willing to donate a living donor kidney. He was financially secure through income and health insurance coverage.

Mr. Morgan presented to the emergency department with a 2-day history of not feeling well accompanied by nausea and vomiting. He was agitated and slightly confused. He was complaining of moderate-to-severe chest pain diffused over the precordium. Initial assessment revealed jugular vein distension, scattered crackles bilaterally throughout the lung bases, and pitting peripheral edema bilaterally in the lower extremities. Cardiac monitoring demonstrated sinus tachycardia with a rate of 116 bpm. A pericardial friction rub and an S_3 gallop were auscultated. His wife informed the nurse that Mr. Morgan missed his previous appointment for dialysis and was 8 kg (18 lb) heavier than his dry weight of 74 kg (164 lb). Current vital signs and laboratory results were as follows:

BP	180/110	Temperature	38.7° C (101.6° F [Rectal])
HR	116 bpm	Height	175 cm (5'10")
Respirations	36/min	Weight	82 kg (182 lb)

RBCs	$3.1 \times 10^6/mm^3$	Na^+	136 mmol/L	Creatinine	26.9 mg/dl
WBCs	13,500/mm³	K^+	7.3 mmol/L	Mg	1.3 mEq/L
Hgb	8.5 g/dl	Cl^-	110 mmol/L	PO_4	12 mg/dl
Hct	26%	CO_2	10 mmol/L	BUN	194 mg/dl
Platelets	226,000/mm³	Glucose	95 mg/dl		

pH 7.2* SaO₂ 85%
PaCO₂ 53 mm Hg HCO₃⁻ 10 mmol/L
*At room air.

The physician ordered admission to the medical intensive care unit (ICU) for immediate hemodialysis. Oxygen was administered by a 40% face mask, and continuous arteriovenous hemofiltration dialysis (CAVHD) was initiated via a permanent arteriovenous (AV) fistula in the right forearm. An initial 4-hour dialysis treatment reduced Mr. Morgan's body weight to 76.5 kg (170 lb). Postdialysis assessment revealed the following: alert, oriented to place and person, blood pressure 160/90, heart rate 94 bpm, respirations 26/min. Mr. Morgan was given a diet restricted to 20 g of proteins and 1000 ml of fluids per day. His medication orders included the following:

- aluminum carbonate (Basaljel), two tablets PO t.i.d.
- ferrous sulfate (Iberet), 500 mg PO q AM
- calcium carbonate (Os-Cal), two 250 mg tablets PO t.i.d. with meals

Hemodialysis was continued on a daily schedule of 4-hour sessions, and Mr. Morgan was transferred to the step-down unit. Mr. Morgan's condition progressively improved, and he was scheduled for discharge. Discharge assessment revealed the following:

BP	160/95	Temperature	36.8° C (98.2° F)
HR	92 bpm	Height	175 cm (5'10")
Respirations	20/min	Weight	76.5 kg (170 lb)

RBCs	$4.1 \times 10^6/mm^3$	Na^+	136 mmol/L	Creatinine	12.6 mg/dl
WBCs	12,000/mm³	K^+	5.8 mmol/L	Ca	8.4 mg/dl
Hgb	9.1 g/dl	Cl^-	98 mmol/L	Mg	2.3 mEq/L
Hct	28.1%	CO_2	15 mmol/L	PO_4	3.2 mg/dl
Platelets	226,000/mm³	Glucose	125 mg/dl	BUN	120 mg/dl

pH 7.48* SaO₂ 95%
PaCO₂ 30 mm Hg HCO₃⁻ 25 mmol/L
PaO₂ 135 mm Hg
*At room air.

Mr. Morgan told his physician that he was unwilling to accept the limitations and restrictions in his life imposed by this illness and requested to have a kidney transplant. He informed the physician that he had discussed this at length with his three brothers and three sisters, and each is prepared to undergo testing to determine if a transplant match is possible.

Six Months Later

The donor testing of Mr. Morgan's siblings found a suitable kidney donor for his transplant. Therefore, 6 months following discharge, Mr. Morgan was readmitted to the transplant unit. Clinical and laboratory assessment revealed the following data:

BP	160/95		Temperature	36.8° C (98.2° F)			
HR	92 bpm		Height	175 cm (5'10")			
Respirations	20/min		Weight	76.5 kg (170 lb)			

RBCs	$4.1 \times 10^6/mm^3$	Na^+	136 mmol/L	Creatinine	10.1 mg/dl
WBCs	$12,000/mm^3$	K^+	5.8 mmol/L	Ca	8.4 mg/dl
Hgb	10.4 g/dl	Cl^-	98 mmol/L	Mg	2.3 mEq/L
Hct	31.2%	CO_2	15 mmol/L	PO_4	3.2 mg/dl
Platelets	$226,000/mm^3$	Glucose	125 mg/dl	BUN	90 mg/dl

pH	7.48*	SaO_2	95%
$PaCO_2$	30 mm Hg	HCO_3^-	25 mmol/L
PaO_2	135 mm Hg		

*At room air.

Preoperatively Mr. Morgan was given methylprednisolone (Solu-Medrol), lymphocyte immune globulin (ATG), and azathioprine (Imuran). A right kidney was transplanted during an uneventful surgery. Estimated blood loss was 200 ml. During the procedure Mr. Morgan received 1400 ml of crystalloid IV solution and 3 U of packed red blood cells. He was transferred from the postanesthesia recovery room to the surgical intensive care. He received oxygen via a 40% face mask and dopamine at 2 µg/kg/min for renal perfusion. He had a Jackson-Pratt drain in the right flank and a Foley catheter to straight drainage. The initial postoperative assessment revealed the following clinical data:

BP	138/92		pH	7.36
HR	92 bpm		$PaCO_2$	35 mm Hg
Respirations	22/min		PaO_2	138 mm Hg
Temperature	36.9° C (98.4° F)		SaO_2	99%
CVP	5 mm Hg		HCO_3^-	25 mmol/L

Na^+	131 mmol/L		BUN	90 mg/dl
K^+	4.8 mmol/L		Hgb	11.1 g/dl
Cl^-	92 mmol/L		Hct	33.5%
CO_2	18 mmol/L		WBCs	$12,500/mm^3$
Creatinine	10.1 mg/dl		RBCs	$4.6 \times 10^6/mm^3$
Ca	8.4 mg/dl		Platelets	$235,000/mm^3$
PO_4	3.3 mg/dl			

Over the next 7 postoperative days Mr. Morgan continued to improve. Blood urea nitrogen (BUN) and creatinine levels continued to drop, urine output averaged more than 100 ml/h, and he was hemodynamically stable. Immunosuppression therapy included decreasing doses of methyl-prednisolone, azathioprine 200 mg every day, and ATG 50 mg q12h. On the seventh postoperative day the relevant laboratory data were

BP	138/92	pH	7.36
HR	92 bpm	$PaCO_2$	35 mm Hg
Respirations	22/min	PaO_2	138 mm Hg
Temperature	36.9° C (98.4° F)	SaO_2	99%
CVP	6 mm Hg	HCO_3^-	25 mmol/L
Na^+	135 mmol/L	BUN	32 mg/dl
K^+	4.4 mmol/L	Hgb	12.9 g/dl
Cl^-	92 mmol/L	Hct	36.7%
CO_2	22 mmol/L	WBCs	13,800/mm³
Creatinine	1.9 mg/dl	RBCs	4.6×10^6/mm³
Ca	8.5 mg/dl	Platelets	296,000/mm³
PO_4	3.3 mg/dl		

Intake	2250 ml
Output (urine)	1050 ml
Output (Jackson-Pratt drain)	5 ml
Weight	76.5 kg (170 lb)

The Jackson-Pratt drain was removed. On the eighth postoperative day Mr. Morgan began to complain of not feeling well, had minimal abdominal tenderness on palpation, and complained of nausea. His temperature fluctuated between 38.4° and 38.8° C (101.2° and 101.8° F). Urinary output dropped to an average of 55 ml/h. Furosemide (Lasix) boluses did not improve his urinary output. On the 11th postoperative day laboratory data revealed that his central venous pressure (CVP) was slightly elevated to 10.5 mm Hg and his weight was up to 82 kg (182 lb). His creatinine was 7.1 mg/dl and his BUN was 120 mg/dl. Muromonab-CD3 (Orthoclone OKT3) was started and CAVHD initiated to support renal function for several days. Mr. Morgan's renal function showed progressive improvement. Cyclosporine was added to his immunosuppression therapy regimen. Mr. Morgan's laboratory data were as follows:

BP	138/92	pH	7.36
HR	92 bpm	$PaCO_2$	35 mm Hg
Respirations	22/min	PaO_2	138 mm Hg
Temperature	36.9° C (98.4° F)	SaO_2	99%
CVP	6 mm Hg	HCO_3^-	25 mmol/L
Na^+	135 mmol/L	BUN	31 mg/dl
K^+	4.4 mmol/L	Hgb	9.5 g/dl
Cl^-	92 mmol/L	Hct	28.7%
CO_2	22 mmol/L	WBCs	13,800/mm³
Creatinine	1.9 mg/dl	RBCs	4.6×10^6/mm³
Ca	8.5 mg/dl	Platelets	296,000/mm³
PO_4	3.3 mg/dl		

Intake   2250 ml
Output (urine) 1050 ml
Weight   76.5 kg (170 lb)

On the 28th postoperative day Mr. Morgan was discharged home with the following regimen:

- cyclosporine 100 mg/ml, 2.5 ml b.i.d.
- ranitidine (Zantac), 150 mg hs
- metoclopramide, 10 mg hs
- azathioprine (Imuran), 150 mg/d
- nystatin, 100,000 U/ml, 5 ml swish and swallow q.i.d.

QUESTIONS

Chronic Renal Failure and Renal Transplantation

1. Discuss the pathophysiology involved in chronic renal failure.

2. Discuss the typical laboratory findings in chronic renal failure.

3. Describe the symptoms of uremia that might be manifested by Mr. Morgan.

4. Describe how the relationship between calcium and phosphate is altered in chronic renal failure.

5. Discuss the pathophysiology of aluminum toxicity in chronic renal failure.

6. Discuss the pathophysiology of pericarditis in chronic renal failure. Why was Mr. Morgan particularly prone to this complication?

7. Discuss the different forms of dialysis used in the treatment of renal failure, including the indications and contraindications for each. Support the decision to use CAVHD in treating Mr. Morgan.

8. Identify pharmacologic agents used in the treatment of chronic renal failure and the rationale for their use.

9. Discuss the dietary management of the patient with chronic renal failure.

10. Identify the clinical complications arising from noncompliance that were manifested by Mr. Morgan.

11. List nursing diagnoses appropriate for care of the patient with chronic renal failure.

12. List the nursing diagnoses appropriate for the care of the patient with a permanent AV fistula for dialysis access.

13. List the components of the teaching plan for the patient with chronic renal failure.

14. List the criteria used in the selection of patients for kidney transplantation.

15. Discuss CAVHD and renal transplantation as alternative treatment modalities for Mr. Morgan. Support Mr. Morgan's decision to select renal transplantation as opposed to CAVHD.

16. List the advantages and disadvantages of a living donor vs. a cadaver donor. Why was it imperative that Mr. Morgan receive a living donor kidney?

17. Describe the cadaver kidney preservation process.

18. Briefly describe the surgical process of renal transplantation.

19. Discuss possible postoperative complications.

20. List the nursing diagnoses appropriate to the care of the renal transplantation patient during the recovery period.

21. Discuss the pathophysiology of acute rejection. Describe the clinical manifestations of acute rejection in Mr. Morgan.

22. Discuss the immunosuppressive pharmacologic agents methylprednisolone, muromonab-CD3 (Orthoclone OKT3), and cyclosporine. Why did the physician add muromonab-CD3 and wait several days to begin cyclosporine?

23. List the components of the teaching plan for Mr. Morgan.

QUESTIONS AND ANSWERS

Chronic Renal Failure and Renal Transplantation

1. **Discuss the pathophysiology involved in chronic renal failure.**

   The kidneys are paired organs located in the dorsal abdominal cavity in the retroperitoneal space on either side of the vertebrae column. Their main function is to maintain proper fluid and electrolyte balance and remove metabolic wastes from the body. Fluid balance is achieved by the kidney's ability to concentrate or dilute urine. Electrolyte balance is achieved by the appropriate absorption and secretion of electrolytes within the tubular system of the nephron. Chronic renal failure may develop slowly over a period of months to years or rapidly over a period of many weeks. Irreversible kidney damage occurs when 85% to 90% of renal function is lost. The hallmark of renal failure is azotemia (Alspach, 1991). All body systems are affected by metabolic waste accumulation, fluid overload, and electrolyte imbalances. Initially, as the glomerular filtration rate begins to fall, medication, diet, and fluid restrictions are used to maintain and support system function. However, with the loss of 90% of nephrons, glomerular filtration rate (GFR) will decrease to 5 ml/min (normal GFR 125 ml/min), and symptoms of uremia will become manifested. At this point hemodialysis, peritoneal dialysis, or kidney transplantation will be necessary to control the body's internal environment (Besnier & Testa, 1993).

2. **Discuss the typical laboratory findings in chronic renal failure.**

   Normal Values

Hct	40% to 54% men; 37% to 47% women
BUN	10 to 26 mg/dl
Creatinine	0.6 to 1.2 mg/dl
Na$^+$	136 to 148 mmol/L
K$^+$	3.3 to 4.9 mmol/L

Cl^- 96 to 106 mmol/L
CO_2 (HCO_3^-)   24 to 30 mmol/L
Anion gap   8 to 20 mmol/L

Pertinent laboratory tests include a blood chemistry with particular attention to the complete blood count (CBC), electrolytes, serum creatinine, BUN, and arterial blood gases to establish baseline data. Chronic anemia is common, and it is not unusual to find hematocrits of 20% to 25%. In addition, it is common to find serum potassium levels elevated and serum sodium levels decreased. BUN and serum creatinine levels are markedly elevated in these patients. Patients with chronic renal failure demonstrate some degree of metabolic acidosis and decreased carbon dioxide (HCO_3^-) levels, since nonfunctioning kidneys can no longer produce new bicarbonate (Kelleher, 1992).

3. **Describe the symptoms of uremia that might be manifested by Mr. Morgan.**

   Uremia is a collection of signs and symptoms that are commonly manifested in the presence of markedly elevated BUN and creatinine levels. As described in the following, every body system is affected (Baer & Lancaster, 1992):

   - genitourinary system: decreased urine volume, increased serum urea nitrogen, and increased serum creatinine
   - cardiovascular system: volume overload, pulmonary edema, hypertension, pericarditis
   - neurologic system: encephalopathy, convulsions, altered mental states, memory loss, decreased muscle strength, psychosis
   - hematologic system: anemia, thrombocytopenia
   - gastrointestinal system: anorexia, nausea, vomiting, gastritis, ulcers, uremic fetor (urine breath), constipation
   - integumentary system: yellow, gray-tinged skin; dryness, itching
   - skeletal system: bone demineralization, osteodystrophy, metastatic calcification

4. **Describe how the relationship between calcium and phosphate is altered in chronic renal failure.**

   Normal Values

   Phosphate   2.7 to 4.5 mg/dl
   Calcium   8.4 to 10.2 mg/dl
   Calcium phosphate product   30 to 40 mg/dl

   Approximately 98% of the total body calcium is found within the bone, with the remaining 2% found in the plasma. It is the ionized plasma calcium level that controls the absorption of calcium from the gastrointestinal tract. Vitamin D must be metabolized by the kidney into its active form, 1,25-DHCC, to facilitate calcium absorption from the gastrointestinal tract. Plasma calcium and phosphate exist in a reciprocal relationship so that when phosphate decreases, the calcium level increases. The amount of phosphate excretion by the kidney is directly proportional to the level of phosphate in the plasma. Thus, if the serum phosphate level is elevated, the kidneys increase the excretion of phosphate to maintain the plasma level between 2.7 and 4.5 mg/dl. The parathyroid hormone plays a significant role in maintaining the calcium-phosphate balance. Whenever the serum calcium level decreases, parathormone is released by the parathyroid gland, which causes calcium to be released by the bone and phosphate to be excreted by the kidney. With irreversible damage to the kidney, the complex relationship between calcium and phosphate is severely altered. The kidney can no longer excrete the majority of phosphate necessary to maintain balance, and an elevated plasma phosphorus occurs. The reciprocal relationship results in a decrease in plasma calcium. The state of hypocalcemia is worsened because the kidney cannot metabolize the active form of vitamin D, which reduces calcium absorption from the gastrointestinal tract and impairs calcium mobilization from the bone. The parathyroid glands respond to the decreased plasma calcium levels and release parathormone to stimulate the resorption of calcium by the bone which in turn increases the plasma calcium level. With both the serum calcium and phosphate levels elevated, the calcium phosphate level is markedly elevated. If the calcium phosphate level exceeds 70 mg/dl, calcium phosphate crystals may precipitate in the brain, eyes, myocardium, lungs, and bone. The increased production of parathormone may lead to further bone demineralization (Makoff, 1991).

5. **Discuss the pathophysiology of aluminum toxicity in chronic renal failure.**

Most ESRD patients ingest aluminum through the use of aluminum-containing phosphate-binding antacids such as Basaljel and Amphojel to control serum phosphorus levels. The cation aluminum, normally excreted by the kidney, may accumulate in patients with chronic renal disease resulting in neuropathic, hematologic, and skeletal toxicity. Aluminum toxicity is manifested by convulsions and altered mental states. Aluminum toxicity can further aggravate anemia and bone demineralization. To avoid this complication, calcium salts may be substituted as phosphate binders. However, calcium salts are not as effective as aluminum-containing antacids and can result in hypercalcemia (Lowery, 1991).

6. **Discuss the pathophysiology of pericarditis in chronic renal failure. Why was Mr. Morgan particularly prone to this complication?**

Mr. Morgan had an accumulation of uremic toxins due to noncompliance with the medical regimen. Toxins inflame and irritate the visceral and parietal layers of the pericardium and "rub" instead of gliding smoothly across each other. This pericardial friction rub can be heard on auscultation by placing the stethoscope's diaphragm over the left midsternal to lower sternal border. Other symptoms include chest pain, usually relieved by leaning forward, a low-grade temperature elevation, and hypotension. The most life-threatening complication of pericarditis is cardiac tamponade (Smith, 1993).

7. **Discuss the different forms of dialysis used in the treatment of renal failure, including the indications and contraindications for each. Support the decision to use CAVHD in treating Mr. Morgan.**

There are two major forms of dialysis available for treatment in renal failure, peritoneal dialysis and hemodialysis (CAVHD). Both techniques use diffusion, osmosis, and filtration via a semipermeable membrane to remove excess metabolic waste and excess fluid and electrolytes. However, CAVHD uses an artificial membrane outside the body, whereas peritoneal dialysis uses the peritoneal membrane in the abdominal cavity. Peritoneal dialysis is a common choice in treating chronic renal failure or the chosen route if the patient in acute renal failure cannot tolerate hemodialysis. However, CAVHD is gaining support as the method of choice for treating uncomplicated chronic renal failure (Bosworth, 1992).

8. **Identify pharmacologic agents used in the treatment of chronic renal failure and the rationale for their use.**

The use of aluminum-containing phosphate-binding antacids such as Basaljel and Amphojel to control serum phosphorus levels must be carefully monitored in patients with chronic renal failure to guard against aluminum toxicity. Chronic anemia is common, and it is not unusual to find hematocrits of 20% to 25%. Preparations that contain folic acid such as Iberet-Folate are the drugs of choice in treating anemia associated with chronic renal failure. Calcium replacement through oral preparations such as Os-Cal are also used (Holechek, 1991).

9. **Discuss the dietary management of the patient with chronic renal failure.**

The role of protein in the development of the uremic syndrome has been widely debated. It is generally accepted that a diet containing only

20 g of "high biologic value" is most successful in treating patients with chronic renal failure. This diet (Giordano-Giovannetti diet) is difficult for most patients to comply with because it is unpalatable and monotonous. Usually patients can tolerate the diet for only a few months and then they progress to 60 g of protein. An adequately hydrated individual can comfortably excrete 1500 to 2000 ml of urine per day. The patient should be instructed to consume fluids to maintain urine output at this volume. Sodium intake should be adjusted until the patient's sodium level is in balance and the patient is adequately hydrated and without edema. Peripheral edema, hypertension, and congestive heart failure are potential complications that must be monitored. Sodium is usually restricted to 2 g along with 2 g of potassium ("Morbidity and Mortality," 1993).

10. **Identify clinical complications arising from noncompliance that were manifested by Mr. Morgan.**

Mr. Morgan had an accumulation of uremic toxins due to noncompliance with his medical regimen. Mr. Morgan experienced nausea and vomiting, agitation, and confusion. In addition, he had chest pain, described as moderate to severe in intensity and diffusely located over the precordium. Pulmonary overload was revealed through neck vein distension, crackles scattered bilaterally throughout the lung bases, and pitting peripheral edema bilaterally in the lower extremities. He had a weight gain of 8 kg (18 lb). Cardiac monitoring demonstrated sinus tachycardia with a rate of 116 bpm. A pericardial friction rub and an S_3 gallop were auscultated. These symptoms are consistent with pericarditis. Laboratory values revealed metabolic acidosis, hyperkalemia, hyponatremia, hyperphosphatemia, hypocalcemia, and anemia.

11. **List nursing diagnoses appropriate for care of the patient with chronic renal failure.**

> ➤ fluid volume excess related to noncompliance with prescribed medical regimen
> ➤ noncompliance with medical regimen related to limitations of disease
> ➤ alteration in self-image related to skin changes and changes in lifestyle
> ➤ impaired gas exchange related to pulmonary edema
> ➤ alteration in nutrition: less than body requirements related to nausea and vomiting
> ➤ high risk for infection related to impaired defense barriers

12. **List nursing diagnoses appropriate for the care of the patient with a permanent AV fistula for dialysis access.**

➤ high risk for infection related to impaired defense barriers
➤ alteration in self-image related to skin changes (Galpin, 1992)
➤ high risk for alteration in cardiac output related to uremic pericarditis and patency of the access

13. List the components of the teaching plan for the patient with chronic renal failure.

- compliance with components of medical regimen such as dialysis schedule and diet and fluid restriction
- prevention of infection
- regular exercise
- maintenance of dialysis access: should be taught how to check for patency of the access and signs and symptoms of infection
- prevention of complications
(Gorrie, 1992)

14. List the criteria used in the selection of patients for kidney transplantation.

Renal transplantation is considered a viable alternative for treatment of ESRD when the individual does not have other medical problems that could increase the risks associated with the procedure. The usual age range for candidates of renal transplantation is 4 to 60 years. In patients older than 60 years, as with Mr. Morgan, the risk of complications increases, and older persons are considered carefully on an individual basis. A thorough body systems assessment is performed before the person is considered for transplantation (Ignatavicius & Bayne, 1991).

The number of patients awaiting organ transplantation has increased dramatically in the last 5 years because of the advances made in transplantation procedures. Currently, 18,000 individuals are awaiting vital organs for transplantation in the United States (United Network for Organ Sharing [UNOS] Update, 1989). All potential organ recipients are entered into the national computer system through the United Network for Organ Sharing (UNOS). A point system has been instituted to allow equitable distribution of this scarce resource. Blood type compatibility between donor and recipient is mandatory.

Five criteria have been established for potential kidney recipients. First, priority is given to the potential recipient with the best antigen match. Second, consideration is given to how long the individual has been waiting compared to other potential recipients in the same locale. Priority is also given to potential recipients who have preformed antibodies to major histocompatibility complex (MHC) antigens because the presence of these antibodies can limit the number of kidneys for which the potential recipient would be eligible. Priority is also given to potential recipients who are medical emergencies. The most common circumstance that qualifies a renal patient as an emergency for transplantation is the inability to maintain AV access for hemodialysis. The final criterion has to do with logistic factors based on the ease and rapidity with which the transplantation can be performed (Clochesy, Breu, Cardin, Rudy, & Whittaker, 1993).

Organs from living related donors provide the highest rates of renal graft survival. General physical criteria for donors include the absence of systemic disease and infection, no history of cancer, absence of hypertension and renal disease, and adequate renal function as evidenced by diagnostic studies. In addition, living-related donors must express a clear understanding of the associated surgery and a willingness to give up a kidney. Some transplant centers also require a psychiatric evaluation to determine the motivation of the donor.

15. Discuss CAVHD and renal transplantation as alternative treatment modalities for Mr. Morgan. Support Mr. Morgan's decision to select renal transplantation as opposed to CAVHD.

CAVHD and renal transplantations are alternative treatment modalities for Mr. Morgan. It is up to the individual to determine which type of therapy is best suited to his/her physical condition and lifestyle. Mr. Morgan has no active malignancy or infectious process. He has a strong support system, with siblings willing to donate a living donor kidney. He is financially secure through income and health insurance coverage. Although Mr. Morgan has had difficulty with complying with the medical regimen of CAVHD because of transportation and distance to the health care facility, he is willing to comply with the medical regimen following transplantation, since these problems will be eliminated.

Conservative medical management of ESRD with dialysis is costly. Although transplantation procedures are expensive, the current success rates have made transplantation a cost-effective treatment option when compared with traditional medical management. For example, a patient undergoing CAVHD costs the federal government, through Medicare, about $40,000 per year. The cost of a kidney transplant is approximately $40,000 for the first year and $5000 yearly for follow-up care. If the transplant functions for 5 years, the cost is $60,000 as opposed to $200,000 for 5 years of CAVHD (Clochesy et al., 1993). Since Mr. Morgan was employed on a full-time basis before beginning dialysis and plans to return to work after the transplantation, other financial considerations are the potential earning power and the discontinuation of any disability benefits previously required.

One of the major obstacles to a successful renal transplant is finding a suitable donor. Blood relatives make the most compatible donors and result in an approximate 90% success rate for the patient (Clochesy et al., 1993). Mr. Morgan had three brothers and three sisters consenting to be a donor if a transplant match was possible. The probability for finding a suitable donor and achieving a successful transplant were favorable. It is imperative that Mr. Morgan receive a living donor kidney because the more similar the tissue antigens of the donor are to those of the recipient, the more likely it is that the transplant will be successful and immunologic rejection will be avoided.

Renal transplantation could also eliminate the lifestyle restrictions for the patient. Mr. Morgan was required to report to a community-based hemodialysis clinic 75 miles from his home three times each week. Approximately 24 hours each week were required for travel and treatment time. By choosing renal transplantation, Mr. Morgan hoped to alleviate the inconvenience and discomfort of the frequent dialysis therapies.

16. **List the advantages and disadvantages of a living donor vs. a cadaver donor. Why was it imperative that Mr. Morgan receive a living donor kidney?**

Cadaver organ donors are previously healthy individuals who have suffered irreversible brain injury of a known cause. The most common causes of injury are cerebral trauma from motor vehicle accidents or gunshot wounds, intracerebral or subarachnoid hemorrhage, primary brain tumor, and anoxic brain damage resulting from drug overdose or cardiac arrest. The brain-dead donor must have effective cardiovascular function and must be supported on a ventilator to preserve organ viability. The donor must be free of extracranial malignancies, sepsis, and communicable diseases including hepatitis, syphilis, tuberculosis, and human immunodeficiency virus (HIV) (Clochesy et al., 1993). The age range of most suitable donors is newborn to 65 years. Age is generally less important than the quality of organ functions (Clochesy et al., 1993).

Cadaver Donor Kidney

a. Advantages
   (1) Success rate of transplantation has improved to 85% to 90%.
   (2) Cadaver kidneys can maintain viability for as long as 72 hours after removal from the donor.
   (3) Average cost of transplant is $40,000 (same as living donor transplant).
b. Disadvantages
   (1) Potential organ recipient is placed on a national registry (UNOS) to allow equitable distribution of scarce organ supply.
   (2) Organ recipient may die while waiting for a kidney because of limited supply and great demand.
   (3) Few kidneys are available for transplantation, and surgery must be done as kidneys become available.
   (4) Recipients' physical and psychological health may not be optimal.

Living Related Donor Kidney

a. Advantages

    (1) Recipient is not placed on the national registry to wait for a kidney.

    (2) A living related donor provides the highest rate of renal graft survival (90%).

    (3) Average cost is $40,000, and it is more cost effective over the long term than CAVHD is.

    (4) Current research favors donor-specific blood transfusion, in which blood from the kidney donor is transfused into the recipient. This has improved graft survival, especially of organs from living donors.

    (5) Surgery can be scheduled electively to optimize patient's state of health. The organ suffers less ischemia, since it is not transported.

b. Disadvantages

    (1) Kidney removal from a living donor requires greater surgical care and is a delicate procedure lasting 3 to 4 hours.

    (2) Donors experience more pain than recipients.

    (3) Small risk of complications or death to donor.

    (4) Donor must have annual physical examinations for life to assess the function of the remaining kidney.

    (5) There is a psychological impact to both the donor and recipient.

It was imperative that Mr. Morgan receive a living donor kidney because the success rate at age 67 years is greater; the transplantation can be scheduled electively so that the state of his health can be optimal at the time of surgery; and the ischemic time will be lessened because the need for transport time is eliminated.

17. Describe the cadaver kidney preservation process.

The cadaver donor nephrectomy is conducted as a sterile autopsy in the operating room. All arterial and venous vessels are carefully preserved (Ignatavicius & Bayne, 1991). The aorta and vena cava are cannulated from below and ligated above the renal arteries and veins. The cadaver kidneys are flushed with a cold Ringer's lactate solution containing heparin 10,000 U/L. Once the transplantable kidney has been surgically removed, it is preserved in a sterile, iced electrolyte solution and transported to a transplant center. Kidneys can maintain viability for as long as 72 hours before they must be transplanted (Clochesy et al., 1993).

Preservation by Perfusion

The kidneys are perfused with a cold (6° to 10° C) solution at low flow, low pressure to provide the kidney with nutrients and oxygen and to remove products of metabolism. The kidneys can be preserved in this process for up to 72 hours (Southard & Belzer, 1988).

Preservation by Cold Storage

A high-potassium, low-sodium solution that resembles the electrolyte balance inside kidney cells is used to flush the kidney, and then the kidneys are stored in this solution in sterile plastic bags at temperatures of 6° C or less. The kidneys can be preserved in this process for up to 30 hours (Collins, 1988).

18. Briefly describe the surgical process of renal transplantation.

After induction of anesthesia, the genitalia and abdominal skin are prepped, and a Foley catheter is placed in the urinary bladder. The bladder is rinsed with a broad-spectrum antibiotic solution and gravity filled to capacity, and the catheter is clamped until the urinary tract reconstruction portion of the operation begins. Usually, the kidney graft is placed extraperitoneally in the contralateral iliac fossa through a Gibson incision on the same side from which it was removed from the donor. The renal artery is attached to the hypogastric or internal iliac artery, and the renal vein is anastomosed to the external iliac vein. Mannitol, 0.5 to 1 g/kg, is infused during and immediately after renal revascularization to act as an osmotic diuretic. The urinary tract reconstruction is by tranvesical or extravesical ureteroneocystostomy. The recipient's own nonfunctioning kidney is usually not removed unless it is infected, greatly enlarged, or causing medically uncontrollable hypertension (Clochesy et al., 1993).

19. Discuss possible postoperative complications.

Numerous potential complications are associated with renal transplantation. Vascular complications nearly always require surgical intervention. Stenosis of the renal artery may occur, which is evident by the presence of hypertension, auscultation of a bruit over the artery anastomosis site, and decreased renal function. To correct stenosis of the renal artery the involved artery must be surgically resected and the kidney anastomosed to another artery. Other vascular problems include vascular leakage and thrombosis, both of which require an emergency nephrectomy.

Wound complications include hematomas, abscesses, and lymphoceles. Genitourinary tract complications such as ureteral leakage, ureteral fistulas, ureteral obstruction, calculus formation, bladder neck contractures, scrotal swelling, and graft rupture may also necessitate surgical intervention (Ignatavicius & Bayne, 1991). The most common and most life-threatening complication of renal transplantation is rejection. In tissue rejection, a reaction occurs between the antigens in the transplanted kidney and the antibodies and cytotoxic T cells in the recipient's blood. These immunologic substances treat the transplanted kidney as a foreign invader and cause tissue destruction, thrombosis, and eventual necrosis of the tissue (Ignatavicius & Bayne, 1991).

20. **List the nursing diagnoses appropriate to the care of the renal transplantation patient during the recovery period.**

   ➤ altered tissue perfusion: renal
   ➤ impaired skin integrity
   ➤ altered urinary elimination: retention/diuresis
   ➤ altered comfort: pain
   ➤ high risk for infection related to immunosuppression
   ➤ high risk for fluid volume excess related to renal failure
   ➤ high risk for fluid volume deficit related to diuresis
   ➤ alteration in nutrition: less than body requirements related to nausea and vomiting and postoperative pain
   ➤ noncompliance with medical regimen related to limitations of disease
   ➤ alteration in self-image related to changes in lifestyle
   ➤ knowledge deficit related to self-care activities

21. **Discuss the pathophysiology of acute rejection. Describe the clinical manifestations of acute rejection in Mr. Morgan.**

   The types of rejection are hyperacute, acute, and chronic. Hyperacute rejection occurs within 48 hours after transplant surgery. There is no treatment of this type of rejection, and after recognition of the problem, the rejected kidney is removed quickly to prevent further complications. Clinical manifestations include elevated temperature, elevated blood pressure, and pain at the transplant site (Ignatavicius & Bayne, 1991). Acute rejection usually occurs between 7 and 14 days after surgery but may occur up to 2 years after transplantation. The most common manifestations of acute rejection include oliguria or anuria, temperature greater than 37.8° C (100° F), enlarged and tender kidney, fluid retention, increased blood pressure, chronic fatigue, and changes in urinalysis and blood chemistry laboratory values. Acute rejection can be halted with early recognition and immediate administration of increased dosages of immunosuppressive drugs (Ignatavicius & Bayne, 1991).

   Chronic rejection occurs gradually during a period of months to years. The clinical manifestations include gradually decreasing BUN levels and changes in serum electrolyte levels. There is no treatment of chronic rejection, and the patient is conservatively managed until renal function deteriorates and dialysis is required (Ignatavicius & Bayne, 1991).

   On the eighth postoperative day, Mr. Morgan began to demonstrate signs and symptoms of acute rejection. He complained of not feeling well, minimal abdominal tenderness on palpation, and nausea. His temperature fluctuated between 38.4° and 38.8° C (101.2° and 101.8° F). Urinary output dropped to an average of 55 ml/h and did not improve with furosemide (Lasix) boluses. On the 11th postoperative day laboratory data revealed that his CVP was slightly elevated to 10.5 mm Hg and his weight was up to 82 kg (182 lb). His creatinine level was 7.1 mg/dl, and BUN was 120 mg/dl.

22. **Discuss the immunosuppressive pharmacologic agents methylprednisolone, muromonab-CD3 (Orthoclone OKT3), and cyclosporine. Why did the physician add muromonab-CD3 and wait several days to begin cyclosporine?**

Methylprednisolone (Solu-Medrol)

Methylprednisolone, a corticosteroid, acts as an antiinflammatory agent to prevent the movement of leukocytes into tissue during resection. In addition, methylprednisolone limits antibody production and blocks the antigen-antibody complex formation. Numerous side effects of corticosteroids include infections, gastrointestinal tract bleeding, ulcers, pancreatitis, delayed wound healing, diabetes mellitus, psychosis, cataracts, fluid and electrolyte imbalances, and hypertension (*Physicians Desk Reference*, 1994).

Muromonab-CD3 (Orthoclone OKT3)

Muromonab-CD3 is a monoclonal anti-T-cell antibody that reacts with and blocks the function of all T cells, thereby reversing acute renal allograft rejection. The usual dosage of muromonab-CD3 is 5 mg/d. The drug is administered by intravenous bolus only. Muromonab-CD3 may not be given with any other drug. Side effects include respiratory complications, such as acute pulmonary edema. This drug requires meticulous nursing assessment because it is given intravenously and reactions frequently occur with the first administration. Clinical manifestations of a reaction include fever, chills, dyspnea, and chest pain (*Physicians Desk Reference*, 1994).

Cyclosporine: Cyclosporine is a newer drug used to prevent and treat rejection of renal transplants. Cyclosporine works by interfering with T cell growth and can be given orally or intravenously. If administered orally the drug may be diluted in various liquids but should be taken 1 to 2 hours after meals at the same time each day to maintain a consistent absorption rate and thereby maintain a consistent blood level. The usual dosage of cyclosporine is 6 mg/kg in divided doses every 12 hours. Cyclosporine increases the risk of renal failure and hepatotoxicity.

Nursing responsibilities require observing for nephrotoxicity, hepatotoxicity, and potential malignancy, especially lymphoma. The nurse should monitor blood levels of the drug to ensure they are therapeutic but not toxic. Therapeutic trough levels range between 250 and 350 mg/ml. Six to eight weeks after renal transplantation the dosage is usually decreased to 4 to 5 mg/kg. (*Physicians Desk Reference,* 1994).

Muromonab-CD3 was added to Mr. Morgan's medical regimen on the 11th postoperative day when Mr. Morgan's laboratory values indicated worsening signs of acute rejection. Muromonab-CD3 drug therapy was added to block cytotoxic human T cells and the generation of other T cell functions. The symptoms of renal allograft rejection, such as the ones noted in Mr. Morgan's condition, are subtle and difficult to differentiate from similar symptoms of drug-induced nephrotoxicity. Cyclosporine was not administered immediately to Mr. Morgan because of the impaired renal function. After several days of CAVHD to support renal function Mr. Morgan's creatinine level had dropped to 1.9 mg/dl, and cyclosporine was added to the regimen. Cyclosporine may be added to the medical regimen of acute rejection when the creatinine level is 2.5 mg/dl or less.

23. List the components of the teaching plan for Mr. Morgan.

The individual receiving renal transplantation requires extensive health care teaching. The teaching plan will include information about medication regimens, including dosage, side effects, symptoms of toxicity, and the monitoring of blood levels. The plan should also include clinical manifestations of rejection and symptoms of infection. Education regarding changes in diet and activity level is essential to ensure compliance. Symptoms of vascular complications and self-monitoring of weight, urine output, blood pressure, and edema are an important part of the plan. Finally the individual should be made aware of the existence of support groups and how to network with these groups.

Chronic Renal Failure
and Renal Transplantation

Alspach, J. G. (1991). *Core curriculum for critical care nursing.* Philadelphia: Saunders.

Baer, G., & Lancaster, L. (1992). Acute renal failure. *Critical Care Nursing, 14*(4), 1–21.

Besnier, D., & Testa, A. (1993, June–July). Chronic renal failure. *Solutions Chronicle, 148–149,* 10–13.

Bosworth, C. (1992). SCUF/CAVH/CAVHD: Critical differences. *Critical Care Nursing, 14*(4), 45–55.

Clochesy, J., Breu, C., Cardin, S., Rudy, E., & Whittaker, A. (1993). *Critical care nursing.* Philadelphia: Saunders.

Collins, G. (1988). Kidney preservation by cold storage. In G. J. Cerilli (Ed.), *Organ transplantation and replacement* (pp. 296–311). Philadelphia: J. B. Lippincott.

Galpin, C. (1992). Body image in end-stage renal disease. *Image Journal of Nursing Scholarship, 1*(1), 88–94.

Gorrie, S. (1992). Patient education: A committee. *ANNA Journal, 19*(5), 504 & 506.

Holechek, M. J. (1991). Medication review: An alternative phosphate binder—calcium acetate. *ANNA Journal, 18*(3), 321–322.

Ignatavicius, D., & Bayne, M. (1991). *Medical-surgical nursing,* Philadelphia: Saunders.

Kelleher, R. (1992). Dialysis in the surgical intensive care patient: A case study. *Critical Care Nursing, 14*(4), 72–77.

Lowery, S. (1991). Case management of the anemic patient epoetin alfa: Focus on aluminum management. *ANNA Journal, 18*(1), 56–57.

Makoff, R. (1991). The value of calcium carbonate in treating acidosis, phosphate retention, and hypocalcemia. *Nephrology News Issues, 5*(7), 16, 18–29, & 32.

Morbidity and Mortality of Dialysis. (1993). *National Institutes of Health Consensus, 11*(12), 1–33.

Physicians desk reference. (1994). Oradell, NJ: Medical Economics Data.

Smith, S. H. (1993). Uremic pericarditis in chronic renal failure: Nursing implications. *ANNA Journal, 20*(4), 432–438 & 508.

Southard, J. H., & Belzer, F. O. (1988). Kidney preservation by perfusion. In G. J. Cerilli (Ed.) *Organ transplantation and replacement.* (pp. 312–321). Philadelphia: J. B. Lippincott.

United Network for Organ Sharing (UNOS) Update. (1989). *UNOS releases 1988 transplantation statistics* (Vol. 5, p. 1). Richmond, VA: United Network for Sharing.

13

Subarachnoid Hemorrhage with Aneurysm

Cinda Alexander, MSN, CCRN, CNRN

CASE PRESENTATION

Connie, a 42-year-old white woman, presented to the emergency department with complaints of severe left temporal headaches after collapsing at work. Initially, while at work, Connie was confused and incontinent of urine. After arrival in the emergency department Connie was cooperative, her pupils were equal and reactive, and she was mildly disoriented. She stated that the headaches were "unlike any" she had experienced before. According to Connie's husband, Connie had experienced these headaches for about 3 to 4 weeks. Additional symptoms included nausea, photophobia, and a mildly stiff neck. A computed tomographic (CT) scan of the head without contrast revealed a subarachnoid hemorrhage in the area of the internal carotid artery. Her serum Na^+ is 130 mmol/L, K^+ is 3.6 mmol/L, and Cl^- is 106 mmol/L.

Initial assessment data after admission to the emergency department were

BP	152/78
HR	102 bpm
Respirations	22/min
Temperature	37.2° C (99° F)
SaO_2	92% on room air

Neurologic signs were

- Lethargic, arouses to name
- Pupils equal and reactive
- Follows commands, moves all extremities equally
- Oriented to person only
- Glasgow Coma Scale 14

After admission and evaluation in the emergency department, Connie was stabilized and transferred to the critical care unit (CCU). She was scheduled for an arteriogram the next day. Treatment with aminocaproic acid (Amicar) and nimodipine (Nimotop) was begun. Connie continued to complain of a generalized headache and neck stiffness. Assessment data were

BP	142/80
HR	84 bpm
Respirations	24/min
Temperature	37.2° C (99° F)
SaO$_2$	98% on room air

Neurologic signs were

- Pupils equal and reactive
- Follows commands, moves all extremities equally, grasp equal
- Oriented to person and place
- Lethargic, arouses to name
- Glasgow Coma Scale 13

Connie was stable throughout the night. Her arteriogram study the next morning revealed a left vertebral posterior inferior cerebellar aneurysm. Connie and her family were present when the physician discussed the results of the arteriogram. Her treatment options were explored, and specific questions from the family were answered. Connie's neurologic status remained stable, and the decision to proceed with "early surgery" was made.

Surgery

At 10 AM the following morning, Connie underwent a craniotomy for a clip ligation of the left inferior cerebellar aneurysm.

Postoperative Course

Immediately after surgery Connie's vital signs were stable. She recovered from the general anesthesia, responded to her name, and moved all extremities to command during the initial hour of recovery in the intensive care unit (ICU). Connie continued to show general recovery and recognized her family during the following hours. Several hours after surgery she developed a sudden headache, confusion, and gross weakness in her left hand. Her vital signs were

BP	162/94
HR	110 bpm
Respirations	32/min
Temperature	38.3° C (101° F)

Neurologic signs were

- Pupils equal and reactive
- Follows command all extremities, left grasp weak
- Disoriented, speech inappropriate
- Glasgow Coma Scale 11

A stat CT scan of the head demonstrated postoperative changes associated with the surgery, aneurysm clip artifact, minimal air, and no obvious collection of blood. With no obvious postoperative hematoma, a decision was made to repeat the arteriogram, which demonstrated apparent narrowing of the arteries. It was concluded that Connie was experiencing a vasospasm. Her Na^+ level was 145 mmol/L, K^+ was 3.9 mmol/L, and Cl^- was 109 mmol/L.

After an arterial line and pulmonary artery (Swan-Ganz) catheter insertion, hypervolemic/hyperfusion therapy was initiated and continued over the next 5 days. Connie's neurologic status stabilized and improved with this therapy. Connie was slowly weaned from this therapy, and her neurologic status remained stable for an additional 48 hours. Connie was then transferred to a neurosurgical step–down unit. Neurologically, she was alert and oriented, although easily confused if given multiple instructions. She moved all extremities to command; however, she has continued to demonstrate a mild weakness in her left hand and arm. She was discharged 8 days later to a rehabilitation unit with an anticipated discharge home after rehabilitation therapy.

QUESTIONS

Subarachnoid Hemorrhage With Aneurysm

1. What is the clinical presentation of a subarachnoid hemorrhage?

2. Describe the incidence, mortality, and morbidity associated with acute subarachnoid hemorrhage.

3. How is a subarachnoid hemorrhage diagnosed?

4. Describe the pathophysiology involved and consequences of blood in the subarachnoid space.

5. Give the rationale for Connie's hyponatremia.

6. How is a subarachnoid hemorrhage classified?

7. What therapeutic modalities should be anticipated for this patient following surgery? Give the rationale for each.

8. What parameters require close monitoring for this patient?

9. What are the general complications associated with aminocaproic acid (Amicar) and nimodipine?

10. What are the general "aneurysm precautions" observed for subarachnoid patients who potentially have a cerebral aneurysm?

11. Describe the pathophysiology associated with cerebral aneurysm.

12. Define the different types of aneurysms.

13. What are the secondary injuries associated with a ruptured aneurysm and subsequent subarachnoid hemorrhage?

14. What are the advantages and disadvantages of early vs. late surgical intervention?

15. What nursing care is of particular importance after a craniotomy?

16. Describe the pathophysiology and incidence of rebleeding. When is rebleeding likely to occur?

17. What clinical changes should be anticipated if a patient is experiencing rebleeding?

18. How is rebleeding diagnosed?

19. What is the treatment for rebleeding? What is the duration of treatment?

20. Describe the pathophysiology and incidence of vasospasm? When is vasospasm likely to occur?

21. What causes vasospasm?

22. How is cerebral vasospasm diagnosed? What clinical symptoms should be anticipated?

23. What is the mortality and morbidity of vasospasm and rebleeding?

24. What is the treatment for vasospasm? What additional approaches to the treatment of vasospasm are discussed in the literature?

25. How long is the treatment of vasospasm continued?

26. How long will Connie remain "at risk" for vasospasm or rebleeding?

QUESTIONS AND ANSWERS

Subarachnoid Hemorrhage With Aneurysm

1. **What is the clinical presentation of a subarachnoid hemorrhage?**

   Patients often report feeling sudden, severe, violent headaches, unlike any experienced before. Immediate loss of consciousness, nausea, vomiting, cranial nerve palsies, and focal neurologic deficits such as weakness of an extremity may also be present. Blood in the subarachnoid space produces signs and symptoms of meningeal irritation such as nuchal rigidity or stiff neck, photophobia, blurred vision, nausea and vomiting, headache, and fever. With the initial seepage of blood into the subarachnoid space, there may be a sudden onset of deep coma. In as many as 40% of subarachnoid hemorrhage cases there are prodromal signs or warning symptoms, such as headache, that can indicate that a small leakage of blood has occurred. However, these early symptoms are often ignored or attributed to other causes (Cook, 1991; Hickey, 1992; Nikas, 1991).

2. **Describe the incidence, mortality, and morbidity associated with acute subarachnoid hemorrhage.**

   Subarachnoid hemorrhage occurs in 25,000 to 30,000 North Americans annually; of these, 50% die. One third of these deaths occur before the individual enters the health care system. An additional 30% suffer permanent neurologic damage and disability. The average age of occurrence is 50 years with patients ranging anywhere from 35 to 60 years (Cook, 1991; Hickey, 1992; Manifold, 1990).

3. **How is a subarachnoid hemorrhage diagnosed?**

   Diagnosis is based on history, clinical presentation, and a number of diagnostic procedures. Lumbar puncture may be used to confirm blood in the cerebrospinal fluid (CSF), which circulates in the subarachnoid space. The spinal fluid is bloody grossly and xanthochromic (a yellow discoloration of the CSF) after centrifuge. Lumbar puncture is avoided if there is suspicion of intracranial hypertension because of the risk of brain herniation (Cook, 1991; Romeo, 1993). CT scan within 48 hours of the bleeding episode can demonstrate the blood in the subarachnoid space in 75% to 85% of all patients (Cook, 1991). Magnetic resonance imaging (MRI) may be used to identify the subarachnoid blood and inner structures of the brain. A four vessel cerebral angiography is the mainstay of diagnosis and usually is able to provide a definitive diagnosis of aneurysm or arteriovenous malformation. Cerebral angiography visualizes both intracranial and extracranial vessels. Contrast medium is injected, and a series of radiographic films are recorded (Hickey, 1992; Manifold, 1990; Mason, 1992).

4. Describe the pathophysiology involved and consequences of blood in the subarachnoid space.

Subarachnoid hemorrhage is defined as arterial blood that has extravasated into the subarachnoid space, which normally contains CSF. Subarachnoid hemorrhage as a result of a ruptured aneurysm usually occurs around the circle of Willis at a point of bifurcation of the arterial vessels (Cook, 1991). The amount of blood may range from small amounts of bleeding to large amounts that extend beyond the site of leakage, flooding into cisterns and the ventricular system. Blood is an irritant to brain tissues that initiates an inflammatory response and cerebral edema. Subarachnoid hemorrhage patients are often hypertensive after the initial bleeding probably due to the release of catecholamines into the circulatory vasculature. This hypertension maintains or improves the cerebral perfusion pressure. Fibrin, platelets, and fluid around the point of arterial rupture, usually an aneurysm, seal off the tear (Hickey, 1992). Following a subarachnoid hemorrhage, neurologic injury occurs immediately as a result of blood seeping into adjacent tissues or may be delayed as a result of a secondary event such as rebleeding or vasospasm. Estimates are that 45% of those individuals that survive the initial bleeding will present with transient loss of consciousness. This probably is due to either intracranial hypertension and increased intracranial pressure or transient cardiac arrhythmias as a result of blood around the brain stem (Kirsch, Diringer, Borel, & Hanley, 1989).

5. Give the rationale for Connie's hyponatremia.

According to Segatore (1993) hyponatremia is the most common electrolyte imbalance associated with subarachnoid hemorrhage patients. Hyponatremia is associated with a high incidence of brain ischemia and infarction. The pathogenesis of hyponatremia following subarachnoid hemorrhage remains unclear and is probably due to cerebral salt wasting or the syndrome of inappropriate antidiuretic hormone (Segatore, 1993).

6. How is a subarachnoid hemorrhage classified?

The Hunt and Hess classification system is most commonly used to "grade" the severity of a subarachnoid bleeding episode in terms of clinical presentation and significance. The grades range from grade I (asymptomatic or minimal headache) to grade V (deep coma, extension abnormal, and moribund appearance). Surgical timing may be judged by the presenting grade and clinical progression. The higher grades are associated with a much higher mortality and morbidity (Hickey, 1992; Manifold, 1990).

7. What therapeutic modalities should be anticipated for this patient following surgery? Give the rationale for each.

After stabilization and control of systemic blood pressure, bed rest and aneurysm precautions are instituted. Elastic stockings or antithrombic pumps may be used to counter the effects of bed rest and hemostasis. Normal hydration is supplemented with intravenous therapy. Drug therapy includes the following (Cook, 1991; Hickey, 1992; Kirsch et al., 1989; Sikes & Nolan, 1993):

- *anticonvulsants:* prophylactically to prevent seizures since blood in the subarachnoid space is an irritant to the surrounding tissues
- *steroids:* controversial but may be used if there are signs of increased intracranial pressure, focal neurologic deficits, or cerebral edema
- *calcium channel blocker:* used prophylactically to reduce or minimize the threat of vasospasm
- *antifibrinolytic therapy:* controversial, used to prevent clot lysis at the point of rupture—Agents such as aminocaproic acid or tranexamic acid reduce the risk of rebleeding during the first 2 weeks after rupture. The clot reinforces the wall of the aneurysm. If this therapy is used, it is initiated immediately upon diagnosis of a subarachnoid hemorrhage.
- *analgesics:* to control headache and pain associated with meningeal irritation
- *mild sedative:* possibly used if the patient is agitated and at risk for increasing intracranial pressure due to combativeness
- *stool softener:* to prevent straining at bowel movements and initiation of Valsalva's maneuver, which may trigger increased intracranial pressure

8. **What parameters require close monitoring for this patient?**

Serial evaluation of neurologic signs and vital signs are assessed for signs of complications such as hydrocephalus, increased intracranial pressure, rebleeding, or vasospasm. The nurse also monitors for complications associated with prolonged bed rest. Detailed clinical assessment is paramount in the care of this patient to detect any early changes in neurologic status that may indicate secondary complications.

9. **What are the general complications associated with aminocaproic acid (Amicar) and nimodipine?**

Aminocaproic acid (Amicar) has been associated with an increase in hydrocephalus and vasospasm. Calcium channel blockers are associated with hypotension, which can induce cerebral ischemia in the subarachnoid hemorrhage patient. Calcium antagonists significantly limit the effectiveness of vasopressor drugs used to maintain systemic blood pressure (Kirsch et al., 1989).

10. **What are the general "aneurysm precautions" observed for subarachnoid patients who potentially have a cerebral aneurysm?**

Aneurysm precautions include the following: (Hickey, 1992):

- Place in a quiet room.
- Control the room light to prevent strong, direct light.
- Reading and watching TV may be allowed if these activities do not overstimulate the patient.
- Maintain good oxygen and carbon dioxide exchange; supplemental oxygen is usually ordered.
- Maintain head of bed elevation, generally 20 to 30 degrees to augment cerebral venous drainage.
- Restrict fluid (approximately 1500 to 2000 ml/24 h).
- Maintain bed rest, possibly with bathroom privileges (avoid straining for bowel movements).
- Restrict visitors and discuss with visitors the importance of a calming, supportive environment.
- Nursing care and diagnostic tests should be scheduled to avoid overstimulating the patient.

11. **Describe the pathophysiology associated with cerebral aneurysm.**

Cerebral aneurysms are saccular outpouchings of the walls of a cerebral artery. The cause of a cerebral aneurysm is unclear. However, at least two theories have been identified in the literature. The congenital theory suggests that a congenital weakness exists in the wall of the artery's medial layer allowing an outpouching. The degenerative theory suggests that a local weakness develops in the intima due to hemodynamically induced degenerative changes. In midlife the vessel develops an outpouching of the intimal layer due to hemodynamic stress on the weakened area (usually due to arteriosclerosis). Aneurysms often occur in the area of the circle of Willis at a point of bifurcation or a junction of the arteries. Rupture often occurs in association with physical activities or strain (Cook, 1991; Hickey, 1992).

12. Define the different types of aneurysms.

Classification by shape (Hickey, 1992):

- *berry:* most common, berry shaped with a neck or stem
- *saccular:* saccular outpouching
- *fusiform:* outpouching without a neck or stem
- *traumatic:* associated with head trauma
- *mycotic:* caused by septic emboli
- *Charcot-Bouchard:* microscopic, associated with hypertension and often located in the brain stem and basal ganglia
- *Dissecting:* associated with atherosclerosis; blood forced between the intimal layer and medial layer

13. What are the secondary injuries associated with a ruptured aneurysm and subsequent subarachnoid hemorrhage?

Rebleeding

An aneurysm releases additional blood into the subarachnoid space. With each rupture episode, patient mortality increases dramatically. Rarely do patients survive the third episode of a rupture and rebleeding.

Hydrocephalus and Increased Intracranial Pressure

Subarachnoid hemorrhage and subsequent clot(s) in the subarachnoid space may interfere with the flow and reabsorption of CSF via the arachnoid villi. Large clots may mechanically interfere with the flow of blood through the ventricular system, resulting in hydrocephalus and increased intracranial pressure (Hickey, 1992; Kirsch et al., 1989).

Seizures

Seizures following a subarachnoid hemorrhage are more common in younger adults with a ruptured aneurysm and may occur in 10% to 26% of patients. Seizures are often followed by rebleeding probably due to the increased cerebral blood flow and perfusion pressure. Prophylactic anticonvulsant therapy is generally advocated, and often Dilantin (phenytoin) is the drug of choice (Cook, 1991; Kirsch et al., 1989).

Vasospasm

Vasospasm could be defined as a narrowing of the vessels in the area of the subarachnoid hemorrhage. Vasospasm can lead to cerebral ischemia and a cerebral infarct (Kirsch et al., 1989).

Hypothalamic Dysfunction

Hypothalamic dysfunction may be exhibited as hyponatremia due to a "salt-wasting" mechanism and electrocardiogram (ECG) changes as a result of an overstimulated sympathetic system (Cook, 1991; Segatore, 1993).

14. What are the advantages and disadvantages of early vs. late surgical intervention?

Traditionally, surgical repair of the aneurysm is delayed 7 to 14 days to allow cerebral edema to subside and to allow for medical stabilization of the patient. However, during the waiting period, the peak incidence of both rebleeding and vasospasm occurs. The trend now is toward early surgery, defined as within 1 to 3 days, for patients who are good candidates and have a clinical grade of I or II and minimal or no subarachnoid blood visualized on CT scan.

Early surgery allows for the prevention of rebleeding and aggressive treatment with hypervolemia and hypertension for the vasospasm as necessary. Early surgery consists of removal of the subarachnoid clot, which perhaps minimizes the vasospastic reaction to the clot. The reported incidence of vasospasm is somewhat higher for those patients undergoing early surgery (65%) (Manifold, 1990). Early surgery carries a higher risk probably because of the technically difficult nature of surgery on an edematous brain. Miyaoka, Sato, and Ishii (1993) suggest in a retrospective analysis of 1622 cases that early surgery for grade I and II patients was not a major factor in predicting outcome. However, early surgery for grade III and IV patients does appear to provide additional benefits of preventing a rebleeding episode and allowing for aggressive treatment of vasospasm and clot removal at the time of surgery.

15. What nursing care is of particular importance after a craniotomy?

Overall and serial evaluation of neurologic status is critical to detect any changes associated with development of a postoperative intracranial blood clot. Airway maintenance is essential, as these patients often have difficulty controlling their airway because of neurologic deficits. Evaluation of increased intracranial pressure related to cerebral edema is critical, particularly after suctioning or painful procedures. Electrolyte imbalances are also a concern postoperatively for the craniotomy patient because of the diuresis that occurs intraoperatively. As craniotomy patients recover, nutrition and complications of bed rest must be carefully assessed. Postoperative pain, particularly headache, requires attention with judicious use of pain medication (Romeo, 1993).

16. Describe the pathophysiology and incidence of rebleeding. When is rebleeding likely to occur?

Rebleeding occurs when the fibrin-platelet clot is displaced either by hypertension or fibrinolysis. Women, patients in poor premorbid health, patients with elevated systolic blood pressures, and patients with a high clinical grade on the Hunt and Hess scale are more likely to rebleed. Aneurysm patients are at risk for rebleeding until the aneurysm is clipped or treated in some fashion. Peak incidence for rebleeding is 24 to 48 hours following the aneurysm (Cook, 1991; Hickey, 1992; Kirsch et al., 1989; Manifold, 1990).

17. What clinical changes should be anticipated if a patient is experiencing rebleeding?

The clinical presentation of rebleeding is generally quite profound with gradual or sudden deterioration in neurologic status. The patients may complain of an increase in pain associated with a headache. Often there may be sudden onset of nausea and vomiting and rise in systolic blood pressure and intracranial pressure (Cook, 1991).

18. How is rebleeding diagnosed?

The definitive diagnosis of rebleeding is made by a second CT scan and evidence of increasing subarachnoid hemorrhage.

19. What is the treatment for rebleeding? What is the duration of treatment?

Ideally, treatment consists of prevention. The definitive prevention is surgical clip ligation of the aneurysm (Cook, 1991). The efficacy of prophylactic treatment while waiting for surgical intervention is controversial. Antifibrinolytic agents such as aminocaproic acid (Amicar) are administered with the initial diagnosis of subarachnoid hemorrhage to prevent clot lysis. Aminocaproic acid is discontinued intraoperatively once the clip is in place.

20. Describe the pathophysiology and incidence of vasospasm? When is vasospasm likely to occur?

Vasospasm is a narrowing of the arteries in the area of the aneurysm and subarachnoid hemorrhage. The specific cause of vasospasm is debated in the literature. There is a correlation between the incidence of vasospasm and the amount of blood released into the subarachnoid space. The extent of the clot (when located in the basal cisterns and cerebral fissures) should be considered when evaluating the probability of spasm. Subarachnoid clots larger than 5 by 3 mm in the basal cisterns or a layer of blood 1 mm or thicker in the area of the cisterns have a high correlation with spasm (Hickey, 1992; Manifold, 1990). The following have a high incidence of vasospasm: patients presenting with a high clinical grade on the Hunt and Hess scale and patients with hyponatremia, hypovolemia, electroencephalogram abnormalities, increased cerebral blood flow velocity, decreased regional cerebral blood flow, and fibrinogen degradation products >80 µg/ml in the CSF (Sikes & Nolan, 1993). Vasospasm is also associated with a loss of autoregulation, tissue ischemia, and ultimately tissue infarction. The onset of vasospasm is usually 4 to 14 days day after the initial subarachnoid hemorrhage, with a peak around day 7. The threat of vasospasm persists for up to 3 weeks (Cook, 1991; Hickey, 1992; Kirsch et al., 1989).

21. What causes vasospasm?

The cause of vasospasm is still unknown; however, a dominant theory exists. Once the clot in the subarachnoid space begins to break down, spasmodic agents are released, resulting in vasospasm. According to Cook (1991), theories of etiology include the following:

- Biochemical process resulting in contraction of arterial muscle cells
- Release of spasmodic substances during the breakdown of erythrocytes and platelets
- Release of mitogenic substances from platelets, resulting in structural vessel changes
- An inflammatory process resulting in vasculopathy

There is also much interest in the role that oxygen-free radicals may play in the development of vasospasm.

22. How is cerebral vasospasm diagnosed? What clinical symptoms should be anticipated?

With deterioration of neurologic function and no radiographic evidence of rebleeding, a second angiogram provides definitive diagnosis of vasospasm. Other causes of a change in condition such as electrolyte imbalance and development of hydrocephalus must be considered as well. Clinically, patients exhibit a gradual onset of confusion and focal deficits such as limb weakness.

23. What is the mortality and morbidity of vasospasm and rebleeding?

Mortality related to vasospasm is high, approaching 40% to 60%. Among those who survive the initial subarachnoid hemorrhage, 50% of those will develop clinical symptoms of vasospasm, resulting in delayed cerebral ischemia. Morbidity is associated with the degree of cerebral ischemia, infarction, and permanent neurologic injury. Mortality associated with rebleeding is as high as 70% and increases with each episode of rebleeding. Patients rarely survive a third rebleeding event. Morbidity is associated with the location and degree of cerebral tissue injury with each event and can be quite severe (Cook, 1991; Hickey, 1992; Kirsch et al., 1989; Manifold, 1990).

24. What is the treatment for vasospasm? What additional approaches to the treatment of vasospasm are discussed in the literature?

Current modalities of treatment are aimed at increasing cerebral perfusion pressure using hypervolemic/hypertensive therapy and pharmacologic agents to (Hickey, 1992; Sikes & Nolan, 1993):

- dilate cerebral arteries
- improve rheologic findings
- maximize cardiac performance

Guidelines for hypervolemic/hypertensive therapy are as follows (Hickey, 1992):

- central venous pressure >10 mm Hg
- pulmonary capillary wedge pressure 14 to 18 mm Hg
- hematocrit 33% to 35%
- heart rate >70 bpm
- 30% rise in mean arterial blood pressure (130 to 150 mm Hg)

Despite the interest in a variety of drugs to prevent the narrowing of arteriole walls, the results have not been promising. The greatest interest is currently in the use of calcium antagonists. Of the calcium channel blockers available, nimodipine is currently the drug of choice. Nimodipine is more potent than nifedipine (Procardia), is lipid soluble, readily crosses the blood-brain barrier, and perhaps has fewer systemic effects from hypotension.

Nimodipine promotes collateral circulation, reduces platelet aggregation, and blocks calcium influx into single nerve cells, thus promoting an anticonvulsant effect. Nimodipine enhances the cardiac function by reducing afterload. Treatment is initiated within 96 hours of subarachnoid hemorrhage and is continued for 21 days. Typical dosage is 60 mg every 4 hours orally. Currently, intravenous nicardipine is under study as an alternative, since nimodipine is available only in oral form and many subarachnoid patients are unable to adequately swallow because of a depressed neurologic state (Haley, Kassell, & Torner, 1993).

Rheology is the study of blood's ability to flow. Patients with a subarachnoid hemorrhage often have increased blood volume within the brain tissue, suggesting microstagnation. Increased hematocrit, erythrocyte aggregation, platelet aggregation, plasma viscosity, and shear rate affect blood viscosity. The hematocrit is the easiest to manipulate and is done so by hemodilution. Crystalloids and colloids are used in conjunction to provide hemodilution and hypervolemic therapy to increase the cerebral perfusion to the tissues deprived by vasospasm. Plasm protein fraction (Plasmanate), 5% albumin, hetastarch (Hespan), or dextran may also be used (Sikes & Nolan, 1993).

Additional drugs may be used to maximize cardiac performance and promote supported hypervolemic/hypertensive therapy. The mean arterial blood pressure is elevated to the point where the clinical condition of the patient improves and is then titrated down to the point at which neurologic status is maintained. Therapy can be much more aggressive in patients who have clipped or surgically secured aneurysms once the threat of rebleeding has been removed.

Inotropic and vasoconstrictive therapy may be necessary to support the desired elevation in blood pressure. Dopamine (Intropin) (3 to 10 µg/kg/min), dobutamine (Dobutrex) (2.5 to 10 µg/kg/min), and phenylephrine hydrochloride (Neo–Synephrine) (10 to 100 µg/min) are commonly used. Atropine sulfate may be necessary to block vagal bradycardia induced by hypervolemia. Vasopressin (Pitressin) may be used to keep urine output to less than 200 ml/h and to prevent diuresis as a response to hypervolemia. Digitalis (Digoxin) may be necessary for the patient at risk for pulmonary compromise and cardiac failure (Sikes & Nolan, 1993).

Cerebral angioplasty is indicated for patients who do not improve with conventional therapy. This investigative therapy involves temporary balloon dilation of the affected arterial segment(s). Arterial dilation is immediate and permanent. Complete recovery has been reported using this technique (Cook, 1991). Possible use of oxygen–free radical scavengers (lazaroids) is being considered to prevent cellular damage. Intracisternal injection of the drug recombinant tissue plasminogen activator (rtPA) is also under evaluation (Sikes & Nolan, 1993; Zabramski et al., 1991).

25. How long is the treatment of vasospasm continued?

Hypervolemic therapy is maintained until stabilization of the patient's condition and resolution of the acute phase. Calcium antagonists are usually continued for 21 days (Sikes & Nolan, 1993).

26. **How long will Connie remain "at risk" for vasospasm or rebleeding?**

   The risk for rebleeding is present until the aneurysm is surgically treated by clip ligation or clamp of the main feeder artery. In untreated aneurysms after the first year, the risk of rebleeding is cumulative at 3% for each year (Cook, 1991). The risk for vasospasm is present for approximately 21 days.

Subarachnoid Hemorrhage With Aneurysm

Cook, H. A. (1991). Aneurysmal subarachnoid hemorrhage: Neurosurgical frontiers and nursing challenges. *AACN Clinical Issues, 2*(4), 665–674.

Haley, E. C., Kassell, N. F., & Torner, J. C. (1993). A randomized controlled trial of high-dose intravenous nicardipine in aneurysmal subarachnoid hemorrhage. *Journal of Neurosurgery, 78,* 537–547.

Hickey, J. V. (1992). *Neurological and neurosurgical nursing.* Philadelphia: J. B. Lippincott Company.

Kirsch, J. R., Diringer, M. N., Borel, C. O., & Hanley, D. F. (1989). Cerebral aneurysms: Mechanisms of injury and critical care interventions. *Critical Care Clinics, 5*(4), 755–772.

Manifold, S. L. (1990). Aneurysmal SAH: Cerebral vasospasm and early repair. *Critical Care Nurse, 10*(8), 62–70.

Mason, P. J. (1992). Neurodiagnostic testing. *Critical Care Nurse, 12*(6), 64–75.

Miyaoka, M., Sato, K., & Ishii, S. (1993). A clinical study of the relationship of timing to outcome of surgery for ruptured cerebral aneurysms. *Journal of Neurosurgery, 79,* 373–378.

Nikas, D. L. (1991). The neurologic system. In J. G. Alspach (Ed.), *Core curriculum for critical care nursing* (pp. 412–418). Philadelphia: Saunders.

Romeo, J. (1993). Patients with craniotomies. In J. M. Clochesy, C. Breu, S. Cardin, E. B. Rudy, & A. A. Whittaker (Eds.), *Critical care nursing* (pp. 788–793). Philadelphia: Saunders.

Segatore, M. (1993). Hyponatremia after aneurysmal subarachnoid hemorrhage. *Journal of Neuroscience Nurses, 25*(2), 92–99.

Sikes, P. J., & Nolan, S. (1993). Pharmacologic management of cerebral vasospasm. *Critical Care Nurse Quarterly, 15*(4), 78–88.

Zabramski, J. M., Spetzler, R. F., Lee, K. L., Papadopoulos, S. M., Bovill, E., Zimmerman, R. S., & Bederson, J. B. (1991). Phase I trial of tissue plasminogen activator for the prevention of vasospasm in patients with aneurysmal subarachnoid hemorrhage. *Journal of Neurosurgery, 75,* 189–196.

14

Head Trauma
Subdural Hematoma

Cinda Alexander, MSN, CCRN, CNRN

CASE PRESENTATION

Amy, a 27-year-old right-handed woman, was involved in a motor vehicle accident. Amy was an unrestrained passenger in a car that swerved off the road and struck a tree. Amy was ejected from the car and found unconscious by the emergency medical service.

After being placed on a spinal board and in a Philadelphia collar, Amy was transported by helicopter to the nearest emergency room trauma center. Amy was somewhat combative and unresponsive to commands at arrival. Her pupils were reactive bilaterally (left > right). Her respiratory rate was 40/min and labored. Subsequently, an endotracheal tube was placed and mechanical ventilation started. Additional treatment included placement of a subclavian intravenous (IV) line, arterial catheter, and Foley catheter. Initial evaluation of her cervical spine revealed no abnormal findings, and the long spine board and Philadelphia collar were removed. Following are Amy's diagnostic data:

BP   90/40
HR   100 bpm
Respirations 40/min
Temperature 36.7° C (98° F)
Pupils reactive L > R
Glasgow Coma Scale 9

Amy's initial computed tomography (CT) scan of the head revealed a left temporal cerebral contusion with a midline shift of brain structures. The CT scan also revealed a left temporal parietal subdural hematoma.

After surgical removal of the hematoma Amy was transferred to the critical care unit. Intubation and mechanical ventilation continued. An intracranial pressure (ICP) monitoring device was placed. Following are her diagnostic data after surgery.

ICP	25 mm Hg		
BP	130/88	pH	7.48
HR	100 bpm	P_{CO_2}	40 mm Hg
Respirations	12/min	P_{O_2}	434 mm Hg
Temperature	37.8° C (100° F)	HCO_3^-	20.4 mmol/L

Ventilator Settings

V_T 700 ml
Rate   12/min
F_{IO_2} 100%

As Amy recovered from the general anesthesia, she opened her eyes to speech, verbalized incomprehensible sounds, and exhibited abnormal general flexion to obtain a Glasgow Coma Scale score of 8. Over the next 2 hours, Amy's body temperature increased to 38.3° C (101° F). Despite hyperventilation, Amy's ICP remained elevated. Her serum osmolality was 282 mOsm/L, K^+ 3.9 mmol/L, and Na^+ 139 mmol/L. Postoperative orders included the following:

- fluid restriction to maintain patient's osmolality between 305 and 315 mOsm/L
- furosemide (Lasix) 20 mg q6h, IV
- mannitol (Osmitrol) 100 g in 10% to 20% solution over a period of 2 to 6 hours
- phenytoin (Dilantin) 100 mg IV q6h

Amy's ICP remained elevated for more than 72 hours; then gradually Amy stabilized. After 2 weeks in the ICU, Amy was transferred to a neurologic step-down unit and then to a head injury rehabilitation unit.

QUESTIONS

Head Trauma
Subdural Hematoma

1. Where does head trauma rank as a cause of death in the United States? What are the statistics associated with head trauma? Include morbidity and mortality information.

2. What are the leading causes of head injury?

3. What is the rationale for Amy being placed on a long spine board with a Philadelphia collar?

4. What is the Glasgow Coma Scale? How is this scale helpful?

5. What are the types of skull fractures associated with head trauma? What clinical presentations and pathophysiology are pertinent in these types of trauma?

6. What special considerations are necessary for those patients with basilar skull fractures in regard to placement of an endotracheal or nasogastric tube?

7. List and describe the focal injuries associated with traumatic head injury. Include the mechanism of injury and clinical presentation associated with each.

8. List and describe the diffuse injuries associated with traumatic head injury.

9. What is the significance of a midline shift?

10. What are the types of subdural hematomas (SDHs)? Include the pathology and clinical presentation of SDH.

11. What surgical intervention is indicated with SDH?

12. Define intracranial pressure (ICP). What methods are available for monitoring ICP? Describe the potential complications of ICP monitoring.

13. What factors determine when an ICP monitoring device is placed?

14. List and describe possible secondary injuries with head injury.

15. Based on Amy's arterial blood gas results, what ventilator changes should be anticipated? What is the desirable $Paco_2$ range in the presence of increased ICP?

16. What effect does hyperventilation have on cerebral blood flow and increased ICP?

17. Describe the pathophysiology of intracranial hypertension. What is the general cause of increased ICP in patients with acute head injury?

18. What is autoregulation and how does it impact cerebral blood flow and ICP?

19. Given an ICP of 25 mm Hg and blood pressure of 120/72, calculate Amy's cerebral perfusion pressure (CPP). Is the CPP an acceptable value? Discuss the drawbacks of CPP values.

20. Discuss the medical management that should be anticipated for this patient. Include rationale and identify at least one potential complication associated with each.

21. Define and discuss the clinical significance of posturing such as abnormal flexion and abnormal extension.

22. Describe the relevance of controlling hyperthermia in the management of head-injured patients?

23. What nursing management actions are essential to avoid or minimize the effects of secondary injury in this patient?

24. What are the potential extracranial effects of increased ICP?

25. Which cranial nerves must be intact before the patient eats or drinks?

QUESTIONS AND ANSWERS

Head Trauma
Subdural Hematoma

1. **Where does head trauma rank as a cause of death in the United States? What are the statistics associated with head trauma? Include morbidity and mortality information.**

   Head trauma is the third leading cause of death in the United States. It is estimated that over 10 million head injuries occur each year. Approximately 750,000 hospitalizations and 100,000 deaths are associated with head injury. Seventy percent of all trauma-related deaths involve a head injury. Mortality from head injury alone is estimated at approximately 50%. A majority of these deaths occur before the individual enters the health care system. The incidence of head injury is three times greater in males than females, and peak incidence is at age 15 to 24 years (Sullivan, Schefft, Warm, & Dember, 1994; Walleck, 1993).

2. **What are the leading causes of head injury?**

   Motor vehicle accidents are the leading cause of head injury with alcohol or drug intake often associated as a contributing factor. Other causes include shootings, falls, assaults, and sporting accidents (Ammons, 1990).

3. **What was the rationale for Amy being placed on a long spine board with a Philadelphia collar?**

   There is a strong correlation between spinal cord trauma and head trauma or general trauma.

4. **What is the Glasgow Coma Scale? How is this scale helpful?**

   The Glasgow Coma Scale is a standardized scale used to evaluate neurologic response. The scale is divided into three sections designed to assess consciousness, verbal abilities, and motor response. The scores range from 3 to 15, with 15 representing normal function (Hartshorn, Byers, & Goddard, 1993). It is generally accepted that a score of 8 or less constitutes coma. The scale is a useful tool to communicate the patient's neurologic condition after a rapid assessment.

5. **What are the types of skull fractures associated with head trauma? What clinical presentations and pathophysiology are pertinent in these types of trauma?**

   Skull fractures are categorized as linear, depressed, or basilar and may be simple, comminuted, or compound in nature. The presence of skull fracture does not delineate the degree of injury to the brain structures within the skull.

   ### Linear Skull Fracture

   Linear skull fractures can be defined as nondisplaced fractures of the skull. The majority of linear skull fractures are not displaced and do not require intervention unless they extend into a major sinus or across a major vascular channel (Walleck, 1993). If there is a fracture across a major vascular channel, such as the middle meningeal artery in the temporal parietal area, the patient should be carefully evaluated for acute epidural bleeding.

   ### Depressed Skull Fracture

   A depressed skull fracture is characterized by an inward depression of the outer table of the skull. Patients will present with an open laceration in the area of the depression and varying degrees of neurologic alterations based on the degree of brain tissue involvement. Surgical intervention may be necessary to remove bone fragment from the meninges or brain tissue. The area of tissue and compression by the bony fragments can become a source of irritability and seizure focus (Hartshorn et al., 1993). If the fracture is severe, clinical presentation may extend to seepage of cerebrospinal fluid (CSF) and brain tissue from the fracture site.

   ### Basilar Skull Fracture

   A basilar skull fracture is located at the base of the skull. If the fracture is significant, the underlying dura may be torn, which allows direct communication with the subarachnoid space and brain tissue. Infection and meningitis are of major concern with this type of fracture. Clinical presentation may include the following (Walleck, 1993):

   - seepage of CSF from the nose (rhinorrhea)
   - bilateral periorbital ecchymosis (raccoon eyes) if the anterior fossa is involved
   - leakage of CSF from the ears (otorrhea) if the middle fossa is involved
   - ecchymosis of the mastoid sinus (battle sign) if the posterior fossa is involved

6. **What special considerations are necessary for those patients with basilar skull fractures in regard to placement of an endotracheal or nasogastric tube?**

The inherent risk associated with endotracheal intubation and passage of a nasogastric tube is penetration through the fracture site and passage into the brain itself. Precautions would include the use of oral route for intubation and nasogastric tubes to minimize this risk. In addition, the nose should never be suctioned for removal of drainage in patients with basilar skull fractures (Walleck, 1993).

7. **List and describe the focal injuries associated with traumatic head injury. Include the mechanism of injury and clinical presentation associated with each.**

The most common focal injuries associated with head injury include concussion, contusion, and intracranial hematomas (Butterworth & DeWitt, 1989).

Concussion

A concussion is a transient, temporary condition of the brain without any structural damage. The clinical symptoms usually include a brief (generally seconds) loss of consciousness, confusion, and some amnesia. However, concussion can be severe enough to induce brief respiratory arrest, pronounced confusion, and severe amnesia. Concussions can be graded I through IV, with IV being the most severe. Clinical presentation and the lack of adequate supervision at home may necessitate hospitalization (Ammons, 1990).

Contusion

A contusion can be described as bruising of the brain. Contusions can be mild, involving a small portion of the brain tissue and minimal clinical symptoms, or they can be large, usually in the case of impact injuries, where the size increases as a result of edema and may produce significant increases in ICP. Injury to the brain usually results from accelerations and decelerations of the brain within the cranial vault. Contusions tend to occur in the frontal and temporal areas and are commonly associated with skull fractures. The significance of a contusion and severity of the neurologic injury is related to the degree of secondary insults such as edema, hemorrhage, and ischemia (Ammons, 1990; Butterworth & DeWitt, 1989).

Hematomas

Intracranial hematomas are classified as extradural or intradural. Extradural hematomas are referred to as epidural and generally are arterial in nature, usually occurring from a laceration of the middle meningeal artery. The clot forms between the inner table of the skull and the outer dura. Clinical symptoms develop quickly and are manifested as a sudden deterioration of consciousness, a fixed and dilated ipsilateral pupil, and hemiplegia or paresis (Walleck, 1993). Subdural hematomas (SDHs; intradural) form when there is bleeding between the dura and arachnoid layers. SDHs are generally venous in nature and are often from tears of cortical bridging veins but can result from bruising of the cortical tissue as well. The bleeding creates direct pressure and irritation of the cortical tissue. Clinical presentation includes marked depressed level of consciousness, pupillary changes (unequal to dilated and fixed), headache, agitation, confusion, and motor deficits (Walleck, 1993). The degree of symptoms is usually dependent on the location and size of the clot formation.

8. **List and describe the diffuse injuries associated with traumatic head injury.**

    Diffuse axonal injury (DAI) is a shear injury to the white matter with stretching and tearing of the reticular activating fibers. Microscopic focal lesions in the white matter include axon contraction balls throughout white matter, gathering of microglial cells, followed by degradation of long tracts (Butterworth & DeWitt, 1989; Walleck, 1993). Microhemorrhagic or necrotic lesions appear in the corpus callosum and in the dorsolateral part of the upper brain stem (Sahuquillo-Barris, Lamarca-Ciuro, Vilata-Castan, Rubio-Garcia, & Rodriguez-Pazos, 1988). Clinical presentation includes deep and profound coma, abnormal posturing, increased ICP, hypertension, and hyperthermia. The hallmark of DAI is immediate and prolonged coma without radiographic identification of a specific cause (Walleck, 1993).

9. **What is the significance of a midline shift?**

    A midline shift on CT scan or magnetic resonance imaging (MRI) indicates the delicate structures of the central portion of the brain, such as the ventricles and brain stem, have been displaced laterally. Brain tissue displacement is poorly tolerated and leads to areas of ischemia, diffuse edema, and shearing of structures (Walleck, 1993).

10. **What are the types of subdural hematomas (SDHs)? Include the pathology and clinical presentation of SDH.**

    SDHs are classified as acute, subacute, and chronic, with mortality ranging from 52% to 90% (Walleck, 1993; Wilberger, Harris, & Diamond, 1991).

Acute SDH generally occurs within 48 hours of the initial injury. Clinical presentation is usually progressive, with possible headache, symptoms of increased ICP, pupillary and motor changes, and marked coma.

Subacute SDH develops 2 to 24 days after the initial injury. SDHs are often difficult to diagnose and are strongly indicated by failure to regain consciousness after head trauma (Hickey, 1992).

Chronic SDH can develop from minor head trauma. Often chronic SDH is associated with the elderly population because of cerebral atrophy, which can result from a minor fall or bump of the head. In the chronic state the blood clot becomes encased within a membrane. Clinical symptoms generally are subtle and vague with progressive confusion, drowsiness, headache, seizures, and hemiparesis. Symptoms associated with chronic SDH may not become apparent until several weeks to months after the initial injury (Hickey, 1992). Persons with alcoholism are prone to chronic SDH formation as a result of frequent falls and changes in clotting factors associated with alcoholism.

11. What surgical intervention is indicated with SDH?

Small SDHs can be treated medically, as they can be reabsorbed if there is no evidence of significant increased ICP or shifting of brain structures. Acute SDH is surgically treated by craniotomy and removal of the clot. Subacute SDH may require a craniotomy flap or may be treated by burr holes if the clot has degenerated into a thick viscous liquid. Chronic SDH is treated with burr holes and placement of a temporary drain. Persistent chronic SDH may require a craniotomy flap to remove the membrane flap (Walleck, 1993).

12. Define intracranial pressure (ICP). What methods are available for monitoring ICP? Describe the potential complications of ICP monitoring?

ICP is a dynamic state of equilibrium that exists among the three components within the cranial vault: blood, brain, and CSF. Any increase in one component necessitates a decrease in another component for the dynamic equilibrium to remain constant; otherwise, an increase in ICP occurs (Monro-Kellie doctrine).

There are a variety of methods to measure ICP, including catheters and transducer setups that measure pressure from the epidural area, subdural area, subarachnoid space, tissue, and intraventricular spaces. The major complication associated with ICP monitoring is infection. Generally, the more invasive the method, the greater risk of serious consequences of infection. Other complications associated with ICP monitoring include hematoma and migration of the catheter or device (Alspach, 1991).

13. What factors determine when an ICP monitoring device is placed?

Indications for an ICP monitor are somewhat controversial. General guidelines for placement include the following (Butterworth & De-Witt, 1989):

- a Glasgow Coma Scale score of 8 or below
- intradural hematomas or contusions
- demonstrated cerebral edema on CT scan
- midline shifts

14. List and describe possible secondary injuries with head injury.

Secondary insults precipitated by brain trauma include hypoxia, hypercapnia, hypotension, and cerebral edema or intracranial hypertension.

Hypoxia

Brain injury often leads to irregular and inadequate respiratory efforts. Early management of the airway at the scene of injury and aggressive respiratory support is critical. Hypoxemia contributes to neurologic damage, as the brain compensates for a deceased oxygen supply by increased cerebral blood flow. This offers a luxury perfusion to the uninjured tissue and contributes to increased cerebral blood volume, thus increasing ICP (Walleck, 1992).

Hypercapnia

Carbon dioxide is a potent cerebrovasodilator that will increase cerebral blood flow and contribute to increased intracranial hypertension.

Hypotension

Hypotension is often the result of multisystem injury and overall blood loss. The mean arterial pressure (MAP) must be sufficient to maintain cerebral perfusion. Hypotension contributes to general cerebral hypoperfusion (Walleck, 1992).

Intracranial Hypertension

Cerebral edema associated with head trauma may be local or diffuse. Cerebral edema exaggerates the amount and severity of neurologic injury and leads to increased ICP. Intracranial hypertension is a major complication and the most frequent cause of death associated with brain injury. Most of the care of head injured patients is aimed at control of ICP (Bouma, Muizelaar, Bandoh, & Marmarou, 1992; Walleck, 1992). Wilberger, Harris, and Diamond (1991) found that control of increased ICP after removal of an SDH was a variable more critical to outcome than operative timing of the removal of the clot.

15. **Based on Amy's arterial blood gas results, what ventilator changes should be anticipated? What is the desirable PaCO$_2$ range in the presence of increased ICP?**

   Ventilator changes to reduce the PaCO$_2$ include increasing the rate (frequency) or tidal volume. Decreasing the FiO$_2$ to minimize the effect of oxygen toxicity is also indicated.

16. **What effect does hyperventilation have on cerebral blood flow and increased ICP?**

   Hyperventilation assists with the reduction of carbon dioxide, a potent cerebrovasodilator. With a reduction of PaCO$_2$ there is vasoconstriction of the cerebral blood vessels, decreased cerebral blood volume, thus decreased ICP. Target levels for PaCO$_2$ are generally 25 to 27 mm Hg. Severely lowered PaCO$_2$ levels have a potential for ischemia and infarction (Walleck, 1993).

17. **Describe the pathophysiology of intracranial hypertension. What is the general cause of increased ICP in patients with acute head injury?**

   Normal ICP is 0 to 15 mm Hg. There may be some variations associated with the type of monitoring device used. Intracranial hypertension is defined as a sustained increase in ICP above 15 mm Hg caused by the following conditions:

   - conditions that increase brain volume such as hematomas or cerebral edema
   - conditions that increase cerebral blood flow, including hyperemia and hypercapnia
   - conditions that increase CSF volume such as increased production of CSF, decreased absorption, and obstruction hydrocephalus

   Cerebral edema is a common complication of moderate to severe head injury that results in increased ICP. The state of increased pressure is further complicated by hypotension, resulting in deceased oxygenation to the tissues, and hypercapnia, resulting in cerebrovasodilation (Hickey, 1992; Walleck, 1992).

18. **What is autoregulation and how does it impact cerebral blood flow and ICP?**

   Walleck (1993) describes autoregulation as the automatic change in cerebral blood vessels in response to varying systemic pressures to maintain a continuous perfusion pressure gradient to the tissues without wide fluctuation of flow. The reflex maintains constant perfusion in spite of wide variations in systemic mean arterial pressure (MAP). When autoregulation is disrupted, as may be the case in traumatized brain tissue, that area of tissue is dependent on systemic pressure for perfusion.

19. **Given an ICP of 25 mm Hg and blood pressure of 120/72, calculate Amy's cerebral perfusion pressure (CPP). Is the CPP an acceptable value? What are the drawbacks of CPP values?**

To calculate MAP:

$$\frac{Syst + (2 \times Diast)}{3} = MAP \qquad Systolic + \frac{(2 \times Diastolic)}{3} = MAP$$

To calculate CPP: MAP − ICP = CPP

$$120 + \frac{(2 \times 72)}{3} = 88 \ (MAP) \qquad 88 - 25 = 63 \text{ mm Hg (CPP)}$$

Controversy exists over the "minimal" acceptable CPP value. Generally, 60 mm Hg is considered to be the lowest acceptable value. Once ICP rises and CPP begins to fail, cerebral tissue is deprived of sufficient blood flow, and ischemia and infarction occur. If the ICP rises too high, the brain tissue herniates, followed by ischemia and infarction. If the herniation process continues without intervention, death caused by brain stem compression is usually the result (Hickey, 1992; Kirsch, Diringer, Borel, Hart, & Hanley, 1989; Walleck, 1993).

20. **Discuss the medical management that should be anticipated for this patient. Include rationale and identify at least one potential complication associated with each.**

Hyperventilation

Hyperventilation is induced to decrease the $PaCO_2$ and promote vasoconstriction of cerebrovasculature, thereby decreasing cerebral blood flow and ICP. However, severe reduction of $PaCO_2$, below 20 mm Hg, can cause hypoxia and tissue ischemia or infarction (Alspach, 1991).

Osmotic Diuretics

Osmotic diuretics decrease brain edema by creating a vascular gradient promoting movement of water from brain tissue into the vascular compartment. Hyperosmolarity and renal failure are potential complications of this treatment. Mannitol is the drug of choice because of its rapid onset of action (Walleck, 1989).

Loop Diuretics

Loop diuretics, such as furosemide (Lasix), are often used in combination with osmotic diuretics. The benefits probably relate to the ability of loop diuretics to reduce total body fluid, preventing acute pulmonary edema and congestive heart failure that can be a complication of osmotic therapy (Walleck, 1989).

Fluid Restriction

Fluid restriction remains controversial in the care of head-injured patients. Too much fluid restriction may result in severe dehydration. The patient's osmolality is the best guide for fluid therapy with a goal of 305 to 315 mOsml/L (normal 280 to 300 mOsml/L) (Walleck, 1989).

Glucocorticosteroids

The use of steroids in the management of cerebral edema associated with head injury remains controversial. The two most commonly used glucocorticosteroids are dexamethasone (Decradon) and methylprednisolone (Solu–Medrol). Steroids are still used widely in the treatment of brain tumors. Steroids may exert a stabilizing effect on the cell membrane. Side effects associated with large doses of steroids include decreased resistance to infection and gastrointestinal hemorrhage (Walleck, 1989).

Barbiturate Coma Therapy

Barbiturate coma therapy is still considered for use in uncontrolled ICP associated with cerebral edema. Barbiturates lower ICP; however, the mechanism is not well understood. Barbiturates are associated with numerous complications, including hypotension and decreased cardiac output (Kirsch et al., 1989; Walleck, 1993). An ICP monitoring device must be used during barbiturate therapy so that the nurse can evaluate the patient's neurologic status, since the patient is in a drug-induced coma.

Seizure Control

Posttraumatic epilepsy occurs on 5% to 20% of head-injured patients. The more severe the injury, the greater the likelihood of seizure activity. According to Dupuis and Miranda-Massari (1991), risk factors to assess include intracranial hematoma, focal neurologic deficits, posttraumatic amnesia lasting more than 24 hours, depressed skull fracture, and age under 5 years. Dilantin (phenytoin) is the drug of choice in seizure control. Diazepam (Valium) is useful in short-term management as well.

21. Define and discuss the clinical significance of posturing such as abnormal flexion and abnormal extension.

Posturing, such as abnormal extension and abnormal flexion, are often associated with abnormal brain stem function. The presence of abnormal posturing does not clearly predict outcome after acute head injury. However, it does emphasize the need for close neurologic monitoring, as the brain has been severely compromised (Hartshorn et al., 1993).

22. **Describe the relevance of controlling hyperthermia in the management of head-injured patients?**

    Hyperthermia increases metabolic activity in the brain tissue, resulting in a greater oxygen demand. This leads to an increase in cerebral blood flow and production of carbon dioxide in a brain already compromised with cerebral edema and increased ICP (Walleck, 1992).

23. **What nursing management actions are essential to avoid or minimize the effects of secondary injury in this patient?**

    Walleck (1992) outlines the following guidelines for patient care.
    Patient Positioning: Patient position should always promote venous drainage from the brain. The head, neck, and chest are maintained in alignment to prevent obstruction of the jugular veins and twisting of the neck. The head of the bed is usually elevated. According to Feldman et al. (1992), elevation of the head at 30 degrees significantly reduces ICP without compromising cerebral blood flow and CPP.
    Ventilation: Airway management and pulmonary toilet are important protocols to manage head-injured patients and prevent pulmonary complications.
    Hyperventilation and Oxygenation: Hyperventilation and oxygenation before and after pulmonary suctioning can minimize the negative effects of suctioning. Caution must be observed to avoid overhyperventilation, which may lead to $PaCO_2$ below 25 mm Hg.
    Maintenance of Blood Pressure: Hemodynamic stability is critical in the head-injured patient to avoid wide fluctuation in MAPs. Appropriate treatment of hypotension with IV fluids and pharmacologic agents and ongoing assessment of MAP are indicated.
    Normothermia: Monitoring and maintenance of normal body temperature are necessary to avoid the effects of a hypermetabolic state on ICP.
    Neurologic Assessment: Ongoing assessment of the neurologic function of the patient is paramount to detect subtle changes that may indicate deterioration of the patient's condition. Serial evaluation and collaboration among caregivers are critical to ensure that any changes in status are noted.
    Physical Care: There has been much interest in the literature as to the effects of personal care such as bathing, oral hygiene, and range of motion on ICP. Individualization based on patient response is necessary to determine those activities that are well tolerated and those to be avoided. Generally, it is accepted that physical activities should be spaced to allow the patient recovery time and avoid compounded effects on the ICP.

24. **What are the potential extracranial effects of increased ICP?**

    According to Bloomfield (1989), the following are major extracerebral effects of traumatic brain injury:

Pulmonary Effects

Hypoxia: Hypoxia occurs as a result of ventilation-perfusion ($\dot{V}/\dot{Q}$) mismatch or pulmonary shunt.

Noncardiogenic Pulmonary Edema: Cerebral ischemia triggers a response of sympathetic discharge that alters capillary permeability in the lungs and creates an increase in atrial pressure.

Adult Respiratory Distress Syndrome (ARDS): ARDS is a common complication of head-injured patients, resulting in an increase in dead space, decrease in pulmonary compliance, and formation of hyaline membrane.

Aspiration Pneumonitis: Head-injured patients are often unable to guard their airway because of a depressed level of consciousness, leaving them at risk for aspiration.

Fat Emboli: Fat emboli are often associated with long bone fractures seen in multiple trauma patients.

Pulmonary Contusion: Pulmonary contusion frequently accompanies head injury when created by multiple trauma.

Cardiovascular Effects

Hyperdynamic Cardiovascular Response: Hyperdynamic cardiovascular response is a cardiovascular effect associated with head trauma, a state of elevated cardiac output, increased heart rate, and increased blood pressure.

Posttraumatic Hypertension: Posttraumatic hypertension is precipitated by increased sympathetic activity, resulting in increased systolic blood pressure associated with the Cushing's phenomenon.

Gastrointestinal Effects

Pancreatitis: Pancreatitis is a gastrointestinal effect secondary to blunt trauma to the abdomen that may be difficult to diagnose because of the patient's decreased level of consciousness.

Stress ulceration: Stress ulceration may be present as erosive gastritis or gastrointestinal bleeding resulting from increased acidity.

Electrolyte and Metabolic Derangements

Hyponatremia: Hyponatremia is associated with diarrhea, vomiting, gastric suction, and syndrome of inappropriate antidiuretic hormone (SIADH).

Hypernatremia: Hypernatremia usually represents water loss and may also be the result of diabetes insipidus (DI).

Potassium Deficits: Deficiencies may be related to inadequate potassium replacement, diuretics, or alkalemia.

Thyroid and Adrenal Malfunction: Trauma to the hypothalamus and pituitary glands results in thyroid and adrenal malfunction.

Nutrition

Autocatabolic State: Autocatabolic state is an effect of increased ICP caused by stress-related hypermetabolism and gluconeogenesis.

Coagulation Abnormalities: Disseminated intravascular coagulation (DIC) is the most common coagulopathy associated with severe head trauma, especially with acute SDH and contusions. The cause of DIC is a high thromboplastic activity of brain tissue.

25. Which cranial nerves must be intact before the patient eats or drinks?

It is essential that the nurse evaluate the following cranial nerves before the patient eats or drinks:

- cranial nerve V (trigeminal): chewing
- cranial nerve VII (facial): facial muscles
- cranial nerves IX, X (glossopharyngeal and vagus): gag and swallowing
- cranial nerve XII (hypoglossal): tongue

Only if these cranial nerves are intact bilaterally can the patient take nourishment by mouth (Walleck, 1993).

References

Head Trauma Subdural Hematoma

Alspach, T. (1991). *Core curriculum for critical care nursing* (4th ed.). Philadelphia: Saunders.

Ammons, A. (1990). Cerebral injuries and intracranial hemorrhages as a result of trauma. *Nursing Clinics of North America, 25*(1), 23–31.

Bloomfield, E. L. (1989). Extracerebral complications of head injury. *Critical Care Clinics, 5*(4), 881–891.

Bouma, G. J., Muizelaar, J. P., Bandoh, K., & Marmarou, A. (1992). Blood pressure and intracranial pressure–volume dynamics in severe head injury: Relationship with cerebral blood flow. *Journal of Neurosurgery, 77,* 15–19.

Butterworth, J. F., & DeWitt, D. S. (1989). Severe head trauma: Pathophysiology and management. *Critical Care Clinics, 5*(4), 807–819.

Dupuis, R. E., & Miranda-Massari, J. (1991). Anticonvulsants: Pharmacotherapeutic issues in the critically ill patient. *AACN Clinical Issues, 2*(4), 639–655.

Feldman, Z., Kanter, M., Robertson, C. S., Contant, C. F., Hayes, C., Sheinberg, M. A., Villareal, C. A., Narayan, R. K., & Grossman, R. G. (1992). Effect of head elevation on intracranial pressure, cerebral perfusion pressure, and cerebral blood flow in head-injured patients. *Journal of Neurosurgery, 76,* 207–211.

Hartshorn, J. C., Byers, V. L., & Goddard, L. (1993). Nervous system injury. In J. Hartshorn, M. Lamborn, & M. I. Noll, (Eds.). *Introduction to critical care nursing* (pp. 246–267). Philadelphia: Saunders.

Hickey, J. V. (1992). *Neurological and neurosurgical nursing.* Philadelphia: J. B. Lippincott.

Kirsch, J. R., Diringer, M. N., Borel, C. O., Hart, G. K., & Hanley, D. F. (1989). Medical management and innovations. In K. A. Gould (Ed.), *Critical care nursing clinics of North America* (pp. 143–151). Philadelphia: Saunders.

Sahuquillo-Barris, J., Lamarca-Ciuro, J., Vilata-Castan, J., Rubio-Garcia, E., & Rodriguez-Pazos, M. (1988). Acute subdural hematoma and diffuse axonal injury after severe head trauma. *Journal of Neurosurgery, 68,* 894–900.

Sullivan, T. E., Schefft, B. K., Warm, J. S., & Dember, W. N. (1994). Closed head injury assessment and research methodology. *Journal of Neuroscience Nursing, 26*(1), 27–29.

Walleck, C. A. (1989). Controversies in the management of the head-injured patient. In K. A. Gould (Ed.), *Critical care nursing clinics of North America* (pp. 67–72). Philadelphia: Saunders.

Walleck, C. A. (1992). Preventing secondary brain injury. *AACN Clinical Issues, 3*(1), 19–27.

Walleck, C. A. (1993). *Patients with head injury and brain dysfunction* (pp. 677–706). Philadelphia: Saunders.

Wilberger, J. E., Harris, M., & Diamond, D. L. (1991). Acute subdural hematoma: Morbidity, mortality, and operative timing. *Journal of Neurosurgery, 74,* 212–218.

15

Epidural Hematoma

Laura S. Platt Smith, MSN, RN
Cinda Alexander, MSN, CCRN, CNRN

CASE PRESENTATION

David Peters, age 24 years, was driving home from a party late at night when he lost control of his car and hit a tree. On impact his head hit the windshield. A witness to the accident stated that Mr. Peters was unconscious for at least 5 minutes but was awake when the paramedics arrived on the scene at 3 AM.

On arrival at the emergency department (ED), Mr. Peters was awake and restless with little memory of the accident. He was slightly combative with the ED staff, and his breath was reported to smell of alcohol. A small laceration was observed on his left temple. Skull x-rays identified a left-sided temporal fracture. Vital signs were as follows:

BP 128/80
HR 88 bpm
Respirations 22/min
Temperature 36.6° C (97.8° F)

Mr. Peters was admitted to a medical-surgical unit for observation. He remained alert and oriented throughout the night with no changes noted in his neurologic status. However, at 7 AM the assessment revealed that Mr. Peters was very irritable and did not know the date or time. By 8 AM, he became drowsy and was mumbling incoherently. The physician on call was notified and a stat computed tomography (CT) scan was ordered, which revealed a left-sided epidural hematoma (EDH).

Emergency Surgery

Mr. Peters was immediately taken to the operating room where a craniotomy was performed to remove the clot. He tolerated the procedure well and was admitted to the neurologic intensive care unit postoperatively.

Postoperative Course

Postoperatively, Mr. Peters was drowsy but arousable to voice. Pupils were equal and reactive. A large head dressing was in place with no signs of drainage noted. An arterial line was placed, and a peripheral intravenous (IV) line of 5% dextrose in lactated Ringer's solution (D_5LR) was infusing at 100 ml/h. Mr. Peters was also receiving oxygen at 3 L/min via nasal cannula. Diagnostic data were

BP	90/60 (arterial line)	pH	7.35
HR	92 bpm	PaO_2	82 mm Hg
Respirations	24/min	$PaCO_2$	35 mm Hg
Temperature	37.7° C (99.7° F)	SaO_2	95%
		HCO_3^-	28 mmol/L

Two days later, Mr. Peters was awake and alert with no neurologic deficits noted. Vital signs remained stable. The arterial line was discontinued, and he was tolerating a regular diet. He was transferred back to the medical-surgical unit and discharged 2 days later.

QUESTIONS

Epidural Hematoma

1. Describe the pathophysiology of EDH.

2. What is the classic clinical picture of EDH?

3. In the event that Mr. Peter's EDH progressed to uncal herniation, what clinical manifestations may have been observed?

4. What diagnostic modalities are used to diagnose a patient with EDH?

5. Discuss the options for surgical intervention in patients with EDH.

6. What pharmacologic agents can be used to decrease intracranial pressure (ICP) and cerebral edema in the patient with EDH or other head injuries?

7. What nursing or patient actions can result in an increased ICP? A decreased ICP?

8. Discuss the nursing responsibilities in the monitoring and assessment of the patient with EDH.

9. What other nursing interventions are required for the patient with EDH?

10. Discuss the rationale for monitoring arterial blood gases in the patient with a head injury.

11. List the nursing diagnoses that may be appropriate for the patient with EDH.

QUESTIONS AND ANSWERS

Epidural Hematoma

1. Describe the pathophysiology of EDH.

EDH is defined as a collection of blood between the inner periosteum of the skull and the dura mater (Ammons, 1990). A majority of EDHs result from arterial bleeding; however, venous bleeding from damage to the meningeal vein or dura sinus is also a potential source (Ammons, 1990). The most common location for an EDH is the temporal fossa. Other sites may include the subfrontal region or occipital-suboccipital area (Ammons, 1990). EDH of the cervical spine is a rare clinical condition that may be traumatic or spontaneous in origin (Mercado, 1989).

A temporal fracture may lead to a laceration of the meningeal artery, as the temporal region is the thinnest portion of the skull. An epidural hemorrhage occurs as a result of the bleeding meningeal artery. An expanding hematoma may lead to cerebral displacement and uncal herniation. The hematoma can push the temporal lobe medially, causing herniation of the uncus and hippocampal gyrus over and through the tentorial notch (Ammons, 1990). The result is a compromised blood supply that suppresses basic stem functions.

2. What is the classic clinical picture of EDH?

According to Clochesy, Breu, Cardin, Rudy, and Whittaker (1993), the classic picture of EDH consists of a loss of consciousness as a direct result of the injury followed by a lucid interval. The lucid interval can last anywhere from a few minutes to hours and is followed by a depression in the level of consciousness. One third of patients diagnosed with EDH develop these classic symptoms (Clochesy et al., 1993). As cited by Alspach (1991), other signs and symptoms of EDH include headache, irritability, restlessness, nausea, and vomiting.

3. **In the event that Mr. Peter's EDH had progressed to uncal herniation, what clinical manifestations may have been observed?**

Signs of herniation include ipsilateral dilation of the pupil, ptosis and deviation of the eye outward, and ipsilateral hemiparesis. As herniation progresses, bilateral pupil dilation and contralateral hemiparesis may be noted. With further deterioration, the patient may experience decerebrate rigidity, bilateral hyperactive deep tendon reflexes, and respiratory difficulties (Manifold, 1986).

4. **What diagnostic modalities are used to diagnose a patient with EDH?**

In the patient with EDH, a CT scan will reveal an area of density that indicates the location and extent of the hematoma (Alspach, 1991). As cited by Clochesy et al. (1993), the CT scan allows for rapid identification of the hematoma so that treatment can be initiated quickly with a resulting reduction in mortality and morbidity for these patients. Smith and Miller (1991) identified the need for clinical vigilance and subsequent examinations, even though the initial CT scan is normal, as the EDH may not have yet developed in the patient. Since as with Mr. Peters the majority of EDH patients have a skull fracture, typically in the temporal area, an x-ray of the head and neck is diagnostically beneficial. Wilberger (1990) identified exploratory burr holes as a potential diagnostic procedure in the event that a CT scan is not immediately available.

5. **Discuss the options for surgical intervention in patients with EDH.**

According to Evans and Billittier (1990), a delay in evacuation of a hematoma increases the morbidity and mortality of patients with intracranial injuries. Evans and Billittier (1990), identified the usefulness of burr hole decompression in patients with severe head injuries whose conditions were deteriorating so rapidly that there was no time for a CT scan to be completed. Burr holes, however, are not a definitive treatment. If blood is successfully evacuated from the burr hole, the patient will require a craniotomy for complete clot removal (Evans & Billittier, 1990). Surgical removal of the clot is necessary to minimize any neurologic deficit by preventing herniation or a shift in brain tissue (Hartshorn, Lamborn, & Noll, 1993). A craniotomy consists of cutting through the scalp and muscle, creating a bone flap to open the dura mater. At this time the clot can be removed and the damaged vessel repaired. A craniotomy may also be used to remove tissue so that the brain has room to swell in the cranium, with the option of replacing the bone flap only after the edema subsides (Aumick, 1991).

6. **What pharmacologic agents can be used to decrease intracranial pressure (ICP) and cerebral edema in the patient with EDH or other head injuries?**

Mannitol, an osmotic diuretic agent, can reduce ICP by removing extracellular fluid from within the brain by the vascular osmotic pressure gradient. As a result, blood flow and ICP are reduced (Clochesy et al., 1993). Mannitol's rapid onset of action makes it the drug of choice for reducing ICP. Hyperosmolality and acute renal failure are complications; therefore, fluid and electrolytes and serum osmolality must be monitored closely (Clochesy et al., 1993).

Furosemide (Lasix) has also been found to be effective in decreasing cerebral edema in head-injured patients. Furosemide acts within the renal tubules by inhibiting the reabsorption of sodium and chloride. Osmotic agents require an intact cellular membrane to pull fluid into the intravascular space; therefore, the fluid may be removed from normal brain tissue instead of injured tissue. In contrast, furosemide (Lasix) can remove fluid from both injured and normal brain tissue (Manifold, 1986).

The use of corticosteroids such as dexamethasone (Decadron) and methylprednisolone (Solu-Medrol) in the reduction of ICP is controversial. According to Clochesy et al. (1993), the use of steroids may be effective in stabilizing the cell membrane, improving cerebral blood flow, and restoring autoregulation. However, the risk of complications such as immunosuppression and gastrointestinal hemorrhage may outweigh the benefits (Clochsey et al., 1993).

Barbiturates such as pentobarbital may be given to decrease ICP through a reduction in cerebral metabolic rate, cerebral blood flow, and systemic blood pressure (Manifold, 1986).

7. **What nursing or patient actions can result in an increased ICP? A decreased ICP?**

As cited by Andrus (1991), the following activities may lead to an increased ICP:

- suctioning: stimulates the cough reflex and Valsalva's maneuver by increasing intrathoracic pressure
- suctioning more than 15 seconds: leads to hypoxia and hypercapnia, leading to increased ICP
- Valsalva's maneuvers: result in decreased cerebral venous drainage, increased cerebral blood flow, and increased ICP; also associated with stimulation of this mechanism: straining on defecation, holding breath, and pulling on side rails or resisting restraints
- positioning in extreme neck flexion, extension, or lateral rotation or flexion of the head: decreases venous drainage from the jugular or vertebral veins and leads to increased ICP

- isometric exercises
- loud noises, painful procedures, nontherapeutic touch
- staff discussing the patient's condition
- seizures
- hyperthermia (increases metabolic rate)
- lack of rapid eye movement (REM) sleep
- spacing activities close together

According to Andrus (1991), the following actions may help to decrease ICP:

- Determine need for suctioning and suction only when necessary.
- Hyperinflate lungs with 100% oxygen before and after suctioning.
- Suction for no longer than 15 seconds, providing several breaths in between; allow a rest period (1 to 3 minutes) between suctioning.
- Record bowel movements and administer stool softeners or other laxatives to prevent constipation and straining.
- Use sandbags or towel rolls to maintain a neutral alignment of the head and prevent head extension or flexion.
- Employ log-rolling techniques when positioning.
- Position head of bed up 30 to 45 degrees.
- Avoid pressing the patient's feet against the foot board (wear high tops).
- Control pain (decrease number of blood or needle sticks); avoid intramuscular injections.
- Use therapeutic touch.
- Avoid speaking loudly about the patient's condition.
- Decrease environmental noises and dim lights.
- Discuss the importance of a therapeutic environment with family members; monitor visitations and notice any agitation of patient; restrict visitors if necessary.
- Play tapes of familiar voices and selective music.
- For temperature more than 37.8° C (100° F) give antipyretic medication or cooling blanket if more than 38.3° C (101° F).
- Allow 30 minutes to an hour between nursing care activities.

8. **Discuss the nursing responsibilities in the monitoring and assessment of the patient with EDH.**

It is beneficial to obtain a thorough patient history including the type of injury involved, level of consciousness at time of injury, baseline vital signs, behavior, and motor function to identify any significant changes in assessment from the baseline.

According to Clochesy et al. (1993), the most reliable indicator of neurologic function is level of consciousness. The Glasgow Coma Scale is the most reliable scale for assessing the level of consciousness by assessing the patient's best eye opening and verbal and motor responses (Reimer, 1989). The scale ranges from 3 to 15. The lower the score, the more severe the head injury. Pupil size and reaction to light should be assessed frequently for changes. Ipsilateral pupil dilation is an indication of herniation from a hematoma, lesion, or edema and is often a late sign.

Blood pressure and heart rate must be assessed frequently to ensure that brain tissues are adequately perfused (Clochesy et al., 1993). Bradycardia, systolic hypertension, and bradypnea are the set of clinical manifestations known as Cushing's triad; however, these are late signs of increased ICP. According to Clochesy et al. (1993), bradycardia, junctional escape rhythms, and idioventricular rhythms can occur in patients with cerebral hemorrhage and increased ICP. Therefore, continuous cardiac monitoring is required. Respiratory patterns must be assessed frequently to identify possible herniation.

Urine output, serum sodium, and osmolarity levels must be monitored to rule out the syndrome of inappropriate antidiuretic hormone (SIADH), which may be a secondary effect of head injury (Reimer, 1989).

9. **What other nursing interventions are required for the patient with EDH.**

For those patients who are immobilized because of ventilator therapy or comatose state, nursing measures must be focused on prevention of complications such as atrophy of muscles and contractures, constipation, skin breakdown, and pulmonary complications. Musculoskeletal complications may be prevented by range of motion exercises and repositioning. Patients should be placed on a bowel regimen that includes a stool softener. Pressure ulcers can be prevented with adequate nutrition and pressure-relieving devices, such as an altering pressure mattress or therapeutic rotating bed. Aggressive pulmonary hygiene with position changes is necessary to prevent atelectasis and pneumonia (Ammons, 1990).

Nutritional support should begin within a few days of the head injury to meet the increase in metabolic requirements. Ammons (1990), identified total parenteral nutrition as having better outcomes than tube feeding for the unconscious patient. Glucose must be administered cautiously since hyperglycemia increases oxygen consumption, carbon dioxide production, and energy expenditure (Ammons, 1990). The patient should also be observed for stress ulcers, especially if receiving steroids (Reimer, 1989). The pH of gastric contents should be assessed daily. Prophylactic histamine$_2$ (H$_2$) antagonists such as ranitidine (Zantac) or piperacillin (Pipracil) are usually given.

The emotional needs of the patient and family must be considered at all times, especially when the outcomes of the injury are unknown.

Head-injured patients tend to experience emotional instability, aggressiveness, depression, and impaired concentration. The nursing staff must continually provide emotional support and education regarding treatments and the plan of care to both the patient and family.

10. **Discuss the rationale for monitoring arterial blood gases in the patient with a head injury?**

According to Clochesy et al. (1993), arterial blood gases must be monitored at least every 6 hours for hypoxemia and hypercapnia. Hypoxemia and hypercapnia lead to cerebral vasodilation, increased blood volume in the brain, and subsequently increased ICP (Ammons, 1990).

11. **List the nursing diagnoses that may be appropriate for the patient with EDH.**

> ➤ alteration in cerebral tissue perfusion
> ➤ high risk for infection
> ➤ impaired gas exchange
> ➤ ineffective breathing patterns
> ➤ impaired physical mobility
> ➤ high risk for fluid volume deficit
> ➤ high risk for fluid volume excess
> ➤ ineffective family coping
> ➤ high risk for injury
> ➤ altered thought processes
> ➤ knowledge deficit
> ➤ ineffective airway clearance
> ➤ impaired verbal communication

Epidural Hematoma

Alspach, J. G. (1991). *Core curriculum for critical care nursing*. Philadelphia: Saunders.

Ammons, A. M. (1990). Cerebral injuries and intracranial hemorrhages as a result of trauma. *Nursing Clinics of North America, 25*(1), 23–32.

Andrus, C. (1991). Intracranial pressure: Dynamics and nursing management. *Journal of Neuroscience Nursing, 23*(2), 85–90.

Aumick, J. (1991). Head trauma: Guidelines for care. *RN, 4,* 27–31.

Clochesy, J. M., Breu, C., Cardin, S., Rudy, E. B. & Whittaker, A. A. (1993). *Critical care nursing*. Philadelphia: Saunders.

Evans, T. C., & Billittier, A. J. (1990). Rationale for burr hole decompression in the emergency management of head injuries. *Topics in Emergency Medicine, 11*(4), 64–68.

Hartshorn, J., Lamborn, M. & Noll, M. L. (1993). *Introduction to critical care nursing*. Philadelphia: Saunders.

Manifold, S. L. (1986). Craniocerebral trauma: A review of primary and secondary injury and therapeutic modalities. *Focus on Critical Care, 13*(2), 22–35.

Mercado, R. G. (1989). Traumatic extradural hematoma of the cervical spine. *Neurosurgery, 24*(3), 410–414.

Reimer, M. (1989). Head injured patients. *Nursing, 3,* 34–41.

Smith, H. K., & Miller, J. D. (1991). The danger of an ultra-early computed tomographic scan in a patient with an evolving acute epidural hematoma. *Neurosurgery, 29*(8), 258–260.

Wilberger, J. E. (1990). Emergency burr holes: Current role in neurosurgical acute care. *Topics in Emergency Medicine, 11*(4), 69–74.

16

Gastrointestinal Tract Bleeding

Michael D. O'Grady, MSN, RN

CASE PRESENTATION

At 6 PM James Jones, age 44 years, was transferred from the emergency department (ED) to the intensive care unit (ICU) with a diagnosis of probable gastrointestinal (GI) tract bleeding. The ED history states he had been seen as an outpatient 1 week before because of epigastric pain after drinking alcohol heavily at a New Year party. He stated he had been "hung over and nauseated" for 48 hours and has had severe epigastric pain since the party. He was diagnosed as having gastritis and was sent home with an antiemetic and antacid medication. Although he returned to his job as a commodities trader, he has not felt well since the party. He has been taking two buffered aspirin 2 to 3 times daily in addition to the prescribed medications. He returned to the ED because of nausea, two episodes of vomiting of large amounts, and complaints of extreme weakness. He also experienced dizziness when he stood or sat up abruptly.

Admission vital signs and laboratory data include the following:

BP   96/60 lying flat
HR   126 bpm
Respirations 20/min
Temperature   37.9° C (100.2° F) (tympanic [T])
Hgb   12.5 g/dl
Hct   40%
WBCs   1200/mm³

Emergency Department Record

A 14 gauge nasogastric tube (NGT) was placed in the ED; 350 ml of dark brown "coffee-grounds" liquid returned. The liquid tested positive for guaiac. His stomach was lavaged with 500 ml of normal saline (NS), and the drainage was subsequently clear.

The ICU admission orders were as follows:

1. Monitor electrocardiogram (ECG), vital signs, and intake and output every hour.
2. Maintain bed rest.
3. Nothing by mouth (NPO), except for sips with oral medications.
4. Set NGT to low intermittent suction. If active bleeding occurs, notify physician and irrigate with 30 ml NS q2h and prn until drainage is clear.
5. Give medications orally; clamp NGT for 30 minutes following administration of medication.
6. Give magnesium hydroxide (Mylanta) 30 ml q4h PO.
7. Give cimetidine (Tagamet) 300 mg q6h PO.
8. Give promethazine (Phenergan) 25 mg IM q6h prn for nausea.
9. Give 5% dextrose in lactated Ringers solution (D₅LR) 100 ml/h IV.
10. Schedule for esophagogastroduodenoscopy (EGD) at 7 AM in GI laboratory.
11. Hemoglobin (Hgb) and hematocrit (Hct) at 9 PM.
12. Complete blood count (CBC) and platelet count, prothrombin time, partial thromboplastin time (PTT), chemistry 12, electrolytes, and urinalysis in AM.

Mr. Jones had an uneventful evening. His chart reflected the data shown in Table 16–1.

At midnight his NGT was clamped to administer medication. When the NGT was unclamped at 12:30 AM, 100 ml of bloody drainage had returned. He became restless and anxious. His skin was pale gray and moist. Oxygen was started by nasal cannula at 4 L/min. Vital signs at 12:30 AM were as follows:

BP	84/50
HR	136 bpm
Respirations	20/min

Table 16–1   Vital Signs and Flow Sheet Data

Time	HR (bpm)	Respirations (/min)	BP (mm Hg)	
1900	112	16	104/64	
2000	115	18	100/60	Temperature 37.9° C (100.2° F)
2100	120	20	98/60	
2200	128	20	100/60	Hgb 12.3 g/dl Hct 36%
2300	128	20	96/54	Sleeping
0000	132	20	92/50	Temperature 36.7° C (98° F) (T) voided 120 ml amber

The physician was called, and the following orders were received:

1. Lavage NGT with saline until clear.
2. Stat Hgb and Hct.
3. Type and crossmatch for 2 U of packed red blood cells. Type and screen for an additional 4 U of packed red blood cells.
4. Have surgeon on call. Place a triple lumen subclavian IV line.
5. Measure central venous pressure (CVP) q1h; if below 10 mm Hg, give a 500 ml NS IV fluid challenge. Repeat fluid challenge once if needed.
6. Place a Foley catheter and measure urine hourly.

The orders were carried out. No urine was obtained from the catheter. Laboratory data at 1 AM read as follows:

CVP 8 mm Hg
Hgb 11 g/dl
Hct 31%

At 1:30 AM after two 500 ml fluid challenges, Mr. Jones' CVP was 12 mm Hg, and he had urine output via catheter. IV lines were ordered to infuse D₅LR at 50 ml/h in the peripheral line and NS at 150 ml/h in the central line. His chart reflected the data shown in Table 16–2.

At 7:10 AM Mr. Jones was transported to the GI laboratory for the EGD. The gastroenterologist found diffuse gastritis with a 2 cm duodenal ulcer. A biopsy specimen taken from the gastric wall was tested for *Helicobacter pylori*. No clots were visible, and the ulcer was not actively bleeding. Histologic testing of the biopsy specimen confirmed *H. pylori* infection, and the laboratory ran a culture and sensitivity screening.

Pharmacologic treatment for *H. pylori* was instituted along with histamine receptor antagonists and supplemental antacids. Mr. Jones' physicians elected to treat him conservatively with medication, and Mr. Jones progressed well. He was released from the ICU to the step-down unit in 24 hours and discharged home after 3 days. His medical treatment continued at home with follow-up by physician appointments.

Table 16–2   Vital Signs and Flow Sheet Data

Time	HR (bpm)	Respirations (/min)	BP (mm Hg)	CVP (mm Hg)	Urine Output (ml)	
0200	120	20	84/50	10	30	
0300	116	20	90/58	12	75	
0400	112	20	94/62	12	90	
0500	110	18	96/64	12	94	
0600	110	18	98/62	13	80	
0700	104	18	98/64	12	68	Hgb 10.1 g/dl Hct 28%

Gastrointestinal Tract Bleeding

1. Identify predisposing conditions to GI tract bleeding and list three specific to Mr. Jones.

2. What is the incidence and mortality of GI tract bleeding?

3. Discriminate between the characteristics of upper and lower GI tract bleeding.

4. What complication did Mr. Jones demonstrate?

5. Explain the action and potential complications of antacid treatment.

6. Explain the action and side effects of histamine receptor antagonists.

7. Which factors determine whether blood products will be administered to a patient with GI tract bleeding?

8. Mr. Jones' Hgb and Hct dropped dramatically from admission to 7 AM. Discuss the drop in Hgb and Hct in relation to Mr. Jones' blood loss.

9. If Mr. Jones had been actively bleeding, what other medical procedures could be done to stop the bleeding?

10. What are the indications and types of surgical procedures for upper GI tract bleeding?

11. Identify six nursing diagnoses appropriate for Mr. Jones.

12. What is the incidence of *H. pylori* infection in gastritis and duodenal ulcer?

13. What is the treatment of choice for *H. pylori* infection?

QUESTIONS AND ANSWERS

Gastrointestinal Tract Bleeding

1. **Identify predisposing conditions to GI tract bleeding and list three specific to Mr. Jones.**

   Causes of acute upper GI tract bleeding include gastric and duodenal ulcers, erosive gastritis, esophageal varices, Mallory-Weiss tears, esophagitis, and duodenitis. Mr. Jones' predisposing factors included gastritis secondary to acute alcohol ingestion, aspirin intake, and a stressful job as a commodities trader. Men are diagnosed with peptic ulcers three to four times more frequently than women (Clochesy, Breu, Cardin, Rudy, & Whittaker, 1993).

2. **What is the incidence and mortality of GI tract bleeding?**

   One quarter of a million Americans are affected by acute GI tract bleeding each year with a mortality rate reported at 20%. In high-risk populations the mortality may be as high as 44% (Clochesy et al., 1993; Grove & Klofas, 1990).

3. **Discriminate between the characteristics of upper and lower GI tract bleeding.**

   Bleeding below the ligament of Treitz is defined as lower GI tract bleeding. Upper GI tract bleeding is characterized by hematemesis or melena. Lower GI tract bleeding is characterized by hematochezia (passage of bright red blood from the rectum). In cases of massive rapid upper GI tract bleeding the patient may exhibit both hematemesis and hematochezia. Bleeding below the ligament of Treitz seldom results in vomiting of blood. Vomiting of blood or coffee-ground emesis is a reliable indication of upper GI tract bleeding (Clochesy et al., 1993).

4. **What complication did Mr. Jones demonstrate?**

   Mr. Jones demonstrated hypovolemia due to blood loss. His tachycardia, vital sign changes, drop in urine output, skin color changes, and restlessness indicated moderate to severe hemorrhagic shock (Gardner & Messner, 1992; Hartshorn, Lamborn, & Noll, 1993).

5. Explain the action and potential complications of antacid treatment.

Antacids work by chemical neutralization of stomach (hydrochloric) acid. By increasing the pH of the stomach, antacids decrease the erosion of the stomach and duodenum by gastric acid. Long-term use of antacids may lead to metabolic alkalosis, increased serum sodium levels (sodium bicarbonate antacids), hypercalcemia and renal impairment (calcium carbonate antacids), constipation, phosphate depletion (aluminum-containing antacids), diarrhea and hypermagnesemia (magnesium-containing antacids). Administration of antacids and histamine$_2$ (H$_2$) blockers must be staggered to allow for maximum absorption of both drugs (Clochesy et al., 1993).

6. Explain the action and side effects of histamine receptor antagonists.

H$_2$ receptor antagonists inhibit the action of histamine on the receptor sites of the parietal cells by competing for the sites. They reduce the amount and concentration of gastric secretions. Examples include ranitidine (Zantac), cimetidine (Tagamet), and famotidine (Pepcid). Side effects include confusion, lethargy, seizures, hypotension, hepatotoxicity, thrombocytopenia, gynecomastia, and male impotence (Clochesy et al., 1993).

7. Which factors determine whether blood products will be administered to a patient with GI tract bleeding?

Blood administration is based on the level of shock, the response to IV fluid replacement, and changes in the Hgb and Hct levels. Unstable vital signs after infusion of 2 L of crystalloid fluid replacement indicate the need for blood replacement. An Hgb below 10 mg/dl and Hct below 25% are also used as indicators for blood replacement. The amount of bloody drainage and the presence of active bleeding also increase the requirement for blood replacement. The changes in Hgb and Hct are not immediate. A drop in these levels may not occur for hours because of the compensatory mechanisms in the vascular system (Grove & Klofas, 1990; Lockhart & Hoelsken, 1993).

8. Mr. Jones' Hgb and Hct dropped dramatically from admission to 7 AM. Discuss the drop in Hgb and Hct in relation to Mr. Jones' blood loss.

The primary cause of the drop in Hgb and Hct was blood loss. However, some of the effect was caused by fluid replacement diluting the

Hct levels in the blood. Mr. Jones had relative hemoconcentration due to blood loss and compensation by the body. When he received fluid replacement, the Hct and Hgb became diluted and reflected the amount of blood loss (Gardener & Messner, 1992).

9. **If Mr. Jones had been actively bleeding, what other medical procedures could be done to stop the bleeding?**

   Several different therapies may have been used to stop GI tract bleeding (Clochesy et al., 1993; Grove & Klofas, 1990):

   - Iced saline lavage may have been used. However, the effectiveness of this treatment is not clear. The most recent evidence suggests that iced saline is no more helpful in halting bleeding than tepid saline.
   - The use of Ewald, Cantor, or the Sengstaken-Blakemore tubes to apply direct pressure to bleeding esophageal varices has been largely replaced by other therapies.
   - Vasopressin infusion acts to constrict arteries and contract the bowel, thus reducing blood flow and stimulating the formation of thrombus. Vasopressin is normally used for massive GI hemorrhage.
   - Endoscopic electrocoagulation is frequently used to treat bleeding during endoscopic examination.
   - Transcatheter embolization using angiography to identify and embolize a bleeding artery may also be used. Substances such as Gelfoam, cyanoacrylate glue (Crazy Glue), coils, clots, and polyvinyl alcohol may be used. Ischemia or infarction may occur if there is inadequate collateral circulation.
   - Photocoagulation by lasers is also increasingly being used as a treatment modality for GI tract bleeding. It is more expensive than electrocoagulation and has similar results.

10. **What are the indications and types of surgical procedures for upper GI tract bleeding?**

    Indications for surgical interventions are persistent bleeding after medical treatment, presence of neoplasm or malignancy, perforation of obstruction, and recurrence of ulcers.

    Surgical interventions range from oversewing the ulcer site to gastric resection. Billroth I or II indicate partial resection of the stomach. Intractable ulcer disease and bleeding may be treated with a total gastrectomy.

    Vagotomy may be done in conjunction with or separate from the above operations. Vagotomy reduces the gastric secretions by eliminating the vagal stimulation to the stomach (Clochesy et al., 1993).

11. Identify six nursing diagnoses appropriate for Mr. Jones.

> ➤ actual fluid volume deficit related to blood loss, active bleeding, decreased circulatory volume
> ➤ altered tissue perfusion related to decreased oxygen transport, increased oxygen demand, metabolic acidosis
> ➤ high risk for injury related to hemorrhage, nasogastric intubation, altered consciousness
> ➤ anxiety related to fear of death, hemorrhage, treatments
> ➤ knowledge deficit related to contributing factors, diet, medications, alcohol intake, lifestyle, and treatments
> ➤ alteration in nutrition: less than body requirement related to NPO status and NGT suctioning (Clochesy et al., 1993)

12. What is the incidence of *H. pylori* infection in gastritis and duodenal ulcer?

H. pylori is almost universal in cases of gastritis and duodenal ulcer. It is seen in more than 90% of these cases. *H. pylori* was first identified in 1983. It is recognized as the major causative factor in environmental (nonautoimmune) gastritis and peptic ulcer (Fennerty, 1994).

13. What is the treatment of choice for *H. pylori* infection?

H. pylori eradication therapy usually consists of bismuth and two antibiotics. Eight tablets of bismuth with tetracycline 2 g and metronidazole 750 mg daily for 2 weeks has been recommended as the treatment. Current therapy may substitute omeprazole, amoxicillin, or clarithromycin for the previously mentioned antibiotics. These newer antibiotics have high rates of eradication and are tolerated better by patients. Antibiotics may also be prescribed without bismuth. Recurrence of ulcers after healing is less than 10%, and reinfection rates are 1% to 2% per year after treatment. Prevention of *H. pylori* infection and gastric ulcer is currently under investigation (Fennerty, 1994; Forbes et al., 1994).

REFERENCES

Gastrointestinal Tract Bleeding

Clochesy, J. M., Breu, C., Cardin, S., Rudy, E. B., & Whittaker, A. A. (1993). *Critical care cursing*. Philadelphia: Saunders.

Fennerty, M. B. (1994). *Helicobacter pylori. Archives of Internal Medicine, 154,* 721–727.

Forbes, G. M., Glaser, M. E., Cullen, D. J. E., Warren, J. R., Christiansen, K. J., Marshall, B. J., & Collins, B. J. (1994). Duodenal ulcer treated with *Helicobacter pylori* eradication: Seven-year follow-up. *Lancet, 343,* 258–260.

Gardener, S., & Messner, R. (1992, December). Upper GI bleeds. *RN,* 42–47.

Grove, K. L., & Klofas, E. S. (1990). Acute gastrointestinal hemorrhage. *Topics in Emergency Medicine, 12*(2), 9–16.

Hartshorn, J., Lamborn, M., & Noll, M. L. (1993). *Introduction to critical care nursing*. Philadelphia: Saunders.

Lockhart, J., & Hoelsken, R. (1993, March). Abdominal hemorrhage. *Nursing 93, 33.*

17

Acute Pancreatitis

Ann H. White, MSN, MBA, RN, CNA

CASE PRESENTATION

Jan, a 43-year-old woman, presented to the emergency department with acute abdominal pain. This pain had been present for approximately 2 days but had increased in severity over the last 6 hours. The pain was localized to the upper left abdominal quadrant with some radiation to the back. She had vomited three times in the last 6 hours with no relief of pain. Jan's brother, who accompanied her to the emergency department, reported Jan drinks heavily and has a past history of intravenous (IV) drug use. Her brother reported she no longer uses IV drugs but has continued to drink at least a fifth of hard liquor a day. Jan admitted to having a past problem with alcohol and drug use but stated she is now clean. Jan agreed to blood work being drawn, including a blood alcohol and drug screening.

Vital signs and laboratory results obtained in the emergency department follow:

BP   134/76
HR   68 bpm
Respirations 24/min
Temperature 38.6° C (101.4° F) (tympanic)

Complete blood count		Na$^+$	141 mmol/L
WBCs	11 x 10^3/mm^3	K$^+$	3.0 mmol/L
RBCs	4.62 x 10^6/mm^3	Total protein	4.9 g/dl
Hgb	12.3 g/dl	Albumin	2.4 g/dl
Hct	52%	Alkaline phosphatase	120 U/L
Amylase	505 U/L	AST (SGOT)	307 U/L
Lipase	519 U/L	LDH	891 U/L
Glucose	266 mg/dl	Blood alcohol	205 mg/dl
Ca	8.3 mg/dl	Drug screening	results pending

pH	7.35
Pco$_2$	33 mm Hg
Po$_2$	90 mm Hg
HCO$_3^-$	25 mmol/L
Base excess	1
Sao$_2$	91%

While in the emergency department, Jan reported increased pain in the upper left abdominal quadrant. She vomited 100 ml of brown liquid. Her vital signs were as follows:

BP	90/60
HR	100 bpm
Respirations	28/min
Temperature	39.4° C (103° F) (tympanic)

On physical examination, the abdomen was tender with guarding in all abdominal quadrants, and bowel sounds were hypoactive. A nasogastric tube was inserted and an IV started in the emergency department. Jan was transferred to the critical care unit (CCU) with a preliminary diagnosis of acute pancreatitis. The following orders accompanied Jan to the CCU:

- IV of 0.45% NSS with 20 mEq potassium in each bag to run at 125 ml/h
- daily CBC, amylase, lipase, and SMAC 20
- ABGs in the AM
- morphine sulfate 3 mg IV push q2h prn for severe pain
- NPO (no ice chips)
- nasogastric tube to intermittent suction
- blood cultures x 2 if not done in the emergency department
- gentamicin (Garamycin) 80 mg IV piggyback q8h after blood cultures drawn

The laboratory results after the first 24 hours in the CCU are listed below.

CBC				
WBCs	14.6 x 10^3/mm^3	Na$^+$	139 mmol/L
RBCs	3.82 x 10^6/mm^3	K$^+$	3.2 mmol/L
Hgb	10.3 g/dl	Total protein	4.6 g/dl
Hct	42%	Albumin	2.2 g/dl
Amylase	575 U/L	Alkaline phosphatase	139 U/L
Lipase	789 U/L	AST (SGOT)	436 U/L
Glucose	203 mg/dl	LDH	798 U/L
Ca	7.8 mg/dl	Drug screening	results negative

pH	7.22
Pco$_2$	26 mm Hg
Po$_2$	84 mm Hg
HCO$_3^-$	19 mmol/L
Base excess	–6
Sao$_2$	80%

Additional orders received included the following:

1. Change IV to 0.45% NSS with 30 mEq potassium and 1 ampule of 10% calcium gluconate to run at 125 ml/h.
2. Administer oxygen at 2 L via nasal cannula.
3. Repeat ABGs in AM.

Jan's heart monitor revealed a normal sinus rhythm with a prolonged QT interval. Jan's pain subsided after 48 hours, bowel sounds were heard, and she was started on a liquid diet. After 24 hours without pain, Jan was transferred to a medical-surgical unit.

QUESTIONS

Acute Pancreatitis

1. Discuss the pathophysiology of acute pancreatitis.

2. Describe the classic assessment findings that support a diagnosis of acute pancreatitis. Relate Jan's history and physical assessment findings to this description.

3. Compare and contrast hemorrhagic and nonhemorrhagic acute pancreatitis.

4. Jan requested pain medication. What should be the initial nursing actions?

5. Discuss the appropriateness of administering gentamicin (Garamycin) to patients with acute pancreatitis.

6. Discuss significant diagnostic studies that assist in confirming or in monitoring the progress of acute pancreatitis. Relate the diagnostic studies completed on Jan to this discussion.

7. Discuss the dietary management of a patient with acute pancreatitis. What is the purpose of the nasogastric tube and the NPO status?

8. List the nursing diagnoses, outcomes, and interventions appropriate for a patient diagnosed with acute pancreatitis.

9. Identify complications of acute pancreatitis. Based on the change in vital signs, laboratory data, and history, which complication has most likely occurred in this case study?

10. Discuss the prognosis of a patient with acute pancreatitis.

11. Discuss the psychosocial aspects of caring for a patient with acute pancreatitis.

QUESTIONS AND ANSWERS

Acute Pancreatitis

1. **Discuss the pathophysiology of acute pancreatitis.**

Acute pancreatitis results from the premature activation of pancreatic enzymes that cause autodigestion and major cellular destruction of the pancreas and surrounding gastrointestinal structures. The actual pathophysiology is unknown; however, several theories have been proposed to explain the destruction of the pancreatic tissue, none of which are conclusive.

Hennessey (1993) identifies six theories that have been proposed to explain the autodigestion process. The following summarizes these theories:

- Certain substances act as cell toxins, which are believed to alter the metabolic processes of the acinar cells. The acinar cells are responsible for the production and release of pancreatic juice, which contains digestive enzymes. Normally, these enzymes are not activated until they reach the intestines. The hormone cholecystokinin (pancreozymin) stimulates the release of the enzymes through the pancreatic duct system to reach the intestine. Once in the intestine, trypsinogen is converted to trypsin, which activates the other pancreatic enzymes (Hadley & Fitzsimmons, 1990). This theory postulates that the toxic material alters the pancreatic release of these enzymes (Fain & Armato-Vealey, 1988; Krumberger, 1993b).
- Alcohol consumption has been closely associated with pancreatitis. The exact mechanism is unclear. However, alcohol has been found to be irritating to the pancreas. Alcohol causes protein precipitation, which may lead to obstruction of the ducts. Alcohol also produces spasms in the sphincter of Oddi, which leads to further obstruction of the duct system (Hadley & Fitzsimmons, 1990). If the ducts are obstructed, the release of pancreatic juice is blocked, and the enzymes begin to digest the pancreas. In addition, alcohol has been found to increase the acid levels in the stomach. A lowering of the pH in the stomach is a powerful stimulant for the pancreas to release pancreatic juice (Brown, 1991).

- Ductal hypertension is another theory. This theory focuses on the obstruction in the release of pancreatic juices as a result of distal obstruction of the biliary ductal system. The distal obstruction is commonly caused by gallstones actually blocking the duct or by the resulting edema that forms as a gallstone passes. The resulting ductal hypertension may result in the rupture of small ducts and the release of the enzymes (Hadley & Fitzsimmons, 1990).
- The bile reflux theory is that gallstone(s) may obstruct the flow of bile. As a result, the bile takes the path of least resistance, which is to back up into the pancreatic duct, leading to the activation of the enzymes. This is also referred to as the common channel theory. This theory is being challenged as an increasing number of patients who have pancreatitis but do not have this common channel are found.
- The duodenal reflux theory proposes that the duodenal contents back up into the pancreas. Because of activation on the pancreatic enzymes when they reach the intestines, autodigestion and cell damage begin.
- The final theory is the activation of intracellular protease. As a result there is release of lysosomes that cross the acinar cell wall, activate the enzymes, and lead to release of these activated enzymes into the pancreatic and surrounding tissues.

Other factors that can lead to acute pancreatitis include the use of certain drugs such as thiazides, acetaminophen, tetracyclines, and estrogen-containing contraceptives. Surgical procedures including exploration of the common bile duct, pancreatic biopsy, and an endoscopic retrograde cholangiopancreatography (ERCP) may also predispose the patient to the development of acute pancreatitis (Burrell, 1992).

Whatever the cause, the result is autodigestion and cellular damage in the pancreas and surrounding tissues. Once the cycle is begun, it is perpetuated by the cellular damage. The damage to the pancreatic cells causes cell destruction and death. This results in further release of pancreatic enzymes and destruction of more pancreatic cells due to autodigestion. The cycle continues until medical intervention interrupts the cycle.

2. **Describe the classic assessment findings that support a diagnosis of acute pancreatitis. Relate Jan's history and physical assessment findings to this description.**

History taking should include gathering detailed information regarding gallbladder disease, recent abdominal surgical procedures, alcohol use, and prescription and over the counter (OTC) medication use. Specific medications to inquire about include thiazides, acetaminophen, tetracyclines, and oral contraceptives containing estrogen. The patient should be asked about recent consumption of alcohol or a large meal with high levels of fat. A family history of pancreatic or gall-bladder disease is of interest when completing the history (Ignatavi-cious & Bayne, 1991).

Classic assessment findings include abdominal pain that is almost al-ways severe, persistent, and penetrating (Hadley & Fitzsimmons, 1990). Abdominal pain that differs in intensity is usually not associated with acute pancreatitis (Hennessey, 1993). The pain is typically located in the upper left abdominal quadrant or may be in the midepigastric area and may radiate to the back or flank areas. The onset of pain may be directly associated with consuming alcohol or a large meal with fatty foods. Patients experiencing pain associated with acute pancreatitis pre-fer to sit up or lie in a fetal position to decrease the pain. The pain is made worse by lying supine or walking.

Physical assessment of the abdomen may include decreased or absent bowel sounds. The abdomen may be somewhat distended, guarded, and tender to palpation. This tenderness is noted more in the upper quadrants but may be present in all four abdominal quadrants. Ecchy-motic areas may be noted in the flank and umbilical areas.

Additionally, nausea and vomiting occur. Vomiting without a de-crease in pain is considered a hallmark symptom of acute pancreatitis (Hennessey, 1993). Vomiting, along with the extensive third spacing, may lead to dehydration. As a result, the patient may present with poor skin turgor and dry mucous membranes. With extensive loss of fluid, symptoms of hypovolemic shock may be seen.

Because the respiratory system may be seriously compromised by the development of acute pancreatitis, respirations and lung sounds must be carefully monitored. These include dyspnea, tachypnea, hypoxemia, diminished or absent breath sounds especially in the left base, and re-ferred pain to the shoulder. Adult respiratory distress syndrome (ARDS) is the most serious respiratory problem associated with acute pancreatitis, requiring careful monitoring.

Jan had several assessment findings that supported the diagnosis of acute pancreatitis. Her history of alcohol abuse is definitely a factor. Al-though alcohol abuse and acute pancreatitis are more commonly asso-ciated with men in their 50s, it does not preclude other patients having this clinical picture. Jan also has the abdominal pain and radiation asso-ciated with acute pancreatitis. She vomited without relief of pain, which further supports the diagnosis of acute pancreatitis. Diagnostic criteria for acute pancreatitis are listed in Table 17–1.

3. **Compare and contrast hemorrhagic and nonhemorrhagic acute pancreatitis.**

The literature states that acute pancreatitis has two stages. The first stage is nonhemorrhagic or acute interstitial or acute edematous pan-creatitis. In this stage the activated enzymes are released, causing cel-

Table 17–1   Diagnostic Criteria for Acute Pancreatitis

Laboratory Value	Pancreatitis
Serum analyses	Elevated
Serum isoamylase	Elevated
Urine analyses	Elevated
Serum lipase	Elevated
Serum triglycerides	Elevated
Hematocrit	Elevated or decreased
Sodium	Decreased
Potassium	Decreased
Calcium	Decreased
Magnesium	Decreased
Glucose	Elevated
Albumin	Decreased
WBC count	May be elevated
Bilirubin	May be elevated
BUN	May be elevated
Liver enzymes	May be elevated
Arterial blood gases	Hypoxemia and metabolic acidosis

lular damage. Typical symptoms have been described in the previous answer.

The second stage is referred to as hemorrhagic or necrotizing pancreatitis and is considered the more serious form. This stage is characterized by necrosis of the pancreatic tissue with bleeding into the surrounding tissue. The patient may have all the symptoms of nonhemorrhagic pancreatitis plus two additional signs of hemorrhagic pancreatitis: Turner's sign and Cullen's sign (Fain & Armato-Vealey, 1988). Turner's sign is the presence of ecchymotic areas seen in the flank areas. Cullen's sign is the presence of ecchymosis around the umbilical area. The bleeding into the tissue is thought to be the result of damage caused by circulating trypsin to the intravascular structures (Fain & Armato-Vealey, 1988). Both signs are grave indications of the progression of the disease (Fain & Armato-Vealey, 1988).

4. **Jan requested pain medication. What should be the initial nursing actions?**

A call to the physician is the most appropriate action to ensure the most effective pain medication is given.

Opiate analgesics (morphine) are widely used for the relief of acute pain. However, in this case, morphine is not the drug of choice to manage pancreatic pain. Because morphine causes biliary colic and spasms of the sphincter of Oddi, meperidine (Demerol) is usually ordered for a patient with acute pancreatitis (Spencer, Nichols, Lipkin, Henderson, & West, 1993). Krumberger (1993a) reported the use of meperidine, levorphanol, or fentanyl with success. These drugs do not induce spasms of the sphincter of Oddi, which are believed to be the cause of the pain. However, recent studies with morphine have found that patients achieve significant pain relief with minimal effect on the sphincter of Oddi (Krumberger, 1993a).

Pain management is an important component of treating patients diagnosed with acute pancreatitis. Not only does the patient experience a great deal of discomfort, severe pain increases the metabolic activity in the body. This increase in metabolic activity further increases the release of pancreatic enzymes, which is detrimental because of the pathology occurring in the pancreas. The use of a patient-controlled analgesia (PCA) pump or the scheduled use of analgesics every 2 to 3 hours has been suggested to maintain pain control (Hennessey, 1993).

5. **Discuss the appropriateness of administering gentamicin (Garamycin) to patients with acute pancreatitis.**

The use of antimicrobials in the treatment of mild to moderate forms of acute pancreatitis has not been supported by research findings or clinical trials. Antimicrobials are sometimes ordered if an infection is suspected or in severe cases of acute pancreatitis (Hennessey, 1993). Typically, antimicrobials are only ordered once an infection has been confirmed through culture and sensitivity or when additional clinical symptoms, such as an elevation in temperature, are present. The initial antimicrobials of choice are gentamicin or piperacillin (Pipracil) until the results of the culture and sensitivity are obtained.

6. **Discuss significant diagnostic studies that assist in confirming or in monitoring the progress of acute pancreatitis. Relate the diagnostic studies completed on Jan to this discussion.**

Specific laboratory studies to assist in confirming the diagnosis of acute pancreatitis include serum and urine amylase levels, isoamylase levels, serum lipase levels, complete blood count, SMAC 20 (electrolytes, blood sugar, liver enzymes, blood urea nitrogen [BUN]), arterial blood gases, and culture and sensitivity of blood and any drainage.

Serum and urine levels of amylase are usually elevated. The serum amylase level is elevated within the first 24 to 48 hours after the onset of symptoms. However, many other disease processes can also cause an elevation, and this elevation may not be reflective of the extensiveness of the disease process. Isoamylase levels are more specific but many laboratories are unable to perform these types of tests because they do not have the equipment required. Brown (1991) reported that an elevation in the isoamylase P_4 is indicative of acute pancreatitis. Krumberger (1993b) reported that a patient with an elevated serum amylase three times the normal level (60 to 160 Somogyi U/dl) with the symptoms associated with acute pancreatitis should be considered to have acute pancreatitis. Krumberger (1993b) further reported that clinical studies are being conducted on the other enzymes, including trypsin, elastase, and phospholipase A, but have not been found any more reliable than amylase and lipase. Serum lipase levels are also elevated during the first 24 to 48 hours of the onset of symptoms and remain elevated for 5 to 7 days. Lipase is predominantly found in the pancreas; however, other disease processes can cause this elevation.

Nonspecific abnormal laboratory findings include an elevated white blood cell (WBC) count due to the infection. Hematocrit may be elevated initially because of third space fluid losses but later may decrease because of hemorrhaging. Sodium, potassium, calcium, and magnesium levels may be decreased because of vomiting and the saponification of fats. The blood sugar may be elevated if the islets of Langerhans are affected by the disease process and are unable to produce insulin. The BUN may be elevated because of dehydration. Liver enzymes will also be elevated if biliary tract disease is involved.

ABG determinations are imperative because of the respiratory compromise associated with acute pancreatitis. Serial ABGs should be drawn to monitor development of metabolic acidosis and hypoxemia. A culture and sensitivity should be taken of the blood and any other drainage to gather information about the infectious process. The sensitivity will identify any antimicrobials that must be started.

Radiologic testing that may be useful in the diagnosis of acute pancreatitis includes flat plates of the abdomen, ultrasound, computed tomography (CT) scan, or magnetic resonance imaging (MRI) with specific detail to the pancreas. Flat plate of the abdomen may aid in identifying an ileus of the small bowel, which is present in 10% to 55% of patients with acute pancreatitis (Stewart, 1989). Ultrasound, CT scan, and MRI are more commonly used today. Specific detail of the involved pancreas and surrounding structures may be well defined with the use of these radiologic tests. If the patient is obese, the CT scan and MRI are typically the tests of choice.

The final diagnostic tool to consider is an electrocardiogram (ECG), or telemetry. If the patient with acute pancreatitis has a low calcium level, the rhythm strips must be monitored carefully. Low calcium may lead to a prolonged QT interval, with the potential for R on T phenomenon and torsades de pointes or ventricular tachycardia. Correction of the calcium level should prevent the occurrence of dysrhythmias.

7. **Discuss the dietary management of a patient with acute pancreatitis. What is the purpose of the nasogastric tube and the NPO status?**

The initial strategy of diet management is to minimize pancreatic secretions. It was believed that placing a nasogastric tube connected to suction should indirectly decrease the release of pancreatic secretions by preventing the release of secretin (Hennessey, 1993). Secretin must have an acid environment to be released. With the nasogastric suction removing gastric secretions, it was thought that the acid environment would not be created. However, recent clinical studies have not demonstrated this to be true. Today, nasogastric suction should be used only in the case of vomiting, gastric distension, ileus, or an altered mental status.

The patient will be assigned NPO (including no ice chips) status for a period of time until the pain subsides, bowel sounds are clearly present, and the serum amylase levels are normal. Diet intake should begin gradually, starting with clear liquids and progressing to more solid food based on patient tolerance. As the diet is advanced, fat, cholesterol, and triglycerides should be kept to a minimum. If an increase in pain develops, the patient should return to an NPO status. An increase in pain indicates the release of enzymes into the tissue and the resulting autodigestion has begun again. Returning to the NPO status attempts to rest the pancreas and decrease or minimize pancreatic secretions.

Nutritional support is imperative during this time. The patient with acute pancreatitis requires aggressive therapy to meet metabolic and healing needs without stimulation of the pancreas. Total parenteral nutrition (TPN) should be considered for patients with moderate to severe pancreatitis. Composition of the TPN is dependent on the patient's clinical picture and laboratory values. Typically, an amino acid and glucose base is used with essential minerals and vitamins. Electrolyte replacement is dependent on the laboratory values. The inclusion of insulin in the TPN solution is dependent on the production of insulin by the pancreas and the blood sugar levels. Lipid preparations are not used in the patient with pancreatitis, as this will lead to an increase in the release of pancreatic enzymes (Krumberger, 1993a).

8. **List the nursing diagnoses, outcomes, and interventions appropriate for a patient diagnosed with acute pancreatitis.**

Hennessey (1993) developed a nursing care plan for the patient with acute pancreatitis. Although specific nursing diagnoses must be identified based on the patient's clinical picture, Hennessey's plan provides the basis for care. One additional nursing diagnosis has been added by the author to complete the nursing care plan for a patient with acute pancreatitis (Black & Matassarin-Jacobs, 1993; Briones, 1991). See Table 17–2 for nursing diagnoses, outcomes, and interventions.

9. **Identify complications of acute pancreatitis. Based on the change in vital signs, laboratory data, and history, which complication has most likely occurred in this case study?**

Common complications associated with acute pancreatitis include hypovolemic shock, which can lead to renal failure, pulmonary insult

Text continued on page 252

Table 17–2 Nursing Diagnoses, Outcomes, and Interventions for Acute Pancreatitis

Nursing Diagnoses	Outcome Criteria	Nursing Interventions
➤ Fluid volume deficit causing hemodynamic instability related to fluid, plasma, albumin, and blood losses into peritoneum and retroperitoneal space ➤ Dehydration due to nausea and vomiting and fever	Hemodynamic stability (blood pressure, pulse, central venous pressure; pulmonary arterial pressure, adequate peripheral circulation, urine output within normal limits	1. Monitor and record intake and output every hour. 2. Monitor and record central venous pressure, pulmonary arterial pressure. 3. Weigh patient daily. 4. Assess peripheral circulation and level of consciousness. 5. Monitor laboratory values for abnormal hemoglobin and hematocrit, electrolyte imbalance (calcium, magnesium, potassium), and blood urea nitrogen and creatinine. 6. Monitor for signs of bleeding (hemorrhagic pancreatitis: Cullen's sign, Turner's sign, increased abdominal girth). 7. Monitor for signs of hypocalcemia: Chvostek's sign, Trousseau's sign. 8. Monitor vital signs and blood pressure every hour. 9. Monitor for signs of cardiac failure such as dyspnea, chest pain, edema. 10. Provide intravenous fluids and blood products; monitor for signs of fluid overload, such as shortness of breath, edema, abnormal breath sounds (crackles).

Table 17–2   Nursing Diagnoses, Outcomes, and Interventions for Acute Pancreatitis *Continued*

Nursing Diagnoses	Outcome Criteria	Nursing Interventions
➤ Altered comfort; pain related to obstruction of pancreatic duct and diminished blood supply	Pain at tolerable level Vital signs stable	1. Assess patient's pain using pain-rating scale; utilize pain rating to evaluate response to pain management interventions. 2. Instruct patient to tell nurse when pain is present so that interventions can be initiated before the onset of severe pain. 3. Provide analgesics as ordered and before activity or diagnostic procedures; avoid use of morphine because it stimulates spasm of biliary and pancreatic ducts, thus increasing pain; remember to draw blood to determine amylase levels before giving first dose of analgesic to avoid false elevation in amylase. 4. Assist patient to assume a comfortable position to decrease pain; knee-chest or fetal position may provide relief in patients with mild pain. 5. Maintain bed rest and limit activities to reduce metabolic stress. 6. Administer humidified oxygen to avoid hypoxemia and help to decrease respiratory efforts. 7. Administer sedatives as ordered.

Table continued on following page

Table 17-2   Nursing Diagnoses, Outcomes, and Interventions for Acute Pancreatitis *Continued*

Nursing Diagnoses	Outcome Criteria	Nursing Interventions
		8. Eliminate oral intake and maintain nasogastic suction, if ordered, to decrease nausea and vomiting, thereby improving patient comfort. 9. Provide alternative methods of pain control, i.e., back massage, guided imagery, relaxation techniques.
➤ High risk for ineffective breathing patterns related to abdominal distension and pain	Maintains an effective breathing pattern	1. Assess respiratory status every 2 hours. 2. Maintain aggressive pulmonary hygiene. 3. Monitor fluid volume. 4. Place in semi-Fowler's position. 5. Maintain effective pain management.
➤ Impaired gas exchange related to inflammatory process and aggressive fluid therapy, respiratory distress syndrome, atelectasis, microemboli, pain, pleural effusion	Effective breathing patterns with adequate ventilation and oxygenation (PaO_2 and $PaCO_2$ within normal limits) Absence of atelectasis Absence of reduction of pleural effusion, pulmonary edema, microemboli	1. Administer analgesics to relieve pain and allow adequate ventilation. 2. Provide chest physiotherapy and reposition every 1 to 2 hours to prevent atelectasis. 3. Provide oxygen therapy as ordered to prevent hypoxemia. 4. Monitor daily chest x-rays for presence of atelectasis, effusion, edema, and microemboli; review coagulation studies if microemboli are present. 5. Perform respiratory assessments every 1

Table 17–2   Nursing Diagnoses, Outcomes, and Interventions for
Acute Pancreatitis *Continued*

Nursing Diagnoses	Outcome Criteria	Nursing Interventions
		to 2 hours and note presence of tachypnea, dyspnea, or wheezing; identify presence of adventitious breath sounds and absence of normal breath sounds.
		6. Suction whenever necessary and record amount, consistency, and color of secretions.
		7. Monitor arterial blood gas results for hypoxemia, hypercapnia, or acidosis.
➤ High risk for tissue injury related to pancreatic inflammation, peritonitis, formation of pseudocyst, formation of abscesses, bleeding, formation of fistulas	Absence of resolution of peritonitis Absence of fever, pseudocyst, abscesses	1. Administer antibiotics as ordered if causative organism(s) has been identified; preventive antibiotics are not indicated.
		2. Monitor vital signs, especially increases in temperature, and monitor for increase in white blood cell count.
		3. Observe for signs of pseudocyst: upper abdominal pain, mass, tenderness, fever, deterioration, or no improvement in condition.
		4. Observe for signs of abscess: abdominal pain, distension, tenderness, fever, leukocytosis, tachycardia, and hypotension.
		5. Assess for paralytic ileus and fluid accumulation; auscultate bowel sounds every shift.

Table continued on following page

Table 17–2 Nursing Diagnoses, Outcomes, and Interventions for Acute Pancreatitis *Continued*

Nursing Diagnoses	Outcome Criteria	Nursing Interventions
		6. Observe for respiratory distress resulting from ascites or abdominal mass; check breath sounds, presence of cough, sputum production, shallow breathing, elevated diaphragm, and fluid accumulation.
		7. Monitor arterial blood gases for early signs of hypoxemia.
		8. Provide skin care for draining fistulas; use skin barrier to protect skin from pancreatic enzymes; monitor fistula output.
		9. Prepare patient for surgery if an abscess forms.
➤ Alteration in nutrition and metabolic status related to pancreatic dysfunction with altered production of digestive enzymes, insulin, and glucagon; decrease or absence of oral intake; alcoholism; abnormal metabolism	Normal nutritional status Weight gain or maintenance Positive nitrogen balance	1. Eliminate oral intake during acute phase of illness.
		2. Assess nutritional status and general appearance for a. Poor skin turgor b. Lethargy c. Anorexia d. Dry, flaky, discolored skin e. Sunken eyeballs f. Decreased muscle mass and decreased muscular control g. Tremors, twitching
		3. Monitor a. Serum amylase b. Urine amylase c. Lipase d. Glucose

Table 17–2   Nursing Diagnoses, Outcomes, and Interventions for Acute Pancreatitis *Continued*

Nursing Diagnoses	Outcome Criteria	Nursing Interventions
		4. Provide nutritional support as ordered: a. Peripheral nutritional solutions b. Total parenteral nutrition c. Jejunal feedings 5. Monitor laboratory results to prevent complications of nutritional support: a. Electrolyte imbalances b. Hyperglycemia c. Hyperosmolar hyperglycemic nonketosis 6. Provide oral care every 4 to 8 hours. 7. Monitor nasogastric output. 8. Maintain ongoing assessment of nutritional status and therapy including a. Daily weights b. Intake and output c. Nutritional laboratory data (albumin, transferrin, total lymphocyte count) d. Nitrogen balance e. Altered mental status f. Skin turgor g. Muscle atrophy or weakness 9. Monitor fistula drainage and record output every shift.
➤ Anxiety (patient or family) related to insufficient knowledge of disease process, treatment, and diagnostic procedures	Reduction in patient's or family's anxiety with information about disease process, treatment, and diagnostic procedures Patient and family participate in care planning process	1. Assess patient's or family's reason for and level of anxiety. 2. Provide information to patient and family about disease process, treatment(s), and diagnostic procedures.

Table continued on following page

Table 17–2 Nursing Diagnoses, Outcomes, and Interventions for Acute Pancreatitis *Continued*

Nursing Diagnoses	Outcome Criteria	Nursing Interventions
		3. Include patient and family in care planning process.
		4. Evaluate reduction in patient's or family's anxiety.
➤ Knowledge deficit related to change in lifestyle, care, and diet needs	Increased patient knowledge of disease and thus better compliance with treatment regimen	1. Develop client teaching plan.
		2. Include significant others in plan.
		3. Allow verbalization of concerns regarding care and change in lifestyle.
		4. Return demonstration of information understood.
		5. Encourage group support such as AA.

Adapted from Hennessey, K. (1993). Patients with acute pancreatitis. In J. M. Clochesy, C. Breu, S. Cardin, E. B. Ruby, & A. A. Whittaker (Eds.), *Critical care nursing* (pp. 1022–1024). Philadelphia: Saunders.

electrolyte imbalances, pancreatic pseudocyst, and pancreatic abscess (Brodrick, 1991). Krumberger (1993a) also identified hematologic and retinal complications. Most of these complications are lethal if not treated immediately.

Hypovolemic shock commonly occurs as a result of third spacing. Fluid shifts from the vascular system to the intraperitoneal and retroperitoneal spaces as a result of the injury to the abdominal structures from the activated enzymes. Thompson (1992) also reported the release of kinins as a result of the inflammation. These kinins cause vasodilation and increased capillary permeability. As a result, a large amount of plasma and protein leave the vascular system, adding to the potential for hypovolemic shock. Hypovolemia can be extensive, with as much as 4 to 6 L of fluid shifting into the abdomen with severe pancreatitis (Krumberger, 1993a). Further loss of fluid in the vascular system results from decreased dietary intake of protein, thus affecting the oncotic pressure. Patients usually do not take anything by mouth and may experience vomiting, which also add to the loss of fluid in the vascular system. Without aggressive replacement therapy, renal failure may result because of hypoperfusion of the kidneys.

Pulmonary complications are common in patients with acute pancreatitis, including the development of atelectasis, acute lung injury, and pleural effusion. The most serious pulmonary complication is ARDS. Factors that impact the development of respiratory complications include splinting, minimal movement, and decreased coughing during episodes of severe pain. In addition, abdominal distension related to fluid shifting leading to decreased diaphragmatic effort can also depress respirations (Krumberger, 1993a). Seepage of pancreatic fluid can also result in the development of pleural effusion, typically on the left side (Brodrick, 1991). Assessment findings indicating pulmonary complications include adventitious breath sounds, tachypnea, diminished breath sounds, and dyspnea.

Electrolyte imbalances include losses of sodium, potassium, calcium, and magnesium. Sodium and potassium loss is the result of third spacing. Calcium deficits are not clearly understood but are believed to be the result of the pancreatic enzymes' damaging fats. This leads to saponification and chelation of the calcium, resulting in hypocalcemia. The parathyroid glands do not respond to the decrease in circulating calcium as expected, resulting in low serum calcium levels. The saponification of calcium may also result in the chelation of magnesium, thus lowering the serum magnesium as well. Assessment findings include neuromuscular irritability and prolonged QT intervals with hypocalcemia. Another concern is the development of hyperglycemia, which occurs when the pancreatic cells are no longer able to produce insulin.

A pancreatic pseudocyst is the development of necrotic pancreatic tissue, fluid, debris, enzymes, and blood encapsulated in a fibrous tissue (Krumberger, 1993a). A pseudocyst usually resolves by itself but must be monitored through the use of a CT scan or MRI. The cyst may begin to obstruct abdominal structures, or it may rupture, leading to hemorrhagic shock. Assessment findings indicating the development of a pseudocyst include abdominal pain, nausea and vomiting, weight loss, and anorexia after the acute episode of pancreatitis has subsided.

A pancreatic abscess forms in approximately 4% to 10% of the patients with acute pancreatitis (Brodrick, 1991). They usually develop 2 to 4 weeks after an episode and are the result of necrosis of tissue and translocation of gastrointestinal bacteria such as *Escherichia coli, Pseudomonas, Staphylococcus,* and *Klebsiella* (Brodrick, 1991). Assessment findings that indicate the formation of an abscess include an elevated temperature, abdominal pain, vomiting, and possibly a palpable mass in the abdomen. A pancreatic abscess typically requires a surgical procedure for incision and drainage. Antibiotic therapy may also be ordered.

Hematologic complications may result from altered levels of fibrinogen and factor VIII. These alterations are thought to be a result of the activation of certain enzymes in the pancreas. A final complication is the development of sudden loss of vision. This is referred to as *Purtscher's angiopathic retinopathy* and is believed to be the result of complement–induced embolization of leukocyte aggregates (Krumberger, 1993a). These lesions typically resolve in 1 to 3 months.

Based on Jan's clinical picture, the most likely complication is hypo-volemic shock. However, with the elevation in temperature a possible source of infection must be evaluated.

10. Discuss the prognosis of a patient with acute pancreatitis.

One method to predict the outcome of an episode of acute pancre-atitis is to use the guidelines established by Ransom in 1974 (Black & Matassarin-Jacobs, 1993; Stewart, 1989). Eleven criteria were identi-fied by Ransom to help predict the prognosis of patients with pancre-atitis. Five of the criteria are evaluated in the emergency department. The remaining six are evaluated during the first 48 hours after treat-ment is begun.

The five criteria used in the emergency department include (Black & Matassarin-Jacobs, 1993)

(1) age >55 years
(2) WBC >16 x 10^3/mm^3
(3) blood glucose >200 mg/dl
(4) LDH >350 U/L
(5) AST(SGOT) >250 U/L

The six criteria used during the first 48 hours include

(1) hematocrit decreases >10%
(2) BUN >5 mg/dl above baseline
(3) calcium levels <8 mg/dl
(4) arterial Po_2 <60 mm Hg
(5) base deficit increases >4 mmol/L
(6) estimated fluid sequestration >6000 ml

Patients with one or two of the above criteria require supportive care with an expected complete recovery. Patients with three or four of the criteria require more extensive care and have a potential mortality of 15%. Patients with five or six criteria require intensive care, and the mortality rate reaches 50%. Patients with seven or more of the criteria are a medical challenge with an estimated 100% mortality rate (Black & Matassarin-Jacobs, 1993). According to Krumberger (1993a), the Ran-som criteria have a 96% accuracy rate.

Based on the Ransom guidelines, Jan is found to have 6 of the 11 criteria including a blood glucose level of more than 200 mg/dl, LDH more than 350 U/L, and AST more than 250 U/L in the emergency department. After 24 hours her calcium levels dropped below 8 mg/dl; the hematocrit dropped more than 10 percentage points, and the base deficit rose more than 4 mmol/L. Based on this criteria, Jan requires treatment in the ICU and must be monitored closely.

11. **Discuss the psychosocial aspects of caring for a patient with acute pancreatitis.**

Once a patient has experienced the pain of acute pancreatitis, that patient never wants to experience the pain again. If the acute pancreatitis is due to consumption of alcohol, the patient must stop drinking alcohol to decrease the episodes of acute pancreatitis. Counseling of the patient and significant others must be encouraged and supported by the nursing staff.

With other causes of acute pancreatitis, such as biliary obstruction due to gallstones, patients usually have surgery and decrease the possibility of further episodes of acute pancreatitis. However, they must realize the need to be cautious regarding high-fat diet and alcohol consumption.

REFERENCES

Acute Pancreatitis

Black, J. M., & Matassarin-Jacobs, E. (1993). In J. Luckmann & K. C. Sorensen (Eds.), *Medical-surgical nursing: A psychophysiologic approach* (4th ed., pp. 1743–1750). Philadelphia: Saunders.

Burrell, L. (1992). *Adult nursing in hospital and community settings.* Norwalk, CT: Appleton & Lange.

Briones, T. (1991). The gastrointestinal system. In J. G. Alspach (Ed.), *Core curriculum for critical care nursing* (4th ed., pp. 774–780). Philadelphia: Saunders.

Brodrick, R. L. (1991). Preventing complications in acute pancreatitis. *Dimensions of Critical Care Nursing, 10*(5), 262–270.

Brown, A. (1991). Acute pancreatitis: Pathophysiology, nursing diagnoses, and collaborative problems. *Focus on Critical Care, 18*(2), 121–130.

Fain, J. A., & Armato-Vealey, E. (1988). Acute pancreatitis: A gastrointestinal emergency. *Critical Care Nursing, 8*(5), 47–48 & 52–61.

Hadley, S. A., & Fitzsimmons, L. (1990). Acute pancreatitis: A potential life–threatening emergency. *Topics in Emergency Medicine, 12*(2), 39–47.

Hennessey, K. (1993). Patients with acute pancreatitis. In J. M. Clochesy, C. Breu, S. Cardin, E. B. Ruby, & A. A. Whittaker (Eds.), *Critical care nursing* (pp. 1009–1025). Philadelphia: Saunders.

Ignatavicious, D. D., & Bayne, M. V. (1991). *Medical-surgical nursing: A nursing process approach.* Philadelphia: Saunders.

Krumberger, J. M. (1993a). Acute pancreatitis. *Critical Care Nursing Clinics of North America, 5*(1), 185–202.

Krumberger, J. M. (1993b). Gastrointestinal alterations. In J. Hartshorn, M. Lamborn, & M. L. Noll (Eds.), *Introduction to critical care nursing* (pp. 410–418). Philadelphia: Saunders.

Spencer, R. T., Nichols, L. W., Lipkin, G. B., Henderson, H. S., & West, F. M. (1993). *Clinical pharmacology and nursing management* (4th ed.). Philadelphia: J. B. Lippincott Company.

Stewart, C. (1989). Acute pancreatitis. *Emergency Care Quarterly, 5*(3), 71–83.

Thompson, C. (1992). Managing acute pancreatitis. *RN, 55*(3), 52–57.

18

Peritonitis

Lynn Rodgers, MSN, RNC, CCRN, CNRN

CASE PRESENTATION

Ginny Graber, age 40 years, came to the emergency department with severe left lower abdominal pain. The day before her admission she felt nauseated and had abdominal distension, which she attributed to having had no bowel movement for 4 days. Mrs. Graber had been diagnosed with diverticulosis and stated she only has a bowel movement twice a week. She often takes a laxative, which she had done the day before her emergency department visit. She had had no results from the laxative, was still quite nauseated, and had vomited one time. Her last menstrual period was 3 weeks ago. She is 165 cm [5′6″] tall and weighs 74 kg (165 lb).

Physical Assessment

Mrs. Graber was lying on her back with her knees flexed. Her face was flushed, and she was quietly crying, obviously in great distress. Bowel sounds were absent. Her abdomen was slightly distended, firm, and rigid. Rebound tenderness existed over the left lower abdominal quadrant, although her entire abdomen was painful to light palpation. Breath sounds were clear, but respirations were shallow. Mrs. Graber's diagnostic data were

BP	96/50 lying; 84/46 standing
HR	112 bpm lying; 128 bpm standing
Respirations	28/min
Temperature	38.7° C (101.6° F) (Oral)

RBCs	$3.8 \times 10^6/mm^3$	Hct	48%
WBCs	$19,000/mm^3$	Creatinine	1.6 mg/dl
Hgb	12.6 g/dl	BUN	50 mg/dl

Na⁺	148 mmol/L	Amylase	60 U/L
K⁺	3.6 mmol/L	HCG	negative
Cl⁻	107 mmol/L	Urinalysis	normal findings

Na$^+$ 148 mmol/L   Amylase   60 U/L
K$^+$ 3.6 mmol/L   HCG   negative
Cl$^-$ 107 mmol/L   Urinalysis normal findings

Immediate Treatment

- Lactated Ringer's solution (LR) was started at 150 ml/h via an 18 gauge intravenous (IV) catheter.
- Green fluid was aspirated from the nasogastric tube (NGT), which was connected to low continuous suction.
- Immediately after a Foley catheter was anchored, 100 ml of clear, dark urine was returned. Hourly urine specimens were obtained.
- A right subclavian triple lumen central line was inserted. Initial central venous pressure (CVP) and right atrial pressure (RAP) were 1 mm Hg.
- Kidneys, ureters, and bladder x-ray examination (KUB) and upright chest x-ray showed free air under the diaphragm and good location of the CVP line. No pneumothorax was evident. Large distended intestinal loops were obvious.

Further Treatment

- Morphine sulfate 1 to 2 mg IV push was given every 10 to 15 minutes, with a total of 14 mg given in the first 2 hours.
- 2000 ml of LR was infused over the next 2 hours. Breath sounds and orthostatic blood pressure (BP) changes were reevaluated every 15 to 30 minutes. Breath sounds remained clear, and orthostatic changes in BP were less than 6 mm Hg. Urine output was 45 to 50 ml/h. CVP and RAP increased to 4 mm Hg.
- Clavulanic acid/ticarcillin 3.1 g IV partial fill stat was initiated and then ordered every 6 hours.
- A consultation with the enterostomal therapist was held to assess and mark the patient's abdomen for stoma placement, to implement preoperative teaching, and to provide further emotional support to the patient and family.
- An exploratory laparotomy was performed, and the suspected ruptured diverticulum was confirmed. A temporary colostomy was created.

Surgical Intensive Care Unit

After an uneventful recovery room stay, Mrs. Graber was transferred to the surgical intensive care unit (SICU). She received LR at 125 ml/h, oxygen 28% via Venturi mask, and morphine sulfate by patient-controlled anesthesia (PCA) pump. Her CVP readings were 6 to 8 mm Hg, and her urine output was 50 to 70 ml/h. Her NGT remained at low suction. Her lower abdominal incision was well approximated without drainage. Her colostomy was brick red with only a small amount of serosanguineous fluid in the ostomy bag. She had no bowel sounds. Her blood urea nitrogen (BUN) and creatinine dropped to normal levels by the second postoperative day. Her white blood cell (WBC) count peaked at 21,000/mm^3 but also started to drop by the second postoperative day. She was transferred out of the SICU during the afternoon of her second postoperative day in stable condition.

QUESTIONS

Peritonitis

1. What is the function of the peritoneum?

2. Discuss the pathophysiology and causes of peritonitis.

3. What are the clinical signs and symptoms of peritonitis?

4. Explain the abnormalities in Mrs. Graber's admission laboratory results.

5. What are the significant findings of the KUB and chest x-ray?

6. What is the rationale for checking Mrs. Graber's BP in the lying and sitting positions?

7. Discuss the reason fluid resuscitation was initiated in the emergency department.

8. Discuss the rationale for the IV antibiotic chosen for Mrs. Graber.

9. Identify other possible diagnoses that were considered and ruled out for Mrs. Graber.

10. What interventions helped relieve Mrs. Graber's pain? Why?

11. Give the rationale for withholding pain medication immediately after Mrs. Graber's admission to the emergency department?

12. What is the prognosis for patients with peritonitis?

13. What are the primary nursing diagnoses for Mrs. Graber?

QUESTIONS AND ANSWERS

Peritonitis

1. What is the function of the peritoneum?

The peritoneum is a semipermeable serous membrane that lines the abdominal cavity and encloses the abdominal viscera. It is composed of the visceral peritoneum, which covers the viscera, and the parietal peritoneum, which lines the outer walls of the abdominal cavity. The peritoneal cavity is the potential space between these two membranes. The cells of the serosa secrete serous fluid that keep these two outer surfaces moist. This lubrication allows the organs within the abdominal cavity to slide freely against one another. In addition, the peritoneum will react to the presence of chemical or bacterial contaminates with a localized inflammatory reaction (Hole, 1993).

2. Discuss the pathophysiology and causes of peritonitis.

According to Carlson and Geheb (1993), peritonitis is defined as an inflammation of the peritoneum, resulting from chemical or bacterial invasion of the peritoneal cavity. Peritonitis may be classified as primary, secondary, localized, or diffuse, depending on the cause and the severity of the condition. An acute bacterial insult to the peritoneum without any type of perforation to the viscus is considered primary peritonitis. A bacterial infection originating in another area of the body and then transported to the peritoneum by the vascular system is typically the causative agent. Secondary peritonitis can occur with a perforation or rupture of the abdominal viscus, as occurred in Mrs. Graber. Bacterial invasion by the released gastrointestinal contents and severe chemical reaction to released pancreatic enzymes, digestive fluids, and bile initiates the inflammatory insult. Initially, when the peritoneum is contaminated, a localized reaction results in vascular dilation and increased capillary permeability. This allows movement of phagocytic WBCs into the peritoneal cavity. If effective, these polymorphonuclear neutrophil leukocytes (PMNs) ingest or wall off the offending substances, resulting in a contained peritonitis. If these attempts fail, peritonitis progresses. The tissues begin to swell, fibrous exudate develops, and adhesions may form. When the irritant is eliminated, these adhesions may shrink and disappear. Generalized peritonitis is a result of bacterial invasion to a large majority of the peritoneum. This type of infection can affect the entire body and eventually result in bacteremia or septic shock.

Infectious peritonitis can be caused by several different organisms; however, in Mrs. Graber's situation *Escherichia coli* was the identified causative agent. Such organisms can also be the culprits if peritonitis is caused from a rupture of the appendix, perforation secondary to colonic obstruction, toxic megacolon, or traumatic intestinal injury. Pneumococcal peritonitis is a common occurrence in individuals diagnosed with pneumococcal pneumonia. Tuberculous peritonitis is slow to develop and heals causing little or no pain, and gonococcal peritonitis can occur occasionally following massive gonococcemia.

3. What are the clinical signs and symptoms of peritonitis?

Handerhan (1994) reports that the most common symptom of acute peritonitis is abdominal pain. The pain may be localized or diffuse, but the most intense pain is reported in the area of the patient's primary gastrointestinal disorder. This pain frequently is aggravated by movement. Referred pain is common to either the shoulder or thoracic areas. Rebound tenderness, muscular rigidity, and spasm are other major signs of irritation of the peritoneum. Often the patient assumes a side-lying position with knees and hips flexed to decrease the peritoneal irritation. Pain is usually followed by fever (39.4° C [103° F] or higher), chills, extreme weakness, and absolute exhaustion.

As described by Russell (1994) accumulation of serous fluid and inflammatory exudate in the peritoneal cavity causes ascites and abdominal distension. As more intravascular fluid enters the peritoneal cavity, the patient becomes volume depleted. Dehydration is evidenced by dry mucous membranes, poor skin turgor, thirst, tachycardia, orthostatic BP changes, and decreased urinary output. A shallow and rapid breathing pattern develops, decreasing diaphragm excursion and lessening peritoneal irritation and pain. Paralytic ileus occurs frequently in acute peritonitis. Nausea, vomiting, the inability to pass feces and flatus, and the absence of bowel sounds are common findings. Complications are hypovolemic shock, septicemia, organ failure, and mental confusion. Multisystem organ failure is the ultimate result of extensive peritonitis.

4. Explain the abnormalities in Mrs. Graber's admission laboratory results.

Mrs. Graber's complete blood count (CBC) revealed some important information. Her red blood cell (RBC) count was $3.8 \times 10^6/\text{mm}^3$, which could indicate some blood loss. Her WBC count was elevated at 19,000/mm³, with a normal range being 5000 to 10,000/mm³. Her particular laboratory values are important in determining the severity of the infectious process. The hemoglobin level is important for determining the oxygen carrying capacity of the blood. The normal range for women is between 12 and 16 g/dl. Mrs. Graber's hemoglobin result was 12.6 g/dl, which is within the lower limits of the normal range. The normal hematocrit level for women is 40% to 48%. Mrs. Graber's result was 48%, which could be indicative of hemoconcentration resulting from a shift of fluid out of the intravascular space into the peritoneal cavity (Fischbach, 1992).

Normal levels for serum creatinine are between 0.6 and 1.2 mg/dl for women. Mrs. Graber's level was elevated at 1.6 mg/dl. Initial vital signs indicated tachycardia and orthostatic hypotension. This is common in situations where there is blood or volume loss. Elevated creatinine levels could be due to the resulting decrease in kidney function. After catheterization, her urine output of 100 ml of clear, dark urine further indicates a decrease in her kidney perfusion. BUN level is normally 7 to 18 mg/dl. Mrs. Graber's result of 50 mg/dl may indicate a serious condition. Several possible factors causing this condition could be gastrointestinal hemorrhage, shock, dehydration, and impaired renal function. Normal sodium levels are 135 to 148 mmol/L. Mrs. Graber's was 148 mmol/L, which may be increased because of dehydration, insufficient fluid intake, and a shift of intravascular fluid to the interstitial areas. Her potassium level was within normal limits of 3.5 to 5 mmol/L but should be monitored closely for decrease due to fluid loss and sodium conservation efforts by the kidney. Normal blood values for chloride are 98 to 106 mmol/L. Mrs. Graber's slight elevation of 107 mmol/L could possibly be due to dehydration (Fischbach, 1992).

5. What are the significant findings of the KUB and chest x-ray?

The significant radiographic findings that apply to acute abdominal pain are free intraperitoneal air and dilated loops of the intestine (Sleisenger & Fordtran, 1993). Free intraperitoneal air can indicate perforation of a hollow viscus. In Mrs. Graber's case, a ruptured diverticulum was suspected. Dilated loops of the intestine can indicate a paralytic ileus, also common in a ruptured colon. A chest x-ray was performed after central line placement to rule out accidental pneumothorax.

6. What is the rationale for checking Mrs. Graber's BP in the lying and sitting positions?

The rationale for checking Mrs. Graber's BP in the lying and sitting positions was to determine whether she had postural or orthostatic hypotension. According to Jarvis (1993) when a person experiences blood or fluid loss that significantly affects total blood volume, blood pressure responds by decreasing as the patient sits and then stands. With a decrease in blood pressure there is also a compensatory increase in the heart rate. The heart rate increases to maintain a consistent cardiac output. A fall in BP of 10 to 20 mm Hg or more and a rise in the heart rate of 10 to 20 bpm or more is called a postural drop. Mrs. Graber's BP and heart rate did change significantly enough to warrant this diagnosis. Further monitoring of orthostatic hypotension would be indicated if blood and fluid losses were worsening. Another significant measurement from the subclavian line was an initial CVP and RAP of only 1 mm Hg. This is important because it measures the pressure on the right side of the heart. Normal values are 0 to 8 mm Hg. A low reading, such as Mrs. Graber's, could indicate a decrease in blood volume and a "dry" condition intravascularly (Vasquez, Lazear, & Larson, 1992).

7. **Discuss the reason fluid resuscitation was initiated in the emergency department.**

Mrs. Graber was obviously volume depleted as evidenced by the assessment changes discussed. The CVP and RAP were initially 1 mm Hg; after 2000 ml IV fluids, 4 mm Hg; and in SICU, 6 to 8 mm Hg. Mrs. Graber's hypotensive state needed to be corrected as soon as possible to prevent hypovolemic shock (Vasquez et al., 1992). The treatment of choice for hypotension due to a volume deficit is to correct the volume problem rather than constrict the vasculature.

8. **Discuss the rationale for the IV antibiotic chosen for Mrs. Graber.**

Carlson and Geheb (1993) advocate administering IV antibiotics as soon as possible preoperatively once the diagnosis of peritonitis is established. Antibiotics selected must be effective on colonic aerobes and on colonic anaerobes, as is gentamicin. However, selection of a single antibiotic with effectiveness against both aerobes and anaerobes has been more recently advocated. Thus, clavulanic acid/ticarcillin (Timetin) was selected. Antibiotics should be continued throughout the preoperative, operative, and postoperative period for a minimum of 7 to 10 days.

9. **Identify other possible diagnoses that were considered and ruled out for Mrs. Graber.**

A brief review of Mrs. Graber's laboratory work and symptoms in the emergency department indicated that other possible diagnoses needed to be ruled out. These included bowel obstruction, appendicitis, pancreatitis, peptic ulcer, urinary tract stones, ectopic pregnancy, and ovarian cyst (Jess, 1993).

Mrs. Graber presented with severe left lower abdominal pain, nausea, vomiting, and abdominal distension. She had a history of diverticulosis and frequent laxative use. Assessment revealed that she was doubled over in acute pain, her face was flushed, and she was crying. Bowel sounds were absent, and the abdomen was slightly distended, firm, and rigid. Rebound tenderness was noted over her lower left abdominal quadrant with her entire abdomen painful to light tough. Her respirations were shallow.

All of the above signs and symptoms including a WBC greater than $15,000/mm^3$ seemed to indicate appendicitis or possible bowel obstruction. The only symptom that possibly discredited a diagnosis of appendicitis was that the severe pain and rebound tenderness were on the side opposite to the appendix.

Acute pancreatitis is another possible cause for her symptoms. Certainly, the symptoms of nausea, vomiting, elevated temperature, tachycardia, hypovolemia, and hypotension are similar in both diseases, but the location of pain is a key difference. Pancreatic pain is usually felt in the epigastric region or the left upper abdominal quadrant. Abdominal rigidity usually indicates a late sign of pancreatitis, which does not correspond to Mrs. Graber's history. Mrs. Graber's serum amylase was 60 U/L, which is normal and, thus, ruled out pancreatitis. Amylase levels are markedly increased in pancreatitis within 3 to 6 hours after the onset of pain.

Peptic ulcer could also be another consideration because of the sudden onset of constant intense pain. The pain with peptic ulcer is more generalized and has a tendency to be affected by food intake. Signs of hemorrhagic shock that occur with bleeding peptic ulcers were also present. However, lack of blood in the NGT drainage and the lack of history ruled out this diagnosis.

The last diagnosis to be considered is the possibility of a gynecologic complication, such as an ectopic pregnancy, an ovarian cyst, or a urinary tract stone. However, the human chorionic gonadotropin (HCG) test was negative, which rules out a possible pregnancy, and the urinalysis was normal, which rules out urinary tract stones.

10. What interventions helped relieve Mrs. Graber's pain? Why?

Initially, an NGT was inserted, and green drainage was aspirated. This drainage could be very irritating to a ruptured diverticulum and even more irritating to the peritoneum. Decompressing the stomach may also decrease intraabdominal pressure and thus decrease pain. Insertion of a Foley catheter could relieve any further intraabdominal pressure. Morphine sulfate 1 to 2 mg IV push was given at 10 to 15 minute intervals for a total of 14 mg within the first 2 hours of appearance of symptoms. The position of comfort Mrs. Graber assumed also helped to decrease intraabdominal pressure (Carlson & Geheb, 1993).

11. Give the rationale for withholding pain medication immediately after Mrs. Graber's admission to the emergency department.

To obtain an accurate assessment of Mrs. Graber's pain, withholding of all pain medications was necessary. The identification of the exact location of the most severe pain is very important in diagnosing her condition. Pain medication would have masked the signs and symptoms of pain, wasted valuable time, and possibly led to an erroneous diagnosis. When the diagnosis was confirmed, pain medication was given, and other steps were taken to reduce Mrs. Graber's pain (Christou, 1993).

12. What is the prognosis for patients with peritonitis?

Intraabdominal infections carry a significant mortality and morbidity rate in spite of the powerful antibiotics made available over the past 30 years. Survival is most strongly associated with the body's response to the peritoneal contamination rather than the medical interventions performed. Studies indicate mortality rates of 30% to 50%. The risk of death is increased in patients whose peritonitis developed after surgery or trauma compared to patients with peritoneal infection at admission. The risk of death is also increased in patients requiring more than one surgical intervention. Type of surgical procedure performed does not influence the mortality rate. Also, better drainage of the peritoneal cavity does not always help to decrease mortality (Carlson & Geheb, 1993).

Prognosis is dependent on the cause of peritoneal inflammation, amount of time the infection has been present, the body's immunologic response to the infection, the extent of surgical intervention, and body systems involved. Fluid and electrolyte resuscitation, antibiotic therapy, and surgical repair of any perforated viscus are still the most important interventions to prevent death (Sleisenger & Fordtran, 1993).

13. What are the primary nursing diagnoses for Mrs. Graber?

According to Clochesy, Breu, Cardin, Rudy, and Whittaker (1993), the following nursing diagnoses are most applicable in Mrs. Graber's situation:

> ➤ alteration in comfort, pain, and anxiety
> ➤ high risk for infection
> ➤ fluid volume deficit: actual
> ➤ alteration in tissue perfusion
> ➤ anxiety
> ➤ body image disturbance
> ➤ ineffective patient and family coping

Peritonitis

Carlson, R. W. & Geheb, M. A. (1993). *Principles and practices of medical intensive care*. Philadelphia: Saunders.

Christou, N. V. (1993). The prognosis in peritonitis. *Emergency Medicine, 25*(10), 68–70.

Clochesy, J. M., Breu, C., Cardin, S., Rudy, E. B., & Whittaker, A. A. (1993). *Critical care nursing*. Philadelphia: Saunders.

Fischbach, R. T. (1992). *A manual of laboratory diagnostic tests* (4th ed.). Philadelphia: J. B. Lippincott Company.

Handerhan, B. (1994). Investigating peritoneal irritation. *AJN, 94*(4), 71–73.

Hole, J. W. (1993). *Human anatomy and physiology* (6th ed.). Dubuque, IA: William C. Brown Publishers.

Jarvis, C. (1993). *Physical examination and health assessment*. Philadelphia: Saunders.

Jess, L. W. (1993). Acute abdominal pain. *Nursing 93, 23*(9), 34–42.

Russell, S. (1994). Hypovolemic shock: Is your patient at risk? *Nursing 94, 24*(4), 34–39.

Sleisenger, M. H. & Fordtran, J. S. (1993). *Gastrointestinal disease*. Philadelphia: Saunders.

Vasquez, M., Lazear, S. E., & Larson, E. L. (1992). *Critical care nursing*. Philadelphia: Saunders.

19

Esophageal Varices

Linda K. Evinger, MSN, RN, C-OGNP

CASE PRESENTATION

Joseph Hubert, age 59 years, was brought to the emergency department with complaints of dizziness, dyspnea, restlessness, and anxiety. Mr. Hubert currently works as an accountant for a large firm. He is married and has two children living at home. He reported a 2 day history of hematemesis with some bright red blood and large amounts of coffee-ground emesis. Mr. Hubert denied any recent or chronic illnesses and was unable to remember if anyone in his family had ever had problems with gastrointestinal tract bleeding. He did admit to drinking five to six alcoholic beverages almost every day for the past 7 years. Initial assessment revealed cool and clammy skin, distended abdomen with hyperactive bowel sounds, and tachycardia.

Current vital signs and laboratory results are listed below.

BP   92/60
HR   120 bpm
Respirations   28/min
Temperature   36.9° C (98.3° F) (Oral)

Ammonia	60 µg/dl	Glucose	87 mg/dl
LDH	500 U/L	PT	26 s
PTT	85 s	AST (SGOT)	950 U/L
Alkaline phosphatase	165 U/L	ALT (SGPT)	1000 U/L
Total bilirubin	2.5 mg/dl	Albumin	2.3 g/dl

Three hours after arriving in the emergency department, Mr. Hubert was admitted to the intensive care unit (ICU) with an IV of normal saline. Two units of packed red blood cells was administered. Twenty units of vasopressin (Pitressin) in 100 ml of 5% dextrose in water (D_5W) was given intravenously over 20 minutes. A continuous infusion of vasopressin 0.4

U/min was then initiated. Sublingual nitroglycerin was added to the medication regimen. Diagnostic endoscopy, immediately preceded by a saline lavage, was scheduled for the following day. Endoscopy revealed a large esophageal varix (1.5 cm) above the gastroesophageal junction. Only a small amount of bright red blood was observed, so sclerotherapy was performed. A solution of 5% ethanolamine oleate was given by intravariceal injection. Mr. Hubert remained stable following sclerotherapy and was transferred to a medical floor. Subsequent sclerotherapy sessions were scheduled on a weekly basis for 4 weeks.

QUESTIONS

Esophageal Varices

1. Define and discuss the pathophysiology of esophageal varices and portal hypertension.

2. What do Mr. Hubert's laboratory tests indicate about his current health status?

3. Explain how Mr. Hubert's history and laboratory results relate to portal hypertension.

4. Discuss the clinical manifestations of esophageal varices.

5. Identify the diagnostic procedures and nursing implications for esophageal varices.

6. Compare and contrast the treatment options and nursing implications for esophageal varices.

7. Discuss the rationale for Mr. Hubert's vasopressin therapy, management of side effects, and nursing concerns.

8. Identify the relevant nursing diagnoses for Mr. Hubert while he is in the ICU.

9. Discuss the patient/family teaching indicated for Mr. Hubert.

10. What special nursing considerations are prompted by Mr. Hubert's past drinking pattern?

11. Discuss the psychosocial aspects of the care of Mr. Hubert and his family.

QUESTIONS AND ANSWERS

Esophageal Varices

1. **Define and discuss the pathophysiology of esophageal varices and portal hypertension.**

O'Toole (1992, p. 1576) defines varix as "an enlarged, tortuous vein, artery, or lymphatic vessel" and esophageal varices as "varicosities of branches of the azygos vein which anastomose with tributaries of the portal vein in the lower esophagus." Englert and Ruppert (1993, p. 986) define portal hypertension as "increased hydrostatic pressure within the portal venous system." Blood enters the liver through the hepatic artery and the portal vein. The liver is a highly vascular organ that normally offers little resistance to splanchnic blood flow.

Various theories exist to explain the increased resistance that leads to portal hypertension, but no evidence clearly supports one theory. According to O'Toole (1992), the increased pressure is a result of narrowing of the capillaries in the portal vein. Excessive consumption of alcohol can lead to the formation of fibrous tissue around the terminal hepatic venule and adjacent sinusoids, which leads to an increased resistance to blood flow. Inflammatory and occlusive changes can also occur in the hepatic venous system with or without abuse of alcohol. The endothelial lining of the sinusoids can become occluded following injury. This eventually leads to the formation of a basement membrane in Disse's space that causes increased capillaries of the sinusoids to form, resulting in increased resistance to blood flow (Mahl & Groszmann, 1990). Increased resistance results in an increase in portal pressure. The elevated pressure leads to development of a collateral system that carries blood away from the liver. Collateral vessels may be found in the abdominal wall, duodenum, stomach, esophagus, and rectum. According to Krumberger (1993), the most common sites are the esophagus, rectum, anterior abdominal wall, and parietal peritoneum. Normal portal venous pressure is considered to be 2 to 6 mm Hg. A rise in pressure over 10 mm Hg in the portal veins causes the collateral vessels to distend with blood, thus causing enlargement and the formation of varices. Varices usually develop in the esophagus or the upper portion of the stomach. Varices in these areas tolerate high pressures and consequently have a tendency to bleed.

2. **What do Mr. Hubert's laboratory tests indicate about his current health status?**

Mr. Hubert has advanced liver disease. He has experienced blood loss resulting in hypovolemia, which has decreased the hemoglobin level and hematocrit and elevated the white blood cell (WBC) count, platelet count, and blood urea nitrogen (BUN). His sodium and potassium levels were decreased because of the vomiting. His ammonia level was elevated because the diseased liver was unable to convert ammonia to urea for excretion. Lactate dehydrogenase (LDH), aspartate aminotransferase (AST), and alanine aminotransferase (ALT) levels were elevated because enzymes and end products are released into the blood with the destruction of liver cells. The alkaline phosphatase level was increased because of biliary obstruction. The albumin level was low because of impaired liver synthesis. The bilirubin level was elevated because of the liver's inability to conjugate bilirubin, and the prothrombin time (PT) was longer because of diminished synthesis of prothrombin by the liver.

3. **Explain how Mr. Hubert's history and laboratory results relate to portal hypertension.**

Portal hypertension is the primary cause of esophageal varices, which caused the symptoms experienced by Mr. Hubert. Hematemesis is bloody emesis that is either bright red color, indicating fresh bleeding, or a dark, "coffee-ground" color, indicating that blood has been in the stomach where gastric juices have had a chance to act on it. The blood loss accounts for the dizziness, dyspnea, restlessness, tachycardia, and anxiety. Mr. Hubert's admission of long-term heavy alcohol intake would imply cirrhosis as a cause for the portal hypertension. It also would suggest liver disease as a cause for abnormal laboratory test results indicated in question 2. Abdominal distension may be explained by ascites from liver disease. The cool and clammy skin is a sign of shock.

Portal hypertension caused the esophageal varices. The varices, by rupturing, then caused hypovolemia resulting in a decreased hemoglobin and hematocrit, increased BUN, WBC count, and platelet count. The vomiting resulted in the decreased sodium and potassium levels. Increased ammonia, LDH, alkaline phosphatase, AST, ALT, PT, and total bilirubin and decreased albumin also are common in advanced liver disease. Calcium is low because of the decreased albumin and because 50% of the total calcium is protein bound.

4. **Discuss the clinical manifestations of esophageal varices.**

A common symptom of ruptured esophageal varices includes hematemesis, which may be bright red or "coffee-ground" in color. Patients may also report melena (shiny, black, foul-smelling stools caused by degradation of the blood by the stomach acids or intestinal bacteria), mild epigastric pain, and abdominal distress. Pain and discomfort are often absent. Hematochezia (blood in the feces) of bright red or maroon color can occur. Sometimes patients report signs and symptoms of blood loss, which include dizziness, dyspnea, restlessness, and anxiety. Hypotension, tachycardia, decreased level of consciousness, decreased urinary output, and shock may also be present (Hartshorn, Lamborn, & Noll, 1993).

5. **Identify the diagnostic procedures and nursing implications for esophageal varices.**

Barium enema x-ray and endoscopy are both used in the diagnosis of esophageal varices. Endoscopy is preferred over x-ray for patients with an acute bleeding episode, since patients can remain in their own bed. Endoscopy is more accurate than barium x-rays and also allows for immediate sclerotherapy, if applicable. Endoscopy should be performed before x-rays, since barium in the stomach makes immediate endoscopic evaluation difficult (Peterson, 1989). After the patient is hemodynamically stable, gastric lavage is performed to improve visualization. The patient should be reassured that the endoscopy procedure is safe and informed that gagging may occur. However, a local anesthetic may be sprayed in the throat to prevent gagging. A premedication of diazepam, midazolam, or meperidine may be given about 5 minutes before the procedure. A fiberoptic endoscope or gastroscope is used, since it has a fiberoptic light source that enables a clear view of the upper gastrointestinal tract. The patient is instructed to lie on his left side. A rubber mouthpiece is inserted to protect the patient's teeth. The endoscope is inserted into the esophagus and then into the stomach and duodenum. Complications of endoscopy include aspiration, perforation of the esophagus, and rupture of the varices (Englert & Ruppert, 1993). Arteriography is rarely used as a diagnostic tool today because endoscopy provides direct mucosal evaluation. In cases where massive bleeding prevents endoscopy, mesenteric arteriography identifies the bleeding site in 75% of the cases. Arteriographic results are negative if blood loss is less than 0.5 ml/min or if bleeding is venous (Peterson, 1989).

6. **Compare and contrast the treatment options and nursing implications for esophageal varices.**

Endoscopic Injection Sclerotherapy

Englert and Ruppert (1993, p. 987) define endoscopic injection sclerotherapy as "injection of a sclerosing or coagulating substance into varices to stop or decrease the risk of bleeding." Sclerotherapy is currently considered the treatment of choice for an acute episode of esophageal variceal bleeding (Englert & Ruppert, 1993). Agents injected vary, but morrhuate sodium and tetradecyl sulfate are most commonly used. These necrotizing agents work by damaging the endothelium, causing necrosis and subsequent thickening of the varices (Krumberger, 1993). The number of injections is based on the individual, extension of the bleeding area, and the effect of the sclerosing agent on the varices. Injections every 2 to 3 months may be necessary for some patients. During sclerotherapy the patient is kept lying on the left side with the bed elevated to 30 degrees to reduce the risk of aspiration. General anesthesia may not be recommended because of the liver disease. The nurse must closely monitor the patient's respiratory status during and after the procedure. Mortality rate is less than 1%, but complications occur in 10% to 15% of patients. Complications include ulceration of the esophagus, mucosal sloughing, esophageal perforation, stenosis of the esophagus, variceal bleeding, venous embolism, esophageal spasm resulting in substernal chest pain, fever, aspiration pneumonia, and an allergic reaction to the sclerosant (Englert & Ruppert, 1993). Kerber (1993) states that sclerotherapy controls acute episodes of bleeding 90% to 95% of the time. Burnett and Rikkers (1990) report research supporting the use of vasopressin with sclerotherapy.

Intravenous Vasopressin (Pitressin)

Vasopressin, a vasoconstrictor, reduces blood flow to the gut, decreasing portal flow and pressure. Vasopressin is used to control hemorrhaging, but since rebleeding is likely, it is not considered the only treatment needed. Often a loading dose of 20 U in 50 ml of D_5W is given for a period of 30 minutes; then a maintenance dose ranging from 0.1 to 0.5 U/min is begun. No more than 0.9 U/min is considered safe. The patient must be weaned over at least 24 hours when discontinuation is chosen (Englert & Ruppert, 1993). According to Krumberger (1993), the critical care nurse must continuously monitor the patient's electrocardiogram (ECG) and blood pressure. The nurse must be alert for chest pain, dysrhythmias, and other symptoms of coronary artery vasoconstriction. Kerber (1993) suggests that concurrent administration of nitroglycerin may help to decrease the side effects of vasopressin therapy.

Balloon Tamponade

Krumberger (1993) indicates that balloon tamponade may be used if vasopressin therapy is unsuccessful in controlling the bleeding. Several types of tubes may be used for balloon tamponade therapy. The Sengstaken-Blakemore tube (SBT) is a triple lumen tube in which one lumen is for gastric aspiration, one is for inflating the esophageal balloon, and one is for inflating the gastric balloon. Another type is the Minnesota tube, which has one additional lumen for aspiration of the esophagus. A third type is the Linton-Nachlas tube, a triple lumen tube in which one lumen is for gastric aspiration, one is for esophageal aspiration, and the other is for inflation of a large (800 ml) gastric balloon. This particular tube is used for gastric varices. Balloon inflation puts pressure on the varices, which will stop the blood flow. Initially, the tip of the balloon is inserted into the stomach and inflated and clamped. The tube is then withdrawn until resistance is felt causing pressure to be exerted at the gastroesophageal junction. An external traction source may be used via a helmet or the foot of the bed. Traction must be monitored carefully to prevent discomfort, vomiting, and gastric ulceration from too much traction. If bleeding still is not controlled, the esophageal balloon is inflated with pressure from 20 to 45 mm Hg. Tissue damage can occur if the esophageal balloon is left inflated for more than 48 hours. Confirmation of the gastric balloon port below the gastroesophageal junction is done by x-ray. Balloons are usually deflated every 8 to 12 hours to prevent damage to the gastric and esophageal mucosa. Evaluation of the bleeding status of the varices should be done during the deflation time and the nurse must be prepared for rebleeding and hematemesis. When deflating, the esophageal balloon is deflated first to prevent airway occlusion by displacement of the tube upward. Major complications are upper airway obstruction caused by deflation or rupture of a balloon(s), pulmonary aspiration, and esophageal rupture (Englert & Ruppert, 1993). Scissors should be kept at the bedside to facilitate immediate removal of the tube by cutting the lumens if airway obstruction occurs. Suction may be applied above the most proximately located balloon to reduce the possibility of aspiration. Symptoms of esophageal rupture include sudden onset of upper abdominal or back pain which is accompanied with a sudden drop in blood pressure. The nare the tube is inserted in needs to be protected to prevent necrosis.

Portal-Caval Shunt

In a review of treatments of bleeding varices Burnett and Rikkers (1990) noted that surgery to provide a portal-caval shunt was used only as a last resort in cases where all other treatments have failed. The purpose of the surgery is to make a connection between the portal vein and the inferior vena cava (Krumberger, 1993). This diverts blood flow into the vena cava and decreases the portal pressure. A number of procedures exist (end-to-side, side-to-side, splenorenal, mesocaval, portal systemic). Although rebleeding is usually avoided, the long-term survival rates are not good because of the compromised status of the patient before surgery. End-to-side shunts can increase the risk of portal encephalopathy because the blood is diverted away from the liver before it can be detoxified. The splenorenal and mesocaval shunts carry a high rate of thrombosis. Ascites is temporarily increased following these procedures.

Transjugular Intrahepatic Portosystemic Shunt

In 1993, Adams and Soulen reported a new treatment called transjugular intrahepatic portosystemic shunt (TIPS). Catheterization of the hepatic vein is done, preferably through the right internal jugular vein. Using fluoroscopy, a needle is directed into a branch of the portal vein along an intrahepatic tract. The intrahepatic tract is dilated and a stainless steel stent holds it open. The stent is delivered via a balloon catheter. The procedure allows a portosystemic shunt to be placed entirely within the liver. The risks include puncture site bleeding, hematoma formation, reactions to the contrast medium, thrombocytopenia, encephalopathy, disseminated intravascular coagulation (DIC), vascular injury, bile duct trauma, stent migration or thrombosis, and infection. Statistics are promising, but it remains a limited procedure and is not available in all geographic areas.

7. **Discuss the rationale for Mr. Hubert's vasopressin therapy, management of side effects, and nursing concerns.**

   Vasopressin (Pitressin) is a synthetic antidiuretic hormone that can reduce the bleeding in 35% to 60% of patients (Krumberger, 1993). Vasopressin is a vasoconstrictor that lowers portal venous pressure, thereby reducing venous blood flow. The lowered portal venous pressure subsequently lowers pressure in the collateral circulation, which reduces bleeding. Side effects include chest pain, cardiac dysrhythmias, and elevated blood pressure. Nitroglycerin may be given to prevent myocardial ischemia (Englert & Ruppert, 1993). Mr. Hubert must be advised to report any changes or concerns immediately to the nurse.

8. **Identify the relevant nursing diagnoses for Mr. Hubert while he is in the ICU.**

   - altered bowel elimination: diarrhea
   - altered cardiac output: decreased
   - altered comfort: acute pain, nausea, and vomiting
   - altered family processes
   - altered nutrition: less than body requirements
   - altered role performance
   - altered thought processes
   - altered tissue perfusion: gastrointestinal, cerebral, cardiovascular, cerebral, peripheral
   - disturbance in self-concept: body image, self-esteem (long-term or situational)
   - fear

➤ fluid volume deficit
➤ high risk for altered oral mucous membranes
➤ high risk for ineffective breathing pattern
➤ high risk for infection due to invasive procedures
➤ high risk for injury: suffocation
➤ ineffective individual coping
➤ high risk for aspiration
➤ powerlessness
➤ self-care deficit
➤ sleep pattern disturbance

9. Discuss the patient/family teaching indicated for Mr. Hubert.

Teaching areas include those related to procedures, treatments, medications, expectations of therapies, nutrition, alcohol abuse, ICU, and lifestyle changes.

10. What special nursing considerations are prompted by Mr. Hubert's past drinking pattern?

In regard to Mr. Hubert's history of heavy alcohol use, the nurse must discuss the amount of alcohol intake and treatment strategies for elimination of alcohol. Family considerations are of utmost importance in this area. The nurse must offer emotional and psychologic support to Mr. Hubert with relationship to his fears of not surviving and his treatment regimen.

11. Discuss the psychosocial aspects of the care of Mr. Hubert and his family.

Mr. Hubert and his family may or may not have acknowledged that he has a drinking problem. Acknowledging this fact and the changes that will result must be faced as a family because of the impact on the family dynamics. Mr. Hubert may have difficulty changing his drinking behavior if his family does not support him. Possible codependent family members must be evaluated and appropriate referrals made. Alcoholism impacts the entire family, not only the spouse, so consideration of the children is important.

Esophageal Varices

Adams, L., & Soulen, M. C. (1993). TIPS: A new alternative for the variceal bleeder. *American Journal of Critical Care, 2*(3), 196–201.

Burnett, D. A., & Rikkers, L. F. (1990). Nonoperative emergency treatment of variceal hemorrhage. *Surgical Clinics of North America, 70,* 291–305.

Englert, D. M., & Ruppert, S. D. (1993). Patients with gastrointestinal bleeding. In J. M. Clochesy, C. Breu, S. Cardin, E. B. Rudy, & A. A. Whittaker (Eds.), *Critical care nursing* (pp. 945–969). Philadelphia: Saunders.

Hartshorn, J., Lamborn, M., & Noll, M. L. (1993). *Introduction to critical care nursing.* Philadelphia: Saunders.

Kerber, K. (1993). The adult with bleeding esophageal varices. *Critical Care Nursing Clinics of North America, 5,* 153–162.

Krumberger, J. M. (1993). Gastrointestinal alterations. In J. Hartshorn, M. Lamborn, & M. L. Noll (Eds.), *Introduction to critical care nursing* (pp. 386–429). Philadelphia: Saunders.

Mahl, T. C., & Groszmann, R. J. (1990). Pathophysiology of portal hypertension and variceal bleeding. *Surgical Clinics of North America, 70,* 251–266.

O'Toole, M. (Ed.). (1992). *Miller-Keane encyclopedia and dictionary of medicine, nursing, and allied health* (5th ed.). Philadelphia: Saunders.

Peterson, W. L. (1989). Gastrointestinal bleeding. In M. H. Sleisenger & J. S. Fordtran (Eds.), *Gastrointestinal disease: Pathophysiology, diagnosis, management* (Vol. 1, 4th ed., pp. 397–427). Philadelphia: Saunders.

20

Adrenal Crisis

Anne G. Denner, MS, RN

CASE PRESENTATION

Mr. Catt, a 42-year-old man, was admitted to the intensive care unit following surgery for a ruptured appendix. His past history revealed that he has insulin-dependent diabetes mellitus (IDDM). On his admission to the ICU, Mr. Catt's skin was cool and pale and had a slight bronze color. His pedal and tibial pulses were present bilaterally but faint. Breath sounds were clear but slightly diminished bilaterally.

Mr. Catt had taken prednisone 5 mg t.i.d. for the past 3 weeks for treatment of a presumed bout with ulcerative colitis.

After returning from surgery at 3:45 PM, he received an intravenous (IV) infusion of 0.5 normal saline (NS) at 100 ml/h, cefazolin sodium (Ancef) 1 g q6h, and gentamicin (Garamycin) 70 mg q8h.

Postoperative laboratory values and vital signs immediately after surgery at 4 PM were

BP	126/80	Na+	140 mmol/L
HR	80 bpm	Cl–	100 mmol/L
Respirations	18/min	K+	5.0 mmol/L
Temperature	37.8° C (100° F)	Glucose	120 mg/dl

The next morning, however, Mr. Catt complained of feeling so tired and weak that he was almost unable to stand up to urinate. His 6 AM vital signs were

BP 90/60 lying; 65/36 standing	Respirations 24/min
HR 120 bpm	Temperature 38.3° C (101° F)

Blood was sent to the laboratory for electrolyte analysis, and a bolus of 200 ml 0.5 NS was administered. Following this bolus at 6:20 AM, his vital signs were blood pressure 90/60, heart rate 130 bpm, and respirations 20/min. Laboratory results included

Na^+	136 mmol/L
K^+	6 mmol/L
Cl^-	90 mmol/L
HCO_3^-	20 mmol/L
Glucose	60 mg/dl

A second physical assessment of Mr. Catt at this time revealed the following: vague abdominal pain and nausea. He noted that this was not the first time he had experienced these symptoms. He recalled these same feelings about a month ago but thought it was the "flu" or a part of his ulcerative colitis. His incision was checked for hemorrhage but was found to be dry and intact. Mr. Catt's stat electrocardiogram (ECG) showed sinus tachycardia and peaked T waves. At 7 AM another set of electrolytes was ordered in addition to a cortisol level. One ampule of 50% dextrose in water ($D_{50}W$) was given, and Mr. Catt's IVs were changed to D_5W at a rate of 200 ml/h. The 7 AM laboratory results included

Na^+	122 mmol/L
K^+	6.8 mmol/L
Cl^-	88 mmol/L
HCO_3^-	18 mmol/L
Glucose	66 mg/dl
Cortisol	2.6 µg/dl

Mr. Catt was given 4 mg dexamethasone (Decadron) IV as a bolus with an additional 4 mg dexamethasone given q8h until completion of the cosyntropin test. Laboratory data and vital signs at 3 PM were

Na^+	135 mmol/L		HCO_3^-	22 mmol/L
K^+	5.5 mmol/L		Glucose	150 mg/dl
Cl^-	98 mmol/L		BP	110/70
Respirations	20/min		HR	100 bpm
Temperature	38.3° C (101° F)			

A rapid screening test using cosyntropin (Cortrosyn) was ordered. Serum cortisol levels were measured at 30, 60, and 90 minutes to reveal 2.2 µg/dl, 2.6 µg/dl, and 2 µg/dl, respectively. A serum aldosterone level at 90 minutes was 2 ng/dl, while a plasma adrenocorticotropic hormone (ACTH) level was 294 pg/ml.

Mr. Catt's feelings of fatigue soon began to subside, and he was regulated to oral medications within 5 days and discharged.

Adrenal Crisis

1. Mr. Catt has just experienced an adrenal crisis. What are the precipitating factors that have caused his short-term situation? Describe the pathophysiologic mechanisms involved in the precipitation of an adrenal crisis.

2. What are the signs and symptoms characteristic of an adrenal crisis?

3. Differentiate primary adrenal insufficiency from secondary adrenal insufficiency.

4. Describe the components of the axis involving the hypothalamus, anterior pituitary, and the adrenal cortex. What major secretions are produced by each component, and what is the secretion's effect on the other components of the axis (i.e., stimulate or inhibit)?

5. The adrenal cortex secretes both glucocorticoids and mineralocorticoids. Describe the controlling mechanism of the primary mineralocorticoid, aldosterone. How has this mechanism affected Mr. Catt's 7 AM electrolytes?

6. Describe the physiologic functions of endogenous cortisol in the body. Which functions were not being performed as evidenced by Mr. Catt's 6:20 AM and 7 AM laboratory results and vital signs?

7. What other hormones have been shown to interact with the renin-angiotensin-aldosterone system (RAAS) and control aldosterone levels and functions? What other hormones interact with cortisol to affect its physiologic function? What are the effects?

8. Define the stimulation test and the suppression test. Describe the mechanism used in diagnosing Mr. Catt's case. Compare the normal hormone values involved in the hypothalamohypophysial adrenal axis with Mr. Catt's values.

9. Discuss how the diagnosis of Addison's disease is made.

10. What are the goals of treatment for adrenal crisis?

11. What are the primary nursing considerations for patients with adrenal crisis?

12. Identify potential medications for the future treatment of Mr. Catt's Addison's disease. What are their functions and potential adverse reactions?

13. What concepts regarding his disease should Mr. Catt know before leaving the hospital? List the critical events that might precipitate another crisis.

QUESTIONS AND ANSWERS

Adrenal Crisis

1. **Mr. Catt has just experienced an adrenal crisis. What are the precipitating factors that have caused his short-term situation? Describe the pathophysiologic mechanisms involved in the precipitation of an adrenal crisis.**

An adrenal crisis requires some type of trigger or stressor such as surgery, trauma, or infection (Halloran, 1990). Mr. Catt had several factors contributing to his present situation. He evidently had undiagnosed borderline Addison's disease yet had been medicated with prednisone. Prednisone hid and treated the Addison's disease for a few weeks, and its withdrawal helped to precipitate the adrenal crisis. Obviously the stress of the ruptured appendix and resultant surgery were major precipitating factors. Additionally, Reasner (1990) identifies alcohol withdrawal as another precipitating factor. Increased levels of both glucocorticoids (primarily cortisol) and mineralocorticoids (primarily aldosterone) are needed for the body to adapt to the stress (Tepperman & Tepperman, 1988).

Corticotropin-releasing hormone (CRH) from the hypothalamus eventually prompts release of ACTH from the anterior pituitary. ACTH then stimulates release and synthesis of cortisol from the adrenal cortex. Cortisol mobilizes amino acids from skeletal muscle and generally enhances the liver's capacity for gluconeogenesis (Mahan & Arlin, 1992).

The autonomic nervous system's craniosacral outflow also responds to stressors by causing release of norepinephrine (NE) and epinephrine (E), which stimulate hepatic glycogenolysis, lipolysis, and gluconeogenesis (Mahan & Arlin, 1992). These catecholamines also cause vasoconstriction, which in the kidney probably initiates release of renin, which then stimulates the renin-angiotensin-aldosterone system (RAAS). Antidiuretic hormone (ADH, also called vasopressin), is released from the hypothalamus and posterior pituitary during periods of stress. Both aldosterone and ADH attempt to conserve water and electrolytes to sustain sufficient vascular volume (Mahan & Arlin, 1992).

When the adrenal glands are unable to produce sufficient quantities of the needed hormones, fluid and electrolyte imbalances, decreased plasma glucose levels, and hypotension lead to the potentially life-threatening situation of adrenal crisis (Porth, 1994).

2. **What are the signs and symptoms characteristic of an adrenal crisis?**

Severe hypotension and vascular collapse are the hallmarks of the addisonian crisis (McCance & Huether, 1994). Symptoms usually present in adrenal insufficiency are weakness, fatigue, and anorexia. In addition, gastrointestinal symptoms such as nausea, vomiting, abdominal pain or cramping, and diarrhea are often present (McCance & Huether, 1994).

Hypoglycemia, hyponatremia, hypovolemia, and hyperkalemia that occur in primary insufficiency contribute to the symptoms described above. Other symptoms include malaise, personality changes, arthralgias, and myalgias (Chin, 1991; Reasner, 1990). With primary insufficiency, presenting symptoms might include salt craving, coagulopathies, weight loss, vitiligo, and a history of acquired immunodeficiency syndrome (AIDS) or recent surgery (Chin, 1991).

In patients with chronic adrenal insufficiency, hyperpigmentation in the buccal mucosa, skin creases, and nonexposed skin areas may be noted. The hyperpigmentation is caused by excess plasma ACTH levels in the absence of cortisol, the endogenous negative feedback factor for the hypothalamus (Hadley, 1992).

It has been shown that a portion (the first 13 amino acids) of the ACTH molecule is identical to melanocyte-stimulating hormone (MSH). MSH normally increases skin pigmentation (Hadley, 1992). Hadley (1992) also states that it is the heptapeptide sequence (-met-glu-his-phe-arg-try-gly-) that is probably responsible for the melanotropic activity of ACTH.

Patients with secondary insufficiency do not necessarily present with the hallmark signs of hyponatremia, hypovolemia, and hyperkalemia because the secretion of mineralocorticoid is not significantly affected. Additional symptoms, often seen with secondary adrenal insufficiency include cold intolerance and hair loss due to hypothyroidism. Another complaint of decreased libido is related to hypogonadism (Reasner, 1990). Secondary adrenal insufficiency will also lack the hyperpigmentation seen with the primary insufficiency. In the case of secondary insufficiencies, the entire anterior pituitary may be hypofunctioning, producing a variety of symptoms.

A large pituitary tumor may cause the patient to complain of headache and visual field disturbances (Reasner, 1990). See question 3 for further discussion.

3. **Differentiate primary adrenal insufficiency from secondary adrenal insufficiency.**

Adrenal insufficiency may be primary or secondary. Primary insufficiency usually occurs from a progressive destruction of the adrenal gland. Primary insufficiency is uncommon but results in a deficiency of both glucocorticoids and mineralocorticoids. Clinical signs may not by evident until 90% of the gland has been destroyed (McCance & Huether, 1994). Primary insufficiency may be due to an autoimmune or idiopathic atrophy. Adrenal autoantibodies appear in 50% to 70% of the patients who have idiopathic atrophy (McCance & Huether, 1994). As is the case with most autoimmune diseases, Addison's disease is more common in adult women and children (McCance & Huether, 1994).

Although tuberculosis (TB) is a rare cause of Addison's disease in the United States and Europe, it is still a major cause in Japan (McCance & Huether, 1994). Other causes for primary insufficiency include leukemia, amyloidosis, histoplasmosis and sarcoidosis, hemorrhage from trauma, anticoagulation therapy and sepsis, metastasis, and a congenital absence of the ACTH response (Reasner, 1990). Drugs account for a small number of cases of adrenal crisis. Ketoconazole (Nizoral) and aminoglutethimide (Cytadren) may decrease steroid production; phenytoin (Dilantin), barbiturates, and rifampin (Rifadin) cause increased steroid degradation. Each, then, may contribute to an adrenal crisis (Reasner, 1990).

Adrenal hemorrhage leading to adrenal insufficiency is seen as a side effect of medical intervention. Patients receiving anticoagulant therapy (i.e., acute myocardial infarction with anticoagulant therapy) may have concomitant adrenal hemorrhage (Epstein, 1991). The incidence of adrenal hemorrhage from patients with sepsis is variable but is seen more commonly in children with severe meningococcal (Waterhouse-Friderichsen syndrome) or pneumococcal septicemia (Porth, 1994).

Secondary renal insufficiency is usually associated with glucocorticoid deficiency and results from an abnormality in the hypothalamohypophysial adrenal axis function (Hadley, 1992). Secondary insufficiency is associated with reduced or absent ACTH secretion. A common cause of reduced or suppressed ACTH production is prolonged steroid administration for diseases of a nonendocrine origin (Reasner, 1990). Other causes of secondary insufficiency include pituitary tumors and infarction, hypophysectomy, irradiation of the pituitary gland, and infection (McCance & Huether, 1994).

Aldosterone deficiency is uncommon in secondary adrenal insufficiency because aldosterone's release in the body is in response to the RAAS. With normal levels of aldosterone, fluid and electrolyte imbalances are not usually seen with secondary adrenal insufficiency. Exogenous suppression of the hypothalamohypophysial adrenal axis is generally classified as a secondary adrenal insufficiency. Reasner (1990) noted that 30% of patients in one intensive care unit took steroids or had a condition requiring glucocorticoids.

Two rare types of familial hypocortisolism are adrenoleukodystrophy and adrenomyeloneuropathy (McCance & Huether, 1994).

The two types of insufficiency are differentiated using stimulation and suppression tests, which are discussed in question 8. Primary insufficiency is more serious because of the endogenous lack of a portion of the checks and balances of the negative feedback system.

4. **Describe the components of the axis involving the hypothalamus, anterior pituitary, and the adrenal cortex. What major secretions are produced by each component, and what is the secretion's effect on the other components of the axis (i.e., stimulate or inhibit)?**

The hypothalamus produces CRH, which stimulates release of ACTH from the anterior pituitary or adenohypophysis. ACTH is derived from a much larger molecule called proopiomelanocortin (POMC). Included in the fragments cleaved from POMC are ACTH, MSH, β-endorphin, and β-lipotropin (Tortora & Grabowski, 1993). ACTH specifically stimulates the middle region of the adrenal cortex. This region is called the zona fasciculata and secretes mainly glucocorticoids. The inner zone called the zona reticularis is also stimulated somewhat by ACTH, but the zona reticularis secretes only the relatively weak adrenal sex steroids (Hadley, 1992).

ACTH, then, stimulates the zona fasciculata of the adrenal cortex to secrete glucocorticoids, the primary one being cortisol or hydrocortisone (Tortora & Grabowski, 1993). Cortisol accounts for about 95% of the glucocorticoid activity, but the other 5% is stimulated by cortisone and corticosterone. The glucocorticoids provide a negative feedback to the hypothalamus and anterior pituitary to inhibit the production of CRH and ACTH, respectively (Tortora & Grabowski, 1993). This is typical of the negative feedback pattern shown by many other hormones.

5. **The adrenal cortex secretes both glucocorticoids and mineralocorticoids. Describe the controlling mechanism of the primary mineralocorticoid, aldosterone.**

Aldosterone is the primary mineralocorticoid secreted by the outer layer of the adrenal cortex, the zona glomerulosa. Although three different mineralocorticoids are secreted by the adrenal cortex, the most important one is aldosterone, which accounts for about 95% of the mineralocorticoid activity (Tortora & Grabowski, 1993). The other major mineralocorticoid of the adrenal cortex is 11-deoxycorticosterone (DOC) (Biglieri, 1989). Aldosterone plays an important role in the maintenance of extracellular fluid volume and electrolyte balance. It helps to maintain control of blood pressure as a result of the RAAS. The RAAS is stimulated when the body perceives a decrease in normal plasma volume. This decrease in plasma volume is detected by the renal afferent arterioles, which stimulate the juxtaglomerular cells (JG cells) of the juxtaglomerular apparatus (JGA) in the kidney to secrete renin. The JGA consists of JG cells and special chemoreceptor cells of the distal convoluted tubule called the macula densa (Hadley, 1992). Renin converts a plasma protein called angiotensinogen to angiotensin I. The angiotensin I (nonactive form) is converted to angiotensin II by an angiotensin converting enzyme (ACE) found in the lungs. Angiotensin II is one of the most powerful vasoconstrictors known. Not only does angiotensin II cause vasoconstriction, it also stimulates the adrenal cortex to produce aldosterone. The aldosterone causes increased reabsorption of sodium and its accompanying expansion of the extracellular fluid compartment (Tortora & Grabowski, 1993).

How has this mechanism affected Mr. Catt's 7 AM electrolytes?

The 7 AM laboratory results were

Na^+	122 mmol/L
K^+	6.8 mmol/L
Cl^-	88 mmol/L
HCO_3^-	18 mmol/L

Two mechanisms have worked here to complicate the situation. Mr. Catt already had borderline primary adrenal insufficiency or Addison's disease. Note that multiple autoimmune diseases are not uncommon in these types of patients. Mr. Catt's diseases include IDDM, Addison's disease, and ulcerative colitis (McCance & Huether, 1994).

Because of lack of aldosterone, Mr. Catt is hyponatremic. Aldosterone maintains sodium levels and normally does so at the expense of the intracellular cation, potassium. This is why, in the absence of aldosterone, hyperkalemia results. Recall that the sodium-potassium pump is necessary for the transport of those ions. Note that the anions, chloride and bicarbonate, are also reduced to maintain the normal state of a neutral charge. Mr. Catt is also experiencing an abnormal anion gap. This is calculated by subtracting total known contributing anions from cations, which, in this case, gives $122 + 6.8 - (88 + 18) = 23$. When potassium is used, any value over 15 is probably abnormal (Bullock & Rosendahl, 1988).

6. **Describe the physiologic functions of endogenous cortisol in the body. Which functions were not being performed as evidenced by Mr. Catt's 6:20 AM and 7 AM laboratory results and vital signs?**

In 1936 Hans Selye published his paper "A Syndrome Produced by Diverse Nocuous Agents." This syndrome was later referred to as GAS or the general adaptation syndrome. GAS is characterized by three stages: (1) an initial alarm reaction, (2) resistance, and finally (3) exhaustion (Hadley, 1992). These actions describe the sympathoadrenal system's response to stress. Much of the response is brought about by an increase in circulating catecholamines. However, adrenal glucocorticoids are also essential for the body's response to stress (Hadley, 1992).

Glucocorticoids are produced by the zona fasciculata of the adrenal cortex under the regulation of ACTH from the anterior pituitary (Hadley, 1992). Under normal stimuli, cortisol is released in a diurnal pattern, with peaks in the morning and dips in the evenings. Stress alters this secretion rhythm. Glucocorticoids affect carbohydrate, lipid, and protein metabolism. Glucocorticoids increase free fatty acids (FFA) and amino acid release from tissues. Its action is antagonistic to insulin, and excessive secretion of glucocorticoids predisposes persons to diabetes mellitus.

Glucocorticoids also have an effect on reproduction and the nervous system. They are important in the fetal period in imprinting for the fetus (Hadley, 1992).

Cortisol suppresses the inflammatory reaction by inhibiting release of mediators of inflammation such as kinins, histamine, and prostaglandins (Hartshorn, Lamborn, & Noll, 1993). Cortisol also decreases proliferation of T lymphocytes and killer cell activity, as well as decreasing the production of complement. It stimulates appetite, decreases serum calcium, sensitizes the arterioles to the effects of the catecholamines, and increases the glomerular filtration rate (Hartshorn et al., 1993). The effect on the arterioles helps to maintain the blood pressure.

Cortisol assists in the maintenance of normal excitability of the myocardium and central nervous system and helps to maintain emotional stability and personality. Cortisol also aids in insulin production to counterbalance the glucocorticoid–induced effects of hyperglycemia (Chin, 1991).

When the body is exposed to a stressful situation, the hypothalamus senses this stress and secretes CRH. CRH promotes release from the anterior pituitary gland of ACTH, which then stimulates the release of cortisol by the adrenal cortex. Cortisol aids in the body's adaptation to stress in three ways. First, cortisol increases glycogenesis in hepatic tissue. Second, cortisol inhibits the release of kinins, which participate in the antiinflammatory response. Third, cortisol augments the release of catecholamines from the adrenal medulla and increases blood pressure.

Mr. Catt experienced the classic signs of acute adrenal insufficiency (crisis), which include hypotension, dehydration, weakness, and tachycardia. The cardiovascular system was affected by lack of cortisol in that it has lost its vascular tone evidenced by orthostatic hypotension. Mr. Catt's blood pressure dropped to 65/36 when he stood up. Although urine osmolality was unavailable, he was most likely dehydrated because of lack of aldosterone. In addition, even though Mr. Catt had IDDM, his glucose level was only 60 mg/dl because of the low cortisol level.

Reasner (1990) stated that because of the vagueness of the symptoms of acute adrenal insufficiency, a high degree of suspicion would be required to make an early diagnosis. He added that the orthostatic hypotension and tachycardia are almost always present. The hypotension is due to the loss of responsiveness of the vascular system to the catecholamines, whereas the tachycardia is produced in response to the loss of vascular fluids and a drop in cardiac output. This loss stems from aldosterone deficiency, which leads to fluid and electrolyte loss, especially sodium.

7. **What other hormones have been shown to interact with the renin-angiotensin-aldosterone system (RAAS) and control aldosterone levels and functions? What other hormones interact with cortisol to affect its physiologic function? What are the effects?**

Research has confirmed that atrial natriuretic hormone (ANH) is also important in the regulation of aldosterone and sodium and water metabolism (Clinkingbeard, Sessions, & Shenker, 1990). ANH is produced by the atrial cardiocytes and is a polypeptide hormone with 28 amino acids. It produces diuresis and sodium loss (natriuresis) by inhibiting aldosterone, inhibiting release of renin, and release of ADH from the posterior pituitary. Finally, it relaxes vessels, possibly by antagonizing angiotensin II (Hadley, 1992).

Cortisol has "permissive action" with many other hormones (Hadley, 1992). *Permissive action* is a term used in endocrinology to indicate that a hormone "just has to be present in the vicinity for another hormone to carry out its action." This is the role of cortisol with the catecholamines. Cortisol's absence leads to vascular collapse and death. It is essential for synthesis within the sympathetic nerve terminals and for reuptake from the cleft. Cortisol also decreases the rate of degradation by COMT (catechol-*O*-methyltransferase). In addition, cortisol's action on fat mobilization is really its effect on the catecholamines' ability to mobilize fats. Again, cortisol seems to be necessary for the activation of enzymes involved in lipid mobilization (Hadley, 1992).

8. **Define the stimulation test and the suppression test. Describe the mechanism used in diagnosing Mr. Catt's case. Compare the normal hormone values involved in the hypothalamohypophysial adrenal axis with Mr. Catt's values.**

Dynamic tests of endocrine function provide information beyond that obtained from measurements of single hormones or even of hormone pairs.

These tests are based on either stimulation or suppression of endogenous hormone production. The ultimate functional test of endocrine function is to demonstrate a normal response in target tissues to physiologic or stressful stimuli in vivo.

Stimulation tests are used when hypofunctioning is suspected. A tropic hormone is administered to test capacity of a target gland to increase hormone secretion. Response is measured in plasma as an increased concentration of target hormone. One example is where ACTH is given IM or IV when the adrenal cortex is malfunctioning.

Suppression tests are used to assess suspected hyperfunctioning. They also determine if the feedback mechanism is intact. A hormone or other inhibitory compound is administered, and suppression of the target substance is measured. For example, dexamethasone is used to assess hyperfunctioning of the pituitary in the secretion of ACTH.

Several problems exist with this type of testing, including age of the person, need for several subsequent stimulation tests to elicit a normal response, and inherent rhythmicity of cycles. In addition, a variety of drugs might interfere with the dynamic testing.

Several types of stimulation tests are available for testing the hypothalamohypophysial axis. These tests are the consyntropin (Cortrosyn) test and a prolonged ACTH stimulation test, which involves collection of a 24 hour urine sample. During this test the patient who was in a crisis situation is treated with dexamethasone, which does not interfere with the stimulation test. The single dose metyrapone test is useful when secondary adrenal insufficiency is strongly suspected. Metyrapone is an inhibitor of the enzyme needed to convert 11–deoxycortisol to cortisol (Lavin, 1993).

Initial diagnosis of Mr. Catt's problem involves administration of an ACTH stimulation test or cosyntropin (Cortrosyn), which is a synthetic derivative of ACTH. It should rapidly stimulate cortisol and aldosterone production. During the procedure, blood is drawn to determine a base level of cortisol. ACTH and aldosterone can also be drawn. Then 0.25 mg of cosyntropin is injected IV or IM. Repeat samples of blood are drawn at 30, 60, and 90 minutes to determine the diagnosis (Lavin, 1993).

A normal response to ACTH should increase plasma cortisol to at least 6 µg/dl above the baseline. The normal morning level of cortisol is 5 to 23 µg/dl or 138 to 635 nmol/L. The normal value for aldosterone is 0.015 µg/dl or 15 pg/dl. Values for ACTH range from 9 to 52 pg/ml or 2 to 11.5 pmol/L (Davenport, Kellerman, Reiss, & Harrison, 1991). Mr. Catt's cortisol and aldosterone levels are too low, and his ACTH level is too high, indicating a diagnosis of at least acute adrenal insufficiency.

9. Discuss how the diagnosis of Addison's disease is made.

Mr. Catt's diagnosis of Addison's disease is now at least a tempting one because of the following. He already has been diagnosed with IDDM, and he has been treated for ulcerative colitis. Both of these diseases are autoimmune in nature. It is very common for patients to have multiple endocrinopathies, especially if they are of the autoimmune type. Mr. Catt fails to fit one aspect of this syndrome, however; he is male, and most of the persons with multiple endocrine disorders are female.

However, look at some of his laboratory values and presenting signs. His response to the ACTH stimulation test was indicative of an adrenal deficient state. The question is whether it was only temporary, truly acute, and induced by the 15 mg prednisone per day for 3 weeks or whether the prednisone actually was masking the onset of true primary insufficiency. According to Davenport et al. (1991), when the ACTH level exceeds 250 pg/ml (as does Mr. Catt's), primary adrenal insufficiency or Addison's disease is suspected. When the rapid ACTH test results are abnormal, a longer ACTH test should be performed for a conclusive diagnosis.

Mr. Catt's pale bronze skin tone indicates primary adrenal insufficiency. This hyperpigmentation, caused by excess ACTH, accompanies primary states but does not accompany the secondary states or those induced by exogenous steroid administration. Also, Mr. Catt's sodium was extremely low. This indicates that he was having an addisonian crisis of the primary type (Hartshorn et al., 1993). It could also be concluded that Mr. Catt had an ulcerative colitis exacerbation at the same time he was slowly developing Addison's disease.

More than 80% of the adrenal gland must be destroyed before the onset of symptoms of Addison's disease (Davenport et al., 1991). Sometimes, the hyperpigmentation appears before other symptoms appear. The knuckles, knees, elbows, and mucous membranes are the first areas affected by the hyperpigmentation. The patient then complains of fatigue, weakness, irritability, anorexia, and depression.

10. **What are the goals of treatment for adrenal crisis?**

There are three main goals for treatment in the patient with adrenal crisis. The first goal is replacement of fluid volume and correction of electrolyte imbalances. This may require IV administration of as much as 5 L of fluid in the first 12 to 24 hours. Hyperkalemia often responds to volume expansion and glucocorticoid replacement (Hartshorn et al., 1993). Medications should be administered to reestablish high blood levels of the adrenal steroids as the second goal. Hormonal replacement may be dexamethasone (Decadron), 4 mg IV bolus, then 4 mg q8h until the quick ACTH test can be completed (Hartshorn et al., 1993). Another common treatment is 100 mg hydrocortisone (Solu-Cortef) IV push as a bolus with a continuous infusion of hydrocortisone over the next 24 hours. In Mr. Catt's case, fludrocortisone (Florinef) should also be given as a single daily dose of 0.05 to 0.30 mg (Lavin, 1993). The third goal is identification and correction of the underlying illness that leads to increased stress. Once Mr. Catt recovers from his ruptured appendix and the Addison's disease becomes stabilized, the insulin regimen can be readjusted.

Complications seen with glucocorticoid therapy are delayed wound healing, hyperglycemia, metabolic acidosis, and fluid retention (Chin, 1991).

11. **What are the primary nursing considerations for patients with adrenal crisis?**

One nursing diagnosis for the patient in adrenal crisis is fluid volume deficit and electrolyte imbalance. The patient may experience as much as 20% depletion of fluid volume during the crisis. The severity of fluid depletion makes restoration of fluid and electrolyte balance the primary goal (Hartshorn et al., 1993).

During the acute phase of the illness, the severity of symptoms associated with the illness makes emotional support and a calm attitude valuable in helping to reduce stress. Once the crisis is over, knowledge deficit of the disease process and long–term care becomes a nursing diagnosis priority (Alspach, 1991). Exploring the role of stress in precipitating a crisis and ways to avoid emotional and physical stress should occur. Knowledge regarding long-term corticosteroid use is also critical. Medication doses must not be missed, and during times of extreme stress the patient should also consult the heath care provider for possible supplemental doses and should be encouraged to wear a Medic-Alert bracelet (Lavin, 1993).

Alteration in body image in patients with primary insufficiency may also occur, especially with potential hair loss caused by the decreased production of androgens (Epstein, 1991).

12. **Identify potential medications for the future treatment of Mr. Catt's Addison's disease. What are their functions and potential adverse reactions?**

Hydrocortisone succinate (Solu-Cortef) is a glucocorticoid that has effects similar to cortisol (Hartshorn et al., 1993). It is also antiinflammatory and immunosuppressive. In high doses it has mineralocorticoid effects. The initial dose is 100 to 300 mg IV as a bolus, and then 100 mg q8h in a continuous infusion is often prescribed. The main side effects include vertigo, headache, fluid and electrolyte disturbances, hypertension, congestive heart failure, and impaired wound healing. There may also be a tendency toward a cushingoid appearance (Hartshorn et al., 1993).

Cortisone acetate (Cortone) is also used in the treatment of adrenal crisis. It is given as an individualized dosage of 50 mg IV q12h. Its actions are the same as hydrocortisone.

Dexamethasone (Decadron) is used during the cosyntropin test. It is given as a 4 mg IV bolus and then 4 mg IV q8h until the test is complete. Its side effects are the same as those of hydrocortisone (Hartshorn et al., 1993).

Fludrocortisone (Florinef) which is used as a mineralocorticoid. It increases sodium reabsorption in renal tubules, as well as potassium and hydrogen excretion. Its side effects include increased blood volume, edema, and hypertension. It may precipitate congestive heart failure, headaches, and weakness.

13. What concepts regarding his disease should Mr. Catt know before leaving the hospital? List the critical events that might precipitate another crisis.

Mr. Catt's instruction should include the signs and symptoms of insufficiency. His awareness of these facts is essential if he is to cope with Addison's disease as well as the other chronic diseases he has. Patients must adjust their dosage for mild illnesses and must maintain regular contact with their physicians. Patients also must inform all their health professionals of their disease. Patients with Addison's disease should wear a Medic-Alert bracelet. Mr. Catt should obtain and carry with him a traveling kit containing cortisone acetate, prednisone, or deoxycorticosterone acetate for self-injection, and 100 mg vials of hydrocortisone for emergency administration by a physician (Lavin, 1993).

Mr. Catt should have a firm understanding of what type of stressors could potentially precipitate another episode of adrenal crisis. One example is a visit to a dental office. Other stressors include surgery, cold, fever, flu, or even emotional stress. Patients should consult their health care provider if any questions or concerns arise.

REFERENCES

Adrenal Crisis

Alspach, J. G., & Williams, S. M. (1991). *Core curriculum for critical care nursing.* Philadelphia: Saunders.

Biglieri, E. G. (1989). ACTH effects on aldosterone, cortisol, and other steroids. *Hospital Practice, 24*(1), 117–136.

Bullock, B. L., & Rosendahl, P. P. (1988). *Pathophysiology: Adaptations and alterations in function.* Glenview, IL: Scott, Foresman.

Chin, R. (1991). Adrenal crisis. *Critical Care Clinics, 7*(1), 23–42.

Clinkingbeard, C., Sessions, C., & Shenker, Y. (1990). The physiological role of atrial natriuretic hormone in the regulation of aldosterone and salt and water metabolism. *Journal of Endocrinology and Metabolism, 70*(3), 582–588.

Davenport, J., Kellerman, C., Reiss, D., & Harrison L. (1991). Addison's disease. *American Family Physician, 43*(4), 1338–1342.

Epstein, C. D. (1991). Fluid volume deficit for the adrenal crisis patient. *Dimensions of Critical Care, 10*(4), 210–217.

Hadley, M. (1992). *Endocrinology* (3rd ed.). Englewood Cliffs, NJ: Prentice Hall.

Halloran, T. H. (1990). Nursing responsibilities in endocrine emergencies. *Critical Care Nurse Quarterly, 13*(3), 74–81.

Hartshorn, J., Lamborn, M., & Noll, M. L. (1993). *Introduction to critical care nursing.* Philadelphia: Saunders.

Lavin, N. (1993). *Manual of endocrinology and metabolism* (2nd ed.). Boston: Little, Brown.

Mahan, L. K., & Arlin, M. T. (1992). *Krause's food, nutrition and diet therapy* (8th ed.). Philadelphia: Saunders.

McCance, K. L., & Huether, S. E. (1994). *Pathophysiology—The biologic basis for disease in adults and children* (2nd ed.). St. Louis: Mosby–Year Book.

Porth, C. M. (1994). *Pathophysiology: Concepts of altered health states* (4th ed.). Philadelphia: J. B. Lippincott.

Reasner, C. A. (1990). Adrenal disorders. *Critical Care Nurse Quarterly, 13*(3), 67–73.

Tepperman, J., & Tepperman, H. (1988). *Metabolic and endocrine physiology* (5th ed.). Chicago: Year Book Medical Publishers.

Tortora, G. T., & Grabowski, S. R. (1993). *Principles of anatomy and physiology* (7th ed.). New York: Harper Collins College Publishers.

21

Syndrome of Inappropriate Antidiuretic Hormone

Beverly Farmer, MSN, RNC

CASE PRESENTATION

Mr. Strong, a 65-year-old man, was admitted to the neurointensive care unit 2 days ago with the diagnosis of a cerebral aneurysm clipping. His post-surgery recovery was uneventful with stable neurologic and vital signs. His chief complaints were headache and lethargy. On the second postoperative day Mr. Strong was slightly confused as to time and place. The physician was notified and laboratory work was ordered. At the time the laboratory specimens were drawn, Mr. Strong had a tonic clonic seizure and respiratory arrest. An endotracheal tube was placed and ventilator support with the following settings begun:

FIO_2 100%
SIMV rate 16
V_T 750 ml

An arterial line was inserted. Vital signs were

BP 180/100
HR 120 bpm
Temperature 37.2°C (99° F)

He could not follow simple commands; pupils were equal, round, and reactive to light and accommodate (PERRLA); and deep tendon reflexes (DTRs) were diminished. Glasgow Coma Scale at this time was a 13. Laboratory data were

Na^+ 116 mmol/L
K^+ 3.5 mmol/L

Cl⁻   86 mmol/L
Serum osmolality   243 mOsm/kg
Urine osmolality   541 mOsm/kg (serum osmolality + 100)

A pulmonary artery (Swan-Ganz) catheter was inserted to measure fluid and cardiac status. Intravenous (IV) fluids were changed to 3% sodium chloride at 150 ml/h. Furosemide (Lasix) 80 mg IV push was given. Mr. Strong then received demeclocycline (Declomycin) 250 mg q.i.d.

Sixteen hours later, laboratory data were

Na⁺   130 mmol/L
K⁺   3.2 mmol/L
Cl⁻   98 mmol/L
Serum osmolality   275 mOsm/kg
Urine osmolality   400 mOsm/kg

At this time his IV was changed to 5% dextrose in normal saline (D₅NS) at 50 ml/h.

Mr. Strong was extubated within 24 hours. Although he was still weak, his neurologic status had returned to being lucid. Vital signs were

BP   150/90
HR   100 bpm
Respirations   20/min
Temperature   37.3° C (99.2° F)

A 1200 ml/d fluid restriction was prescribed. The demeclocycline (Declomycin) was continued, and furosemide (Lasix) 40 mg b.i.d. was started. After 2 days he was transferred to a medical-surgical unit.

Syndrome of Inappropriate Antidiuretic Hormone

1. Define syndrome of inappropriate antidiuretic hormone (SIADH).

2. Describe the role of ADH in water regulation.

3. Explain the pathophysiology associated with SIADH.

4. Identify the common symptoms associated with SIADH.

5. Explain the effects of SIADH on the major organs.

6. Discuss laboratory studies that are pertinent in diagnosing and treating SIADH.

7. Identify the common causes of SIADH.

8. Discuss the pharmacologic treatment for SIADH.

9. Identify the medical management of SIADH.

10. Describe the role that hemodynamic monitoring would have in the treatment of SIADH.

11. Identify pertinent nursing diagnoses for Mr. Strong.

12. Discuss the nursing care required for Mr. Strong.

QUESTIONS AND ANSWERS

Syndrome of Inappropriate Antidiuretic Hormone

1. Define syndrome of inappropriate antidiuretic hormone (SIADH).

SIADH is a group of symptoms that occurs when ADH (antidiuretic hormone, arginine vasopressin) is secreted in the presence of low plasma osmolality. A decrease in plasma osmolality normally inhibits ADH production and secretion. SIADH is characterized by fluid retention, dilutional hyponatremia, hypochloremia, concentrated urine, lack of intravascular volume depletion, and normal renal perfusion (Ignatavicius & Bayne, 1991).

2. Describe the role of ADH in water regulation.

ADH regulates the body's water balance. It is synthesized in the hypothalamus and stored in the posterior pituitary. When released into the circulation, it acts on the kidney's distal tubules and collecting ducts, increasing their permeability to water. This decreases urine volume because more water is being reabsorbed and returned to circulation. Two mechanisms control ADH release. The first mechanism is serum osmolality (the concentration of electrolytes and other osmotically active particles). When serum osmolality increases, osmoreceptors in the hypothalamus are stimulated, resulting in increased secretion of ADH. Water is reabsorbed, which dilutes the serum and lowers the osmolality.

The second mechanism controlling the release of ADH is blood volume. Baroreceptors in the left atrium are sensitive to changes in pressure. When blood volume rises, pressure on the baroreceptors increases. This stimulus prevents ADH release, so urine output increases and blood volume returns to normal levels. Conversely, a drop in pressure triggers ADH release. The kidney then conserves fluid, and this increases blood volume (Lindamann, 1992).

If too much ADH is released, SIADH results. If not enough ADH is released at the appropriate time, diabetes insipidus (DI) results. DI decreases water reabsorption and results in elevated serum osmolality and a low urine osmolality.

3. Explain the pathophysiology associated with SIADH.

In SIADH, ADH continues to be released in the presence of below-normal serum osmolality, when normally its secretion is inhibited. This results in a simultaneous urine osmolality that is more than that of serum. Dilutional hyponatremia occurs from an increase in tubular reabsorption of water. The retention of water leads to expanded plasma volume. This increase in extravascular fluid causes an increase in the glomerular filtration rate, and reabsorption of sodium and water in the renal tubules is inhibited. The expansion of the plasma volume also inhibits the release of renin and aldosterone (Bowers & Thompson, 1989). Aldosterone is a mineralocorticoid that is released by the adrenal cortex in the presence of angiotensin II. It directly regulates sodium balance because of the sodium–water relationship. Because sodium in solution exerts osmotic pressure (water-pulling effect), water follows low sodium in physiologic proportional amounts. As a result of this sodium-water relationship, aldosterone secretion also indirectly regulates water balance. The primary target tissue for aldosterone is the renal tubular epithelium. Aldosterone secretion is stimulated by a series of events that occurs in response either to decreased sodium levels in the extracellular fluid or to an increased sodium load in the renal tubular fluid (Ignatavicius & Bayne, 1991).

Renin acts enzymatically on the inactive plasma protein angiotensin I. Angiotensin I is further decreased by angiotensin converting enzyme, which seems to be produced in the lung and secreted into the blood. The converting enzyme catalyzes the reaction in which angiotensin I is changed to angiotensin II (Ignatavicius & Bayne, 1991).

Angiotensin II causes massive vasoconstriction of many blood vessels and increases selective blood flow to the kidney. If serum sodium concentration is low and blood volume is above normal, the efferent arteriole is constricted. Efferent arteriolar constriction causes the effective filtration pressure in the glomerulus to be raised, which increases glomerular filtration and urinary output. If serum sodium levels are low and blood volume is normal or low, angiotensin II causes constriction of the afferent arteriole. Blood flow to the glomerulus is then diminished, and effective filtration pressure is low, which decreases glomerular filtration and urinary output.

This action preserves vascular volume while restoring the sodium concentration. At the same time, angiotensin II stimulates the release of the aldosterone from the adrenal cortex (Ignatavicius & Bayne, 1991).

Aldosterone exerts its effects primarily on the distal convoluted tubules of the nephrons. The major effect is the reabsorption of filtered sodium in exchange for excretion of potassium. This effect appears to be mediated via indirect activation of the sodium-potassium pumps in the tubular epithelial membranes. Osmotic water reabsorption passively occurs at the same time in response to sodium reabsorption. This response constitutes a physiologic coping mechanism during volume depletion or sodium depletion states (Ignatavicius & Bayne, 1991).

The release of aldosterone is inhibited in SIADH because of the expansion of plasma volume; therefore potassium levels may fluctuate, since the secretion of potassium is influenced by aldosterone. When sodium is reabsorbed by the kidney under the influence of aldosterone, potassium is usually secreted. However, the aldosterone secretion and sodium reabsorption in SIADH is inhibited; therefore, potassium secretion will be diminished and potassium levels may increase (Clochesy, Breu, Cardin, Rudy, & Whittaker, 1993).

Hypochloremia is also caused by inhibition of aldosterone secretion. Aldosterone indirectly regulates chloride homeostasis through its effect on sodium. Aldosterone causes sodium to be actively reabsorbed by renal tubular epithelium, and chloride follows passively because of the electrical attraction of cations and anions. However, in SIADH, sodium is not being reabsorbed into the circulation but is being secreted into the urine. According to the sodium-chloride relationship, chloride will not be reabsorbed, leading to hypochloremia (Ignatavicius & Bayne, 1991).

The differential diagnosis between hyponatremia caused by SIADH and a modest decrease in serum sodium is that in the latter, sodium is conserved so that urine sodium should be less than 10 to 15 mmol/d. In contrast, in SIADH, the urine sodium is high because of natriuresis (Clochesy et al., 1993).

4. Identify the common symptoms associated with SIADH.

Early symptoms of SIADH include headache, disorientation, weakness, anorexia, muscle cramps, and weight gain. As the serum sodium level decreases the patient experiences personality changes, hostility, sluggish deep tendon reflexes, nausea, vomiting, diarrhea, and oliguria. When the serum sodium level drops below 110 mmol/L, seizures, coma, and death may occur (Collier & Lewis, 1992).

These symptoms are related to water intoxication and will continue to progress unless intervention occurs (Poe & Taylor, 1989).

5. Explain the effects of SIADH on the major organs.

The central nervous, cardiac, and respiratory systems are affected by water intoxication. The primary cause of the central nervous system effects of cerebral edema are due to the shift of the intracellular fluid, leading to symptoms of increased intracranial pressure.

Alterations in cardiac output are associated with the hyponatremia. The pulse is weak and thready, and hypotension may occur. The central venous pressure is low, and neck veins are flat.

Respiratory concerns are secondary to the effects on the central nervous system and cardiovascular system. Gastrointestinal tract involvement is again related to the hyponatremia and is manifested by nausea, vomiting, and diarrhea (Becker, 1990).

6. Discuss laboratory studies that are pertinent in diagnosing and treating SIADH.

Multiple laboratory values are helpful in determining SIADH. The serum sodium level is below normal, as is the serum osmolality. Blood urea nitrogen (BUN), creatinine, hematocrit, albumin, and chloride levels are below normal. Urine specific gravity is increased with very concentrated urine. Urine osmolality is greater than 100% of the serum osmolality. Other diagnostic tests such as complete blood count, chest x-ray, and brain scan may be helpful in identifying the causative factors (Alspach, 1991).

7. Identify the common causes of SIADH.

SIADH is usually the result of a pathologic condition. Cancers, such as bronchogenic, brain, or colon cancer, are often the cause of SIADH. Hodgkin's disease and other lymphomas may be other causative factors. Chemotherapy drugs, as well as many other types of drug therapies, may cause disturbances in the ADH feedback process. Brain injuries, such as hematomas or aneurysms, also comprise a large portion of the underlying pathology of SIADH. Pulmonary disorders such as tuberculosis, asthma, and pneumonia may be additional causative agents (Poe & Taylor, 1989).

8. Discuss the pharmacologic treatment for SIADH.

The standard drug therapy for SIADH includes use of furosemide (Lasix), demeclocycline (Declomycin), or lithium. Furosemide (Lasix) is used to reduce the cardiac workload by producing diuresis. The patient is in danger of developing congestive heart failure. When furosemide is used, the potassium level should be monitored closely.

Demeclocycline (Declomycin) also may be used. Demeclocycline is a tetracycline derivative that interferes with ADH's antidiuretic action and causes nephrogenic DI. The normal dose is 1 g given in four divided doses daily. This drug has the potential for nephrotoxic side effects.

Lithium and phenytoin (Dilantin) may also be used for the same effect as demeclocycline (Declomycin), but the side effects are generally more serious than side effects from demeclocycline (Becker, 1990).

9. Identify the medical management of SIADH.

The primary treatment of SIADH is fluid restriction to reverse hyponatremia. The amount of fluid restriction is driven by the severity of the hyponatremia. As serum sodium levels return to normal, fluid intake may be increased to equal urine output plus insensible loss.

Hypertonic IV fluids should be initiated if there are neurologic symptoms suggesting cerebral edema. A 3% saline solution causes water to be excreted from the cells and reduces the brain cell edema. Once the sodium level returns to normal, a normal saline solution (0.9% NaCl) should be used with a potassium replacement to prevent hypokalemia (Becker, 1990).

10. Describe the role that hemodynamic monitoring would have in the treatment of SIADH.

An arterial line would be helpful in monitoring the patient's blood pressure on an ongoing basis to evaluate cardiac output and peripheral resistance. A pulmonary artery (Swan-Ganz) catheter should be used to evaluate the ability of the heart to handle the volume changes. The right atrial pressure (RAP) measures preload (pressure generated at the end of diastole), which reflects the volume delivered to the heart. The pulmonary capillary wedge pressure (PCWP) measures afterload (resistance to ejection following systole) (Kavanagh, Halperin, & Rosenbaum, 1992).

11. Identify pertinent nursing diagnoses for Mr. Strong.

- ➤ fluid volume excess related to a compromised regulatory mechanism
- ➤ altered thought processes related to cerebral edema
- ➤ alteration in nutrition: less than body requirements related to anorexia, nausea, vomiting
- ➤ high risk of injury related to seizure activity
- ➤ knowledge deficit related to diagnosis and treatment (Lindamann, 1992)

12. Discuss the nursing care required for Mr. Strong.

Continual assessment of Mr. Strong is imperative. Vital signs should be monitored closely. Physical assessment must correlate with the hemodynamics being monitored. Neurologic assessment should be done on an hourly basis during the critical part of the disease process. Seizure precautions should be instituted. Accurate hourly measurement of intake and output provides valuable information. Daily weights are important in assessing fluid status.

Since nutrition may be a problem, skin protection should be incorporated into the care plan. Good oral hygiene is important, since the patient will have fluid restrictions. Teaching Mr. Strong to avoid salty foods should be incorporated into his plan of care.

Preventing nausea and vomiting with use of antiemetics is helpful, since electrolyte balance will be difficult to maintain.

Patient teaching should be an ongoing part of nursing care. The nurse should work with Mr. Strong and his family to assure that there is understanding of the treatment plan, the rationale for the plan, and the outcomes that can be expected (Bowers, 1989).

Syndrome of Inappropriate Antidiuretic Hormone

Alspach, J. G., (1991). *Core curriculum for critical care nursing.* Philadelphia: Saunders.

Becker, K. P. (1990). *Principles and practice of endocrinology and metabolism.* Philadelphia: J. B. Lippincott.

Bowers, A., & Thompson, J. M. (1989). *Mosby's manual of clinical nursing* (2nd ed.). St. Louis: C. V. Mosby.

Clochesy, J. M., Breu, C., Cardin, S., Rudy, E. B., & Whittaker, A. A. (1993). *Critical care nursing.* Philadelphia: Saunders.

Collier, I., & Lewis, S. (1992). *Medical surgical nursing: Assessment and management of clinical problems* (3rd ed.). St. Louis: Mosby–Year Book.

Ignatavicius, D. D., & Bayne, M. V. (1991). *Medical surgical nursing: A nursing approach.* Philadelphia: Saunders.

Kavanagh, B., Halperin, E., & Rosenbaum, L. (1992). Syndrome of inappropriate secretion of antidiuretic hormone in a patient with carcinoma of the nasopharynx. *Cancer, 69*(5), 1315–1319.

Lindamann, C. (1992). SIADH, is your patient at risk? *Nursing 92, 22*(6), 60–63.

Poe, C., & Taylor, L. (1989) Syndrome of inappropriate antidiuretic hormone: Assessment and nursing implications. *Oncology Nursing, 16*(3), 373–381.

22

Diabetic Ketoacidosis

Anne G. Denner, MS, RN

CASE PRESENTATION

Brady, a 39-year-old, 63 kg (140 lb) African-American man, was admitted to the hospital with diabetic ketoacidosis (DKA). After admission to the emergency room, he had multiple episodes of emesis. Brady said he had been vomiting for the past 2 days and admitted to skipping several doses of insulin recently. He mentioned that he had feverish feelings at home and reported an occasional cough.

Brady's assessment revealed the following: pain throughout all abdominal quadrants with "cramping" reported in all four abdominal quadrants. He was extremely lethargic and difficult to arouse at times. He complained of severe thirst. His skin was extremely dry. Electrocardiogram (ECG) showed a sinus tachycardia at 120 bpm. Lungs were clear bilaterally, but respirations were deep and rapid. There was an acetone smell to Brady's breath.

He denied alcohol and illicit drug use and could recall no drug or food allergies. He did report that his father and two aunts have insulin-dependent diabetes.

Brady's psychosocial history revealed the following pertinent information. He works part-time as a janitor and intends to start a second job but only for 2 ½ hours a week. He stated, "I'm on a fixed income, and my medicine runs out sometimes." During the past year, Brady had been admitted to the hospital with the diagnosis of DKA on March 2nd, June 29th, and November 8th. In addition, he had failed to keep his follow-up appointments on July 18th and November 23rd. Brady's diagnostic data are

BP   124/80
HR   122 bpm
Respirations 32/min
Temperature 35.8° C (96.3° F) (Oral)

Hematologic Studies

Hgb	14.5 g/dl	Cl⁻	95 mmol/L
Hct	58%	Creatinine	4.9 mg/dl
Cholesterol	338 mg/dl	BUN	52 mg/dl
Ca^{++}	8.8 mmol/L	Glucose	560 mg/dl
Phosphorus	6.8 mg/dl	Acetone	moderate
Na^+	126 mmol/L	AST (SGOT)	248 U/L
K^+	5.3 mmol/L	CK	34/35 IU/L
LDH	38 U/L		
Alkaline phosphatase	132 U/L		

Arterial Blood Gases

pH	7.19	P_{CO_2}	20 mm Hg
Po_2	100 mm Hg	Sao_2	98% (room air)
HCO_3^-	7.5 mmol/L		

Urine

Specific gravity	1.015	Glucose	4+
Ketones	4+	Nitrates	0
Leukocytes	few	RBCs	many

Home Medications

AM 16 U 70/30 insulin   PM 12 U 70/30 insulin

QUESTIONS

Diabetic Ketoacidosis

1. The hormones involved in intermediary metabolism, exclusive of insulin, that can participate in the development of DKA are epinephrine, glucagon, cortisol, growth hormone, and thyroid hormone. Describe first the pertinent physiology of each hormone and then how each participates in the development of DKA.

2. What is insulin's function in the body? What is the most significant basic defect in the development of DKA? Describe the interplay of factors necessary for the development of DKA.

3. List the classic signs and symptoms for DKA.

4. What is an anion gap? Calculate Brady's anion gap. Why is the anion gap important to calculate and follow in the treatment of DKA?

5. Brady's pH of 7.19 indicates severe acidosis. Discuss Brady's arterial blood gases (ABGs) in regard to acid-base balance.

6. Discuss the possibility of an infection in Brady's case and the effect sepsis or infection would have on a diabetic patient.

7. What are the goals of treatment for DKA?

8. Identify Brady's abnormal laboratory values and describe the treatment modalities used with a patient with DKA in regard to these values.

9. What are four major complications associated with DKA and its treatment?

10. Review Brady's history and laboratory values to determine the diabetic complications to which Brady is most predisposed?

11. Brady's current insulin regimen is 16 U 70/30 in the morning and 12 U 70/30 in the evening. Please discuss Brady's insulin coverage and discuss its adequacy. Include the essential aspects of intensive insulin therapy.

12. What nursing considerations are important in planning Brady's discharge?

QUESTIONS AND ANSWERS

Diabetic Ketoacidosis

1. The hormones involved in intermediary metabolism, exclusive of insulin, that can participate in the development of DKA are epinephrine, glucagon, cortisol, growth hormone, and thyroid hormone. Describe first the pertinent physiology of each hormone and then how each participates in the development of DKA.

Catecholamines, cortisol, glucagon, and growth hormone (GH) are insulin counterregulator hormones. They antagonize insulin by increasing glucose production.

Glucagon is produced by the alpha cells of the pancreas. Glucagon increases blood glucose by stimulating glycogenolysis and glyconeogenesis in the liver. Glucagon is also an antagonist to insulin.

The catecholamines (adrenaline or epinephrine [E]) and noradrenaline or norepinephrine [NE]) are secreted by the adrenal medulla and by adrenergic nerve fibers. E and NE are important mobilizers of stored energy (Alspach, 1991). They mobilize lipid from adipose cells and glucose from extrahepatic sources. E, NE, and glucagon favor the synthesis of glucose by the liver by promoting release of fatty acids, promoting gluconeogenesis, and by inhibiting beta oxidation of fatty acids (Tepperman & Tepperman, 1988).

In the physiologically intact animal, catecholamines inhibit insulin secretion by stimulating α-adrenergic receptors. This tends to accentuate the metabolic actions of catecholamines.

These three hormones oppose the anabolic effects of insulin and activate the enzyme systems for lipolysis and glycogenolysis (Hartshorn, Lamborn, & Noll, 1993). They also promote gluconeogenesis of amino acids; therefore, in cases where there is little or no insulin, the catecholamines and glucagon effectively increase the glucose level, using the uncontrolled mechanisms described above.

Glucocorticoids are produced by the adrenal cortex under the stimulation of adrenocorticotropic hormone (ACTH), which is produced by the anterior pituitary (adenohypophysis). The main glucocorticoid in the human is cortisol. Cortisol's action on intermediary metabolism is best understood if its action is applied in response to stresses such as starvation, disease, or other stimuli that cause significant amounts of ACTH to be secreted (Hadley, 1992). Under these circumstances, cortisol first affects the body's stores of fat. As fat becomes depleted, protein is selected as the next source of energy for the body. The action of glucocorticoids on glucose-6-phosphatase is necessary to provide necessary levels of glucose for the brain.

Cortisol protects the organism against glycogen breakdown until protein wastage is so far advanced that hypoglycemia ensues. At that time, glucagon and the catecholamines stimulate glycogenolysis to ensure sufficient glucose for the central nervous system (CNS; brain and spinal cord).

The interaction of these hormones results in a hyperglycemia that is commonly called steroid diabetes (Catanese, 1991).

Similar mechanisms, if not countered by insulin, will increase the glucose level as seen in DKA. Consider the importance of these diabetogenic mechanisms when the patient with diabetes has an infection or inadvertently omits insulin injections.

GH, which is secreted by the anterior pituitary, has a role in intermediate metabolism because some of its actions are carried out by insulin-like growth factors (IGFs). GH is diabetogenic, but its mode of action is not known (Hadley, 1992). It is stimulatory to insulin secretion but has also been shown to reduce the sensitivity of insulin in the peripheral tissues (Hadley, 1992).

Increased insulin secretion may be indirect and due to the hyperglycemia resulting from reduced glucose uptake by the peripheral tissues. GH promotes growth in that it stimulates transport of amino acids into the cell, incorporation of amino acids into protein, and inhibition of gluconeogenesis.

It has been determined clinically that there is an inverse relation between insulin responsiveness and GH levels. That is, with high exogenous GH doses or in acromegaly, one would expect to find a relative glucose intolerance and an insulin resistance (Catanese, 1991).

The last hormones affecting the body's use of glucose are the thyroid hormones. The thyroid hormones (triiodothyronine [T_3] and tetraiodothyronine or thyroxine [T_4]) are produced in response to thyroid-stimulating hormone (TSH) secreted by the anterior pituitary. TSHs stimulus is thyrotropin-releasing hormone (TRH), which is produced by the hypothalamus. T_3 is the primary thyroid hormone involved in intermediary metabolism. Its main function is focused on respiratory oxygen consumption. At physiologic levels, T_3 is thought to regulate oxygen consumption indirectly by stimulating outward flow of sodium ions. Some dose-dependent net catabolic and anabolic effects on the organism are caused by the thyroid hormones. At lower doses, T_3 favors anabolism and growth in general, as well as lipogenesis and protein synthesis. At higher levels, the effects are catabolic and lead to higher heat production, increased adenosine triphosphate (ATP) generation, and depletion of cellular forms of energy. In cases of thyrotoxicosis, one could anticipate high levels of glucose due to T_3's stimulatory effect on gluconeogenesis and glycogenolysis (Catanese, 1991). In addition, increased lipolysis will increase glycerol and fatty acid fragments, which can effectively raise glucose levels. All these factors, working together and in the absence of insulin, cause DKA to develop.

These same factors may result in insulin resistance seen in severely ketoacidotic patients (Tepperman & Tepperman, 1988). Even low-dose insulin treatment in DKA results in circulating levels of insulin some 4 to 15 times higher than normal. Tepperman and Tepperman (1988) list the factors contributing to insulin resistance as high levels of free fatty acids, presence of high concentrations of counterregulatory hormones, acidosis, and even the hydrogen ion itself. It appears that acidosis interferes with insulin action not only by affecting hormone receptor action but also by inhibiting glycolysis at the 6-phosphofructokinase step.

Other endocrine conditions associated with glucose intolerance include primary hyperaldosteronism, carcinoid tumors, and prolactinomas (Catanese, 1991).

2. What is insulin's function in the body? What is the most significant basic defect in the development of DKA? Describe the interplay of factors necessary for the development of DKA.

The beta cells of the pancreas synthesize insulin. Insulin lowers the blood sugar and may cause hypoglycemia if elevated levels are present by increasing uptake of glucose by muscle, adipose tissue, and liver. It also decreases release of glucose from the liver and increases facilitated diffusion of glucose and related sugars (galactose and xylose) into muscle and adipose tissue. Finally, it increases glycogen formation in liver and muscle by increasing the activity of glycogen synthesis (Hadley, 1992).

Insulin is a protein-sparing hormone. It increases amino acid uptake by muscle and synthesis of proteins from amino acids, especially in the liver. Insulin decreases protein catabolism and is called anabolic because it increases transfer of glucose from blood to the tissues (Hadley, 1992).

Insulin increases fatty acid transport across cell membranes. Insulin decreases lipolysis in adipose and liver tissue and facilitates formation of triglycerides from fatty acids.

The absolute or relative lack of insulin is the most significant basic defect in the development of DKA (Fleckman, 1991). The person with DKA is most often a known diabetic, usually one with insulin-dependent diabetes mellitus (IDDM), who has failed to adequately administer sufficient insulin either due to noncompliance or lack of education. Usually, the patient has omitted his insulin during mild gastrointestinal upset. Occasionally, there is a relative lack of hormones because of increases in some of the counterregulatory hormones (Catanese, 1991). The cause for a relative lack of insulin should be determined, even in cases of known noncompliance such as Brady's. Common causes of relative decreases include sepsis and myocardial infarction. Other causes include infections of the sinuses, teeth, urinary bladder, gallbladder, and perirectal abscesses (Fleckman, 1991). In addition, endocrine disorders such as Cushing's syndrome, acromegaly, thyrotoxicosis, and pheochromocytoma may lead to a relative lack of insulin (Fleckman, 1991). Medications that antagonize insulin also may result in DKA (McCance & Huether, 1994).

3. List the classic signs and symptoms for DKA.

Any person of any age who presents with the following symptoms should be suspected of having diabetes and DKA. These include hyperglycemia, ketosis, altered mental status ranging from drowsiness to coma, weight loss, blurred vision, thirst, excessive urination, enuresis, abdominal pain, nausea, or vomiting (Lorber, 1992a). Other symptoms include tachycardia, orthostatic hypotension, tachypnea, and Kussmaul's respiration. Included also are weakness, anorexia, poor skin turgor, and dry mucous membranes (Graves, 1990). Finally, McCance and Huether (1994) have added pruritus and "fruity" or acetone breath.

Final diagnosis of DKA can be made with the following laboratory values (Fleckman, 1991).

- glucose >250 mg/dl
- pH <7.35
- low HCO_3^-
- high anion gap
- positive ketones

It must be noted that some of the signs of DKA result from the effect that DKA has on hemoglobin function (Tepperman & Tepperman, 1988). It is known that 2,3-diphosphoglycerate (2,3-DPG) regulates the functional activity of hemoglobin. Decreased levels of 2,3-DPG increase the affinity of hemoglobin to oxygen, and the hemoglobin is unable to supply oxygen to the cells. One factor that decreases the level of 2,3-DPG is an inadequate supply of phosphate. Therefore, the combination of acidosis and dehydration results in inadequate perfusion of peripheral tissues. This also applies to the need for phosphate administration during the treatment of DKA. Phosphate enables 2,3-DPG levels to be restored and normalizes hemoglobin function (Tepperman & Tepperman, 1988).

4. What is an anion gap? Calculate Brady's anion gap. Why is the anion gap important to calculate and follow in the treatment of DKA?

The normal anion gap is 12 to 14 mmol/L (Malley, 1990). It is a calculation to determine the presence or absence of substances contributing to the negatively charged group of ions in the body (Yeates & Blaufuss, 1990). These primarily include chloride and bicarbonate but normally may also include albumin. Other substances that can contribute to the anion population include lactic acid as in sepsis or shock, phosphates and sulfates as with kidney failure, and metabolic by-products of ingested substances such as aspirin and antifreeze; however, in the case of DKA, the main contributors to the anion gap are the ketoacids, including β-hydroxybutyric acid and acetoacetic acid (Fleckman, 1991).

Several estimations of the anion gap can be made. One formula for the anion gap (Fleckman, 1991) is

$$Na^+ - (Cl^- + HCO_3^-)$$

Substituting Brady's laboratory values gives

$$126 - (95 + 7.5) = 23.5$$

(The normal anion gap should not be greater than 12.)

A second formula includes the less significant extracellular value for the cation potassium (Yeates & Blaufuss, 1990). That equation is $(Na^+ + K^+) - (Cl^- + HCO_3^-)$. Substituting Brady's values, then gives

$$(126 + 5.3) - (95 + 7.5) = 131.3 - 102.5 = 28.8$$

(Yeates and Blaufuss [1990] consider any value >15 as abnormal.)

Both estimates indicate that Brady's gap is dangerously high and that it must be observed closely during treatment. The proper treatment will allow the anion gap to narrow to within normal limits.

5. **Brady's pH of 7.19 indicates severe acidosis. Discuss Brady's arterial blood gases (ABGs) in regard to acid-base balance.**

6 mmol/L × 1.5 = 9 + 8 = 17 mm Hg (This is the calculated P_{CO_2}.)

Brady's calculated P_{CO_2} of 17 mm Hg is not equal to the last two numbers of the pH value of 7.07; therefore, Brady's disturbance is probably not a pure or simple metabolic acidosis (Fleckman, 1991). However, if you obtain an acid-base map (Malley, 1990) and plot Brady's values of pH of 7.07 and actual P_{CO_2} of 14 mm Hg, these data are consistent with simple metabolic acidosis (Malley, 1990).

It is not uncommon for persons to have mixed disturbances (Malley, 1990). Persons with DKA often have a combination of two or three separate types of acid-base disorders. They may have the anion gap acidosis caused by excretion of β-hydroxybutyrate dehydrogenase and acetoacetate until there is volume depletion and there can be no more excretion (Brody, 1992). If patients are able to maintain some oral intake, they may develop a hyperchloremic nonanion gap acidosis (McCance & Huether, 1994). Finally, they may also have developed a lactic acidosis due to dehydration and poor perfusion (Brody, 1992).

The data given here are insufficient to determine the cause of Brady's possibly mixed acidosis. A blood lactate value (normal is about 1.8 mmol/L or 18 mg/dl) or acetoacetate value might be helpful for positive confirmation (Malley, 1990).

6. **Discuss the possibility of an infection in Brady's case and the effect sepsis or infection would have on a diabetic patient.**

Brady may have some type of acute inflammation in progress. He felt feverish for a few days. The fever could just be a result of the dehydration (Alspach, 1991). If, indeed, Brady did have an infection, neither the infection nor its source could be confirmed because of inadequate laboratory data (no differential available). Plausible sites that must be investigated include the teeth and sinuses. The lungs were clear, but it is possible to have absent crackles and rhonchi in a dehydrated state (Alspach, 1991). No bowel hyperactivity or other gastrointestinal problems were noted. In addition, there were few white cells in the urine, which probably ruled out kidney or bladder infections. He could have had pancreatitis, but, again, there was no increased amylase value that could help to verify that possibility. In addition, there was no tenderness or rebound over the abdomen. However, some of his other enzymes (AST and alkaline phosphatase) were elevated, which could indicate generalized inflammatory responses or tissue degradation. The elevated alkaline phosphatase could, however, be indicative of obstructive liver disease. Again, no laboratory data were present to validate that.

7. **What are the goals of treatment for DKA?**

According to Clochesy, Breu, Cardin, Rudy, and Whittaker (1993), the three goals of managing DKA include improvement of circulatory volume and tissue perfusion, decrease of blood glucose levels, and correction of electrolyte imbalances.

Olefsky, Ellenberg, and Rifkin (1992, p. 1305) stated that the goals of treatment are to "increase the rate of glucose utilization by insulin-dependent tissues, to reverse ketonemia and acidosis, and to correct the depletion of water and electrolytes."

To accomplish either set of these goals, treatment should be categorized in four areas:

(1) administration of insulin
(2) replacement of fluids and electrolytes
(3) treatment of ongoing problems
(4) prevention of complications

Insulin administration reverses the absolute or relative lack of insulin and may include constant or intermittent infusions and subcutaneous or intramuscular boluses. Constant infusion rates result in a smoother metabolic improvement and are associated with a decreased potential for hypoglycemic reactions (Olefsky et al., 1992). Fleckman (1991) notes that insulin administration subcutaneously should be discouraged, since the patient's dehydrated and hypotensive state may result in poor absorption. Many regimens of administration exist, but Fleckman (1991) begins with a modest 10 U dose of regular insulin intravenous (IV) push followed by future administrations via a piggyback line through an infusion pump. Mixing 100 U regular insulin in 100 ml saline results in a solution that minimizes medication errors, since the rate on the pump is the actual number of units being infused per hour. In addition, this size bottle is less likely to be mistakenly altered, which could have disastrous results (Yeates & Blaufuss, 1990).

Fluid replacement should be started immediately for patients with DKA. These patients are dehydrated and hypovolemic and have fluid deficits of 5 to 8 L or more. Therefore, a rapid expansion of intravascular volume is imperative. This can be accomplished by an initial infusion of 1 to 2 L of normal saline in the first 1 to 2 hours (Olefsky et al., 1992). In contrast, Fleckman recommends 500 to 1000 ml NS/h for 4 hours, followed by 250 to 500 ml 0.5 NS/h for the next 4 hours. Clochesy et al. (1993) suggest a bolus of normal saline or lactated Ringer's solution that allows for a gradual resolution of the hyperosmotic state. If the osmolality is altered too rapidly, it might lead to cerebral edema.

Fleckman (1991) and Clochesy et al. (1993) agree that normal saline should be converted to 5% or 10% dextrose in water when the serum glucose is less than 250 mg/dl. However, if cardiovascular or oliguric renal disease exists, caution should be used. To prevent hypoglycemia the dextrose is added to the line when glucose values normalize. This also speeds up resolution of the anion gap by decreasing lipolysis and proteolysis (Yeates & Blaufuss, 1990).

The main electrolyte replacement concern revolves around potassium. The patient often presents, as did Brady, with hyperkalemia. The potassium level represents extracellular potassium and only indirectly reflects the intracellular potassium, which is of far greater significance. The body deficit of intravascular potassium may be much greater. Therefore, potassium should be added to IV fluids when the serum potassium nears 4.5 mmol/L (Yeates & Blaufuss, 1990). However, potassium should not be added to IV fluids of patients who are anuric. This added potassium could result in dangerously high values that could precipitate ventricular dysrhythmias such as Brady's unifocal premature ventricular contractions (PVCs). Clochesy et al. (1993) suggest adding one half of the potassium as the chloride salt and the other half as the phosphate salt, stating that this avoids delivery of excess chloride to the patient and prevents hypocalcemia. This would also prevent the negative effect on 2,3-DPG (Tepperman & Tepperman, 1988).

To prevent complications from treatment of DKA, admission weights and vital signs are obtained, and an indwelling catheter is used for tracking fluids. Blood sugars and potassium levels should be monitored at least hourly. Cardiac monitoring throughout the course of treatment is essential. Hemodynamic monitoring (right atrial pressure, pulmonary capillary wedge pressure) may be necessary in those patients with preexisting cardiac disease to evaluate fluid resuscitation.

8. **Identify Brady's abnormal laboratory values and describe the treatment modalities used with a patient with DKA in regard to these values.**

Brady's sodium was low at 126 mmol/L, and the potassium was high at 5.3 mmol/L. Chloride was low at 95 mmol/L. Sodium and chloride were low because of the vomiting and polyuria. Potassium was high because potassium moves from the intracellular compartment to the extracellular compartment in an exchange for the hydrogen ions (metabolic acidosis). Potassium levels drop as a result of vomiting and polyuria. Once insulin therapy is initiated, potassium returns to the cell.

Brady's calcium was borderline low at 8.8 mmol/L, and his phosphorus at 6.8 mg/dl was high. It has been shown that high phosphate levels can precipitate hypocalcemia and hypomagnesemia (Yeates & Blaufuss, 1990). Therefore, close monitoring of calcium, magnesium, and phosphate is strongly recommended as the electrolyte therapy is instituted (Yeates & Blaufuss, 1990). It is now recommended, however, that phosphate and magnesium levels be allowed to correct themselves, if at all possible. If phosphorus is required, begin phosphorus and potassium therapy simultaneously, using potassium phosphate (Yeates & Blaufuss, 1990). Excessive phosphate repletion could lead to hypocalcemia; therefore, serum phosphate and calcium levels should be carefully observed (Olefsky et al., 1992).

If patients have severe acidosis (pH < 7.0), bicarbonate replacement should be initiated (Olefsky et al., 1992). In severe acidosis the body uses bicarbonate to buffer the high concentration of ketoacids that results when insulin is unavailable to promote glucose entry into the cell (Porth, 1994). Bicarbonate should be administered with extreme caution, since excessive bicarbonate replacement may lead to hypokalemia and may result in rebound CNS acidosis (Olefsky et al., 1992). CNS acidosis "occurs because carbon dioxide is more rapidly diffusible across the blood-brain barrier than is bicarbonate, causing the CNS pH to fall while the peripheral pH is rising. This can lead to stupor and worsening of CNS status at a time when metabolic improvement is occurring" (Olefsky et al., 1992, p. 1306).

Hypomagnesemia occurs in some 25% of persons with diabetes, primarily because of unregulated excessive glucosuria (Zonszein, 1991). Clearly, an inverse relation exists between magnesium levels and glycosuria. In addition, mobilization of fats and protein catabolism are responsible for further magnesium deficits (Zonszein, 1991). Therefore, DKA patients often present with extreme magnesium deficits. However, the magnesium laboratory value was unavailable for Brady.

9. **What are four major complications associated with DKA and its treatment?**

Olefsky et al. (1992) state that the major complications associated with DKA primarily are due to the treatment. These include hypokalemia, late hypoglycemia, rebound CNS acidosis, and CNS deterioration. The authors maintain that with proper treatment the first two can be avoided and the last one is rare.

Hypokalemia is potentially lethal and must be avoided. Brain edema is rare in the adult but occurs more frequently in children. Neurologic signs should be assessed frequently to prevent rebound CNS acidosis.

Hyperchloremic acidosis is due to the replacement of fluid losses with sodium chloride.

10. **Review Brady's history and laboratory values to determine the diabetic complications to which Brady is most predisposed?**

Brady's blood urea nitrogen (BUN) and creatinine were both high, which sometimes occurs in DKA. However, the presence of blood in his urine was undoubtedly associated with the DKA. Brady's creatinine of 4.9 mg/dl could have been caused by ketoacids interfering with the measurement but could also have been reflective of prior damage to the kidneys. If urine output is normal, a creatinine of 2 to 3 mg/dl should normalize rapidly (Fleckman, 1991). No laboratory measure of albumin was given, even though this value would have been helpful. Hypertension and albuminuria have been described as the most sensitive diabetic markers of renal involvement (Lopez-Ovejero, 1992). Brady's blood pressure during the current DKA episode is 124/80, which, although not in the hypertensive range, is relatively high for a person in the dehydrated state. Current therapy for prevention of nephropathy includes administration of angiotensin converting enzyme (ACE) inhibitors such as enalapril (Vasotec) or captopril (Capoten) (Maher, 1992).

11. **Brady's current insulin regimen is 16 U 70/30 in the morning and 12 U 70/30 in the evening. Please discuss Brady's insulin coverage and discuss its adequacy. Include the essential aspects of intensive insulin therapy.**

According to Guthrie (1991), adults should receive insulin 0.5 to 1.5 U/kg/d. Lower ranges are for adults who have hyperglycemia but no ketones, whereas higher dosages are used for patients with DKA. Intensive insulin therapy improves control of diabetes. According to the Diabetes Control and Complications Trial (DCCT), intensive insulin therapy reduces retinopathy, microalbuminuria, and clinical neuropathy and achieves better HbA_{1c} values (Lorber, 1993).

Using the above ranges and calculating Brady's probable needs for insulin reveals the following:

If the lowest value is used (0.5 U/kg/d), then convert 140 lb to kilograms by dividing by 2.2, which yields 63.6 kg x 0.5 U/kg/d = 31.8 U/d of insulin. This is the minimum dose Brady should receive according to the intensive insulin therapy guidelines.

Brady is receiving only 28 U, so he is not receiving sufficient coverage, even if he did not have the possible acute inflammatory process and was taking his insulin. Brady probably should be receiving at least 1 U/kg/d, approximately 64 U. According to intensive insulin therapy regimen, insulin should initially be administered in four injections with 35% being given before breakfast, 22% before lunch, 28% before supper and 15% before bedtime (Guthrie, 1991). Therefore, Brady's injections should be 22 U before breakfast, 14 U before lunch, 18 U before supper, and 10 U at bedtime. This regimen should be accompanied by blood glucose monitoring four times a day (Guthrie, 1991) and compliance with a low-fat, low-sodium, and low-protein diabetic diet. The low-fat diet is suggested because of Brady's high cholesterol. The low-sodium, low-protein diet is beneficial because of Brady's predisposition to nephropathy. Brady's diet should also be a high-fiber diet of approximately 40 g of fiber per day. This amount of fiber will reduce his glucose values as well as his cholesterol and triglyceride levels (Geffner & Lippe, 1993).

After Brady's blood sugars have stabilized, his insulin schedule can be altered so that he receives two thirds before breakfast and one third of his injection before supper (Guthrie, 1991). His 70/30 premixed insulin will continue to work well for this intensive insulin therapy.

For intensive insulin therapy, multiple injections or continuous subcutaneous pumps and multiple blood glucose monitoring (BGM) tests per day are required. Regimens suggest three to five BGM tests per day for intensive insulin therapy, whereas only three are suggested for conventional therapy (Geffner & Lippe, 1993). Several new systems have memory for up to 250 consecutive measurements. These can be off-loaded directly into a physician's computer for analysis. Increased frequency of glycosylated hemoglobins has been changed from the recommended every 3 month interval in conventional therapy to every 6 to 8 weeks in intensive insulin therapy (Geffner & Lippe, 1993).

Exercise is another important aspect of intensive insulin therapy. Patients are encouraged to exercise to prevent hypoglycemia and are further advised to use injection sites most distant from the muscles that will be most active (Geffner & Lippe, 1993).

12. What nursing considerations are important in planning Brady's discharge?

With Brady's cooperation, future complications from IDDM can be reduced 50% to 70% by intensive insulin therapy (Hodge, 1993). The diabetes support team needs Brady's cooperation to maintain strict control over his diabetes. The nurse must work with Brady to develop a health contract that is realistic and geared toward Brady's concept of health. Brady must understand the dangers of elevated glucose levels, know the signs and symptoms of hyperglycemia and hypoglycemia, and be able to verbalize interventions for both. The nurse, dietitian, and Brady should discuss his present eating habits and decide what changes can be made. An exercise plan should also be discussed. Finally, Brady should be informed of local support groups that can help him maintain a regimen of care that will provide an optimum outcome.

It is difficult for people to accept something that threatens their lives, that requires extensive changes in lifestyle, and that imposes a financial burden. The stresses of diabetes are significant (Lorber, 1992b).

REFERENCES

Diabetic Ketoacidosis

Alspach, J. G. (1991). *Core curriculum for critical nursing*. Philadelphia: Saunders.

Brody, G. M. (1992). Diabetic ketoacidosis and hyperosmolar hyperglycemic nonketotic coma. *Topics in Emergency Medicine, 14*(1), 12–22.

Catanese, V. M. (1991). Secondary diabetes. *Practical Diabetology, 10*(2), 8–13.

Clochesy, J. M., Breu, C., Cardin, S., Rudy, E., & Whittaker, A. A. (1993). *Critical care nursing*. Philadelphia: Saunders.

Fleckman, A. M. (1991). Diabetic ketoacidosis. *Practical Diabetology, 10*(3), 1–8.

Geffner, M. E., & Lippe, B. M. (1993). Maximizing management resources to achieve glycemic stability. *Consultant, 33*(4), 55–57, 61–62, 65–66, & 71–72.

Graves, L. (1990). Diabetic ketoacidosis and hyperosmolar hyperglycemic nonketotic coma. *Critical Care Nursing Quarterly, 13*(3), 50–61.

Guthrie, R. A. (1991). New approaches to improve diabetes control. *American Family Physician, 43*(2), 570–578.

Hadley, M. (1992). *Endocrinology* (3rd ed.). Englewood Cliffs, NJ: Prentice Hall.

Hartshorn, J., Lamborn, M., & Noll, M. L. (1993). *Introduction to critical care nursing*. Philadelphia: Saunders.

Hodge, C. (1993). The team approach to intensive insulin therapy. *Practical Diabetology, 12*(3), 13–16.

Lopez-Ovejero, J. A. (1992). Renal involvement in diabetes. *Practical Diabetology, 11*(1), 24–29.

Lorber, D. L. (1992a). Complications of diabetes: Acute glycemic complications. *Practical Diabetology, 11*(2), 12–21.

Lorber, D. L. (1992b). Important considerations: Complications of diabetes—psychosocial problems. *Practical Diabetology, 11*(1), 30–32.

Lorber, D. L. (1993). Metabolic control matters: Implications of the diabetes control and complications trial. *Practical Diabetology, 12*(3), 6–12.

Maher, J. F. (1992). Diabetic nephropathy: Early detection, prevention and management. *American Family Physician, 45*(4), 1661–1667.

Malley, W. J. (1990). *Clinical blood gases: Application and noninvasive alternatives*. Philadelphia: Saunders.

McCance, K. L., & Huether, S. E. (1994). *Pathophysiology—The biologic basis for disease in adults and children* (2nd ed.). St. Louis: Mosby–Year Book.

Olefsky, J., Ellenberg, M., & Rifkin, H. (Eds.). (1992). *Diabetes mellitus—Theory and practice.* New York: Medical Examination Publishing Company.

Porth, C. M. (1994). *Pathophysiology: Concepts of altered health states* (4th ed.). Philadelphia: J. B. Lippincott.

Tepperman, J., & Tepperman, H. (1988). *Metabolic and Endocrine physiology* (5th ed.). Chicago: Year Book Medical Publishers.

Yeates, S., & Blaufuss, J. (1990). Managing the patient in diabetic ketoacidosis. *Focus on Critical Care, 17*(3), 240–248.

Zonszein, J. (1991). Magnesium and diabetes. *Practical Diabetology, 10*(2), 1–5.

23

Multiple System Organ Failure/Multiple Organ Dysfunction Syndrome

Sheila Drake Melander, DSN, RN, FCCM
Sharon West Angle, MSN, RN

CASE PRESENTATION

Mrs. Whitman, a 77-year-old white woman, was admitted to the hospital because of abdominal pain. History on admission revealed that she had an abrupt onset of severe generalized abdominal pain after eating breakfast this morning. She experienced some nausea but no vomiting. The pain remained unremitting, and she was brought to the emergency department and admitted. She complained of having felt a "band" around her stomach for 5 days but felt no pain on the morning of admission. The pain had radiated through to her back, but she also has a history of back pain. She denied any history of heartburn, gallbladder disease, or pancreatitis.

She has a history of intraabdominal carcinomatosis from carcinoma of the ovaries 6 years previously. Review of systems revealed some dyspnea on exertion secondary to her back pain. She complained of dizziness this morning, but she had no complaint of headaches. She denied any chest pain. She has left-sided weakness from an old cerebrovascular accident (CVA).

BP	100/53
HR	82 bpm
Respirations	20/min
Temperature	36.3° C (97.3° F)

She appeared to be in acute distress. Breath sounds were decreased throughout her lungs. Heart tones were normal. The abdomen was flat with absent bowel sounds and tender to palpation. There were no palpable masses or abnormal pulsations.

Admission laboratory data were

WBCs	$4.34 \times 10^3/mm^3$	Glucose	139 mg/dl
Hgb	12.5 g/dl	BUN	39 mg/dl
Hct	38.6%	Creatinine	1.8 mg/dl
Platelets	460,000/mm^3	Bilirubin	0.4 mg/dl
Na$^+$	136 mmol/L	Alkaline phosphatase	56 U/L
K$^+$	4.5 mmol/L	AST (SGOT)	31 U/L
Cl$^-$	101 mmol/L	LDH	140 U/L
CO$_2$	25 mmol/L	Albumin	2.3 g/dl

The patient was given intravenous (IV) fluids and pain medications after admission to the hospital. A computed tomography (CT) scan of the abdomen showed an intraabdominal inflammatory process or a tumor, plus a subdiaphragmatic abscess. A surgical consult was obtained. On day 2 of the hospitalization the patient underwent an exploratory laparotomy for an acute abdomen. Surgery revealed a perforated duodenal ulcer, which was repaired with a Billroth II gastrectomy. Following surgery the patient was admitted to the intensive care unit (ICU). During her initial postoperative period, Mrs. Whitman required dopamine and fluid challenges to maintain her blood pressure. After surgery she received triple antibiotic therapy in response to a temperature elevation, noted immediately after surgery, which continued until postoperative day 10. She received total parenteral nutrition (TPN) postoperatively, and a nasogastric tube (NGT) and duodenostomy tubes set at low suction were placed. Diagnostic data immediately after surgery were

Temperature	38.8° C (101.8° F)
HR	110 bpm
pH	7.41
P$_{CO_2}$	35.6 mm Hg
P$_{O_2}$	123.8 mm Hg
HCO$_3^-$	22.5 mmol/L

Ventilator Settings

F$_{IO_2}$	50%
SIMV rate	10
V$_T$	700 ml

The patient's condition stabilized, and the tubes were removed on the second postoperative day. Dopamine was restarted at 5 μg/kg/min; as Mrs. Whitman's blood pressure stabilized, the dopamine was titrated and then discontinued. On the fourth postoperative day the patient's condition deteriorated, requiring reintubation and mechanical ventilation. The patient's hemoglobin and hematocrit also dropped significantly, requiring a blood transfusion of 2 U packed red blood cells. The patient did not want to be on the ventilator and continuously tried to extubate herself.

Postoperative day 4 diagnostic data were

Temperature	38.9° C (102° F)	Glucose	120 mg/dl
WBCs	14.4 x 10^3/mm^3	BUN	29 mg/dl
Hgb	7.1 g/dl	Creatinine	1 mg/dl
Hct	21.7%	Bilirubin	0.8 mg/dl
Platelets	249,000/mm^3	Alkaline phosphatase	69 U/L
Na$^+$	134 mmol/L	AST(SGOT)	30 U/L
K$^+$	3.8 mmol/L	LDH	142 U/L
Cl$^-$	107 mmol/L	Albumin	1.8 g/dl
CO_2	25 mmol/L		

Triple antibiotic therapy was continued, yet Mrs. Whitman's temperature continued to spike to 38.9° C (102° F) throughout her hospitalization. Multiple cultures were obtained, yet all showed no growth. Diagnostic data were

WBCs	26,000/mm^3	Bilirubin	7.5 mg/dl
Hgb	10.5 g/dl	Alkaline phosphatase	118 U/L
Hct	32.2%	AST	39 U/L
Platelets	561,000/mm^3	LDH	375 U/L
Na$^+$	143 mmol/L	Albumin	1.3 g/dl
K$^+$	4.3 mmol/L	pH	7.37
Cl$^-$	104 mmol/L	P_{CO_2}	56.9 mm Hg
CO_2	36 mmol/L	P_{O_2}	53.4 mm Hg
Glucose	117 mg/dl	HCO_3^-	32.5 mmol/L
BUN	61 mg/dl		
Creatinine	1.1 mg/dl		

Ventilator Settings

F_{IO_2}	60%
SIMV rate	10
V_T	700 ml
PEEP	5 cm H_2O

By postoperative day 10 the patient showed increasing signs of respiratory and liver failure. After consultation with Mrs. Whitman's family and in view of the patient's previous wishes regarding ventilatory support, the ventilator was removed. Mrs. Whitman died shortly thereafter.

Multiple System Organ Failure/Multiple Organ Dysfunction Syndrome

1. Define multiple system organ failure (MSOF)/multiple organ dysfunction syndrome (MODS) and list etiologic factors. What are some theories or hypotheses for the cause of MSOF/MODS?

2. What is the impact of oxygen-free radicals in the development of MSOF/MODS?

3. Discuss some of the paradoxes seen with MSOF/MODS. Establish the significance of vital signs in regard to these paradoxes.

4. What pathophysiologic changes occur with MSOF/MODS?

5. How does MSOF/MODS usually progress in adults? How does progression differ in children?

6. Describe presenting signs and symptoms of the various stages of MSOF/MODS.

7. What are the defining criteria for organ failure/organ dysfunction in each of the different systems? Identify assessment parameters that help in the diagnosis of each type of organ failure/organ dysfunction.

8. List the primary goals of treatment in MSOF/MODS.

9. Describe the importance of nutritional support with MSOF/MODS.

10. What measures are used to prevent gastric complications?

11. What are nursing considerations for the patient with MSOF/MODS?

12. What ethical considerations play a role in the diagnosis of MSOF/MODS?

QUESTIONS AND ANSWERS

Multiple System Organ Failure/Multiple Organ Dysfunction Syndrome

1. **Define multiple system organ failure (MSOF)/multiple organ dysfunction syndrome (MODS) and list etiologic factors. What are some theories or hypotheses for the cause of MSOF/MODS?**

   MSOF is a syndrome that has been described since the mid-1970s separate from single organ failure. It is a simultaneous organ system failure as a result of shock or arrest and is sequential in nature (Huddleston, 1992). The syndrome of MSOF/MODS is defined as a progressive failure of two or more body systems (Huddleston, 1991). MSOF/MODS is usually seen as a complication of multiple trauma, prolonged highly invasive surgical procedures and septic shock, perfusion deficits, shock, and persistent inflammatory foci (Huddleston, 1992; Weil & Pakula, 1992). Most etiologic theories favor a common pathway that creates a systemic reaction as the cause of instead of the result of cardiovascular instability and poor oxygen delivery (Huddleston, 1992). The thought is that this systemic response is the result of a prolonged inflammatory response (Huddleston, 1992). The progressive failure of body systems is precipitated or driven by a large number of mediators in the body and existing clinical conditions (Huddleston, 1992). MSOF/MODS may be a result of an initial injury or insult to the body or of therapeutic interventions (Huddleston, 1992).

   MSOF/MODS is being seen with increasing frequency because patients are surviving longer following severe trauma. Despite advances in the management of severely traumatized or ill patients, the mortality rate remains high, ranging from 60% to 90% and increasing with the number of organs involved. With involvement of three or more systems, mortality approaches 100%. It is estimated that 10% of deaths after multiple trauma and 50% of deaths with acute adult respiratory distress syndrome (ARDS) may be attributed to MSOF/MODS.

MSOF/MODS is the leading cause of death in the surgical ICU patient (Weil & Pakula, 1992).

The following are theories regarding the cause of MSOF/MODS:

(1) Bacterial invasion of the lungs, peritoneum, blood, and other body tissues is uncontrolled.

(2) Systemic host defense activation is overwhelming.

(3) Inflammation is severe with no evidence of sepsis.

(4) The gastrointestinal barrier function is altered.

(5) Injury, shock, and sepsis produce ischemia, which triggers the four preceding events (Bauer, 1990).

The consensus conference of the Society of Critical Care Medicine and the American College of Chest Physicians suggested that the term *multiplesystem organ failure* be abandoned, since it denotes actual organ failure, which is not actually the case, and that the new term *multiple organ dysfunction syndrome* be used (Ackerman, 1994). The new term is considered more appropriate, since organs such as the heart, lungs, and kidneys show signs of dysfunction but do not actually fail. MODS is the result of a systemic inflammatory response system (SIRS), which results from the injury. The SIRS may directly result in MODS or may be a result of sepsis. This term is just being introduced in research articles and possibly will help health care providers better understand the processes involved with MODS or MSOF/MODS. Since this is new terminology, both terms will be used throughout this chapter.

2. What is the impact of oxygen-free radicals in the development of MSOF/MODS?

During critical illness, toxic oxygen metabolites may be produced in excessive amounts and have been implicated as part of the reason for cellular destruction during multisystem organ failure. Normally, antioxidant enzymes are in sufficient numbers to prevent cellular destruction. However, during conditions such as sepsis and multisystem organ failure, patients have depleted their antioxidant defense system and are especially vulnerable to these destructive effects. Oxygen metabolites cause lipid peroxidation and damage to cell membranes, activate the coagulation cascade, and can damage DNA. (Clochesy, Breu, Cardin, Rudy, & Whittaker, 1993; Thelan, Davie, Urden, & Lough, 1994).

3. Discuss some of the paradoxes seen with MSOF/MODS. Establish the significance of vital signs in regard to these paradoxes.

Deitch (1990) describes a set of clinical paradoxes found with MSOF/MODS:

- The organs that frequently fail are not always related directly to the injury or initial insult.
- There is a period of days to weeks between the initial injury or insult and the development of clinical organ failure.
- Although patients may appear to have clinical sepsis with MSOF/MODS, not all have microbiologic evidence of infection or a septic syndrome.
- A septic focus cannot be identified clinically or at autopsy in more than 30% of patients with bacteremia who die of clinical sepsis and MSOF/MODS.
- Identification and treatment of suppurative infections in patients with MSOF/MODS may not improve survival.

Clinical manifestations of SIRS associated with MSOF/MODS are described in Table 23–1.

4. What pathophysiologic changes occur with MSOF/MODS?

Pathophysiologic changes occur in a cascade of events in MSOF/MODS:

a. There is an initial insult or injury to the body.
b. Three main precipitating events or factors lead to the release of mediators in the body:
  (1) Inflammatory immune response (IIR)
  (2) Neuroendocrine activation
  (3) Endothelial damage

Each of these contribute to the primary physiologic changes (Huddleston, 1992).

The neuroendocrine activation is one of the first body defenses to activate with injury. The nervous system releases hormones that stimulate the endocrine system to produce substances that in turn mediate activity within the nervous system. These substances help prepare the body for fight or flight from the initial insult (Huddleston, 1992).

Table 23–1 Clinical Manifestations Associated With Multiple Organ Failure/Multiple Organ Dysfunction Syndrome

Vital Sign	
Temperature	>38° C (100.4° F) or <36° C (96.8° F)
Heart rate	>90 bpm
Respiratory rate	20/min
PaCO$_2$	<32 mm Hg
White blood cell count	>12,000/mm^3 or <4000/mm^3 or >10% immature (band) forms

The IIR normally contains, suppresses, and eliminates infecting organisms and clears damaged tissue of cellular debris and foreign material. However, if this response goes unchecked, there is a domino effect. Current research indicates that a septic focus is essential for the initiation and propagation of MSOF/MODS (McFadden & Sartorius, 1992a, 1992b). Huddleston (1992) states that IIR releases mediators that decrease tissue perfusion and alter cellular oxygen metabolism. This creates by-products of anaerobic metabolism and mediators such as lactic acid, proteases, oxygen-derived free radicals, and catabolic hormones.

Endothelial damage contributes to the activation of the IIR and potential coagulopathies in the patient with MSOF/MODS. Damage to the endothelium increases capillary permeability leading to edema formation and potentiates coagulation abnormalities (Huddleston, 1992).

The next level of pathophysiologic changes occurs in three different areas. The first is a maldistribution of circulating volume due to increased capillary permeability and vasodilation. This leads to vascular fluid leaks into the interstitium and pooling in the periphery, which gives the appearance of edema and decreases vascular volume and blood pressure (Huddleston, 1992).

The second occurrence is an imbalance between oxygen supply and demand due to the increased metabolic demand, tissue damage, and fever. Oxygen supply is limited by the decrease in blood pressure and poor control of tissue perfusion in the microcirculation. Lung abnormalities are seen because of the leaky pulmonary capillary beds (Huddleston, 1992).

The third area of pathophysiologic change is that of abnormal metabolic control: a hyperdynamic and hypermetabolic state that occurs when endocrine activation attempts to compensate for damage and gets out of control. There is an increase in oxygen consumption and carbon dioxide production, which leads to an increased respiratory rate and depth. The protein breakdown from muscle tissue and amino acids is converted into glucose. There is rapid wasting of muscles, and atrophy is evident. If the underlying condition is not reversed, an eventual hypodynamic and decompensated state occurs, leading to organ damage and failure (Huddleston, 1992). With metabolic failure, liver enzyme (AST, ALT, LDH, and Alkaline phosphatase) and bilirubin serum levels rise, plasma protein levels fall, PTT and PT lengthen, and the patient appears jaundiced (Huddleston, 1992).

5. How does MSOF/MODS usually progress in adults? How does progression differ in children?

MSOF/MODS occurs as a syndrome with four distinct clinical stages (Cerra, 1990):

Stage 1   Physiologic shock.
Stage 2   Active resuscitation lasting up to 24 hours.
Stage 3   A hyperdynamic and hypermetabolic state that can last as long
          as 7 to 10 days. During this phase there is evidence of lung in-
          jury.
Stage 4   Liver and renal failure. During this phase the immune system
          also begins to fail (Cerra, 1990).

Failure of the immune system usually begins early and contributes significantly to patient mortality. The longer the syndrome persists, the
greater the mortality. In addition to the above system failures, later
stages produce signs of encephalopathy, coagulopathy, gastrointestinal
tract bleeding, and recurrent infections (Cerra, 1990).

The progression of organ failure in children varies from that seen in
adults. In children organ failure usually occurs in the pulmonary, cardiovascular, and neurologic systems, as compared to the pulmonary,
renal, and hepatic systems in the adult (Czerwinski, 1991).

6. **Describe presenting signs and symptoms of the various stages of
   MSOF/MODS.**

Stage 1 (Early Phase)

During the early phase the patient usually experiences shock and a hypotensive episode, which is usually controlled. The patient appears to
improve for a period of several days.

Stage 2 (False Recovery)

Following this period of recovery the patient begins to display signs of
low-grade fever, tachycardia, dyspnea, and mental confusion. At this
time the chest x–ray may show evidence of patchy infiltrates. Also, coagulopathies and thrombocytopenia may be present. Laboratory values
at this time show normal renal and liver function; however, dyspnea
continues to increase, and intubation and mechanical ventilation may
be necessary.

Stage 3 (Hypermetabolic State)

Following the shock and resuscitation stage, the patient's condition sta-
bilizes but the patient enters into a hyperdynamic, hypermetabolic state
(Cerra, 1990). Cerra (1990) compares this phase to a top athlete running an 8 minute mile; the patient exhibits signs of polyuria, increased
cardiac output, hyperglycemia, hyperlactacidemia, decreased systemic
vascular resistance, leukocytosis, tachycardia, and fever.

Stage 4 (Final and Death)

By the fourth stage the bilirubin starts to climb, is usually more than 3
mg/dl and continues to rise. Renal impairment is seen with elevated

serum creatinine levels. The hyperdynamic and hypermetabolic state continues. Blood glucose and lactate levels continue to rise, and the cardiac output and volume of oxygen utilization continue to increase but with a decrease in systemic vascular resistance. Urinary urea nitrogen excretion increases, and hepatic proteins begin to decrease. There is evidence of increased congestion, coagulopathy, and thrombocytopenia and progression of bacteremia. Inotropic agents and fluids are required to support the blood volume. Preload and polyuria increase. *Candida* organisms, viruses, and cytomegalovirus may be cultured and may be pathogenic. Encephalopathy increases, and gastrointestinal tract bleeding begins. By days 14 to 21 renal failure progresses to the point that dialysis may be needed. By days 21 to 28 death usually occurs (Cerra, 1990).

The above scenario is the most frequently seen clinical picture with MSOF/MODS with two exceptions. First, there may be a primary pulmonary injury where renal and hepatic function do not fail until just a few days before death. Second, MSOF/MODS may continue for the 21 to 28 days described above or may be sudden, with death resulting in a matter of days (Cerra, 1990).

7. **What are the defining criteria for organ failure/organ dysfunction in each of the different systems? Identify assessment parameters that help in the diagnosis of each type of organ failure/organ dysfunction.**

Cardiovascular System

Cardiovascular failure occurs when one or more of the following criteria are met (Knaus & Wagner, 1989):

   (1) A heart rate ≤54 bpm
   (2) Mean arterial pressure ≤49 bpm
   (3) Ventricular tachycardia or fibrillation
   (4) A serum pH ≤7.24 with a $PaCO_2$ ≤49 mm Hg

Cardiovascular assessment includes decreased cardiac output, blood pressure, and ejection fraction. The pulmonary artery pressure, pulmonary capillary wedge pressure, and central venous pressure are increased. In addition, systemic vascular resistance and heart rate may be increased or decreased. Additional findings may include cold and pale skin, weak pulses, narrow pulse pressure, peripheral edema, and cardiac ectopy (Huddleston, 1991).

Pulmonary System

Respiratory failure is dependent on one or more of the following criteria (Knaus & Wagner, 1989):

   (1) Respiratory rate <5/min or ≥49/min
   (2) $PaCO_2$ ≥50 mm Hg

(3) Ventilator dependence or continuous positive airway pressure (CPAP) by the second day of organ failure

Assessment findings may include decreased respiratory depth, increased peak inspiratory pressure, and ventilation-perfusion ($\dot{V}/\dot{Q}$) mismatching. Additional findings may include dyspnea, use of accessory muscles, thick greenish sputum, more than 20% shunting, and infiltrates on chest x–ray (Huddleston, 1991).

Renal System
The presence of one or more of the following findings constitutes renal failure:

(1) Urinary output ≤479 ml/24 h
(2) BUN ≥100 mg/dl
(3) Serum creatinine ≥3.5 mg/dl

Assessment findings might include increased pulmonary capillary wedge pressure and central venous pressure, along with peripheral edema and weight gain (Huddleston, 1991).

Hematologic System
Hematologic failure is based on one or more of the following criteria (Knaus & Wagner, 1989):

(1) WBC <1000/mm^3
(2) Platelets ≤20,000/mm^3
(3) Hematocrit <20%

Additional assessment findings may include pallor and fatigue with evidence of bleeding from the mucous membranes, bruises, thromboembolism, and even disseminated intravascular coagulation (DIC) and systemic infection (Huddleston, 1991).

Neurologic System
Neurologic failure is based on a Glasgow Coma Scale score ≤6 when there is no sedation (Knaus & Wagner, 1989). Physical assessment may reveal a decreased level of consciousness, cerebral perfusion pressure, and respiratory rate. Other assessment findings might include either an increase or decrease in temperature, blood pressure, and heart rate (Huddleston, 1991).

Hepatic System
Liver failure is determined by the presence of one or more of the following criteria (Knaus & Wagner, 1989):

(1) Total bilirubin ≥2 mg/dl
(2) Clinical jaundice

(3) Elevated liver enzymes (AST, ALT, alkaline phosphatase, and LDH)

(4) Serum albumin ≤3 g/dl

Additional assessment findings might include ascites, bleeding from mucous membranes or IV or catheter sites, and bruising (Huddleston, 1991).

Gastrointestinal System

Determination of gastrointestinal failure is based on one or more of the following criteria (Knaus & Wagner, 1989):

(1) Upper or lower GI tract bleeding

(2) Mucosal ulceration or erosion

(3) Diarrhea

(4) Ileus

(5) Bacterial overgrowth identified in a stool culture

Additional findings may include decreased bowel sounds, abdominal distension, and impaction (Huddleston, 1991).

8. List the primary goals of treatment in MSOF/MODS.

There is no definitive therapy for MSOF/MODS. Most treatment is aimed at supporting the failing organ systems. Support may include mechanical ventilation, prophylaxis against gastric stress, dialysis, and aggressive nutritional support (Huddleston, 1992). The other approach is to provide therapy to assist in preventing complications. Three basic principles exist for treatment of MSOF/MODS (Cerra, 1990):

(1) Maintain adequate oxygenation and resuscitation of the microcirculation.

(2) Eliminate or control the source or underlying event. This may include draining of the foci of infection and antibiotic therapy, restoration of perfusion with reversal of lactic acidosis, and fluid resuscitation (Huddleston, 1992).

(3) Offer metabolic and nutritional support (Cerra, 1990). The goal during treatment is to eliminate the flow-dependent oxygen consumption and hyperlactacidemia (Cerra, 1990).

Pulmonary artery monitoring is used to evaluate the resuscitation variables and to adjust blood oxygen content and flow through volume expansion, unloading agents, and inotropic support (Cerra, 1990). Fluid resuscitation is aimed at increasing preload by loading the intravascular volume with IV fluids, both crystalloids and colloids. Crystalloid replacement may consist of three times the amount of volume lost because proteins and fluid do not diffuse into the tissue. If blood loss is significant, blood products should be considered (Huddleston, 1992). The main complication from fluid resuscitation is pulmonary and peripheral edema. Edema is an expected consequence and is not necessarily considered a sign of intravascular volume overload (Huddleston, 1992).

Nutritional support should start 24 to 48 hours after fluid resuscitation. Enteral feedings are preferred over TPN. The goal is to maintain a positive nitrogen balance. Hypercaloric therapy based on 30 to 35 kcal/kg/d is used (Cerra, 1990).

Stress ulcers leading to gastrointestinal tract bleeding are common complications of this syndrome. Stress ulcer complications are prevented by alkalinization with antacids and H_2-receptor blockers such as ranitidine and famotidine (Pepcid).

Because of the high mortality and use of available medical resources, the patient with MSOF/MODS presents many ethical dilemmas. Consideration is given to the role that cost plays in the treatment of the patient with MSOF/MODS, including the cost of rehabilitation if the patient recovers. Because many of these patients are unable to articulate their wishes, the decision to discontinue treatment falls to the family (Huddleston, 1992). The issue of advanced directives and whether they apply in terms of whether MSOF/MODS can be reversed or is versus a terminal condition becomes real. At what point a patient becomes terminal is being questioned.

9. Describe the importance of nutritional support with MSOF/MODS.

Hypermetabolism occurs in MSOF/MODS and results in weight loss, cachexia, and loss of organ function. Nutritional support may not affect the course of the organ failure, but it will prevent nutritional deficits and has proven to result in a reduction of morbidity. The enteral route is the preferred route of nutritional support. Recent guidelines propose that patients should receive 25 to 30 kcal/kg/d with 3 to 5 g/kg/d of glucose. Fat emulsions should be limited to 0.5 to 1 g/kg/d to prevent iatrogenic immunosuppression which is associated with lipid and fat overload (Thelan et al., 1994).

10. What measures are used to prevent gastric complications?

As discussed by Ackerman (1994), the "gut," which was once thought of as a silent organ, now has been cited as the key organ in sepsis. Support of the "gut" by way of nutritional support is vital. Enteral feedings are the suggested route, since parenteral routes carry increased risk for wound infections, sepsis, intraabdominal infections, and pneumonia. It has also been noted that patients who are malnourished and in a hypermetabolic state have immunologic deficits that can further be affected by nutrition. Thelan et al. (1994) suggest "gut" decontamination with enteral antibiotics to prevent nosocomial infections, topical antibiotics in the oral pharynx to prevent colonization, and monoclonal antibodies to assist in fighting endotoxins and passive antibody protection.

11. What are nursing considerations for the patient with MSOF/MODS?

Nursing considerations are varied and may cover the entire list of high-risk or actual problems depending on the organ systems involved. Huddleston (1992) provides an extensive list of nursing diagnoses for the patient with MSOF/MODS, which includes but may not be limited to the following:

- ➤ alteration in tissue perfusion
- ➤ fluid volume deficit or excess
- ➤ impaired gas exchange
- ➤ ineffective airway clearance
- ➤ high risk for infection
- ➤ alteration in nutrition
- ➤ alteration in skin integrity
- ➤ impaired mobility
- ➤ decreased cardiac output
- ➤ anxiety
- ➤ pain
- ➤ hyperthermia or hypothermia
- ➤ impaired communication
- ➤ ineffective family coping

12. What ethical considerations play a role in the diagnosis of MSOF/MODS?

Early in the course of the illness, Mrs. Whitman expressed a desire not to be intubated and to "let me just die." Despite Mrs. Whitman's wishes she received all possible life support interventions. The issue of advanced directives, such as living will and durable power of attorney, will continue to play an important role in today's health care environment. It is important that nurses be prepared to inform patients of the existence of advanced directives and to assist them in developing their own before becoming critically ill and facing the possibility of not having their wishes carried out. Other future ethical considerations for these patients are the rationing of health care dollars and the futility of care. Families and health care workers will face the fact that rehabilitation after recovery in the patient with MSOF/MODS is costly, involving months of rehabilitation before the patient achieves a functional level. Quality vs. quantity of life issues may need to be addressed.

Multiple Organ Failure/Multiple Organ Dysfunction Syndrome

Ackerman, M. (1994). The systemic inflammatory response, sepsis, and multiple organ dysfunction. *Critical Care Clinics of North America, 6*(2), 243–250.

Bauer, A. E. (1990). *Multiple organ failure: Patient care and prevention.* St. Louis: Mosby–Year Book.

Cerra, F. (1990, August 15). The multiple organ failure syndrome. *Hospital Practice,* 169–176.

Clochesy, J., Breu, C., Cardin, S., Rudy, E., & Whittaker, A. (1993). *Critical care nursing.* Philadelphia: Saunders.

Czerwinski, S. J. (1991). Complications of pediatric trauma. *Critical Care Nursing Clinics of North America, 3*(3),479–488.

Deitch, E. A. (Ed.). (1990). Gut failure: Its role in the multiple organ failure syndrome. *Multiple organ failure pathophysiology and basic concepts of therapy.* New York: Thieme Medical.

Huddleston, V. (1991, September). Multisystem organ failure: What you need to know. *Nursing 91,* 34–41.

Huddleston, V. (1992). *Multiple system organ failure: Pathophysiology and clinical implications.* St. Louis: Mosby–Year Book.

Knaus, W. A., & Wagner, D. P. (1989). Multiple system organ failure: epidemiology and prognosis. *Critical Care Clinics, 5,* 221–232.

McFadden, M. E., & Satorius, S. (1992a). Multiple system organ failure in the patient with cancer: Part I: Pathophysiologic perspective. *Oncology Nursing Forum, 19*(5), 719–724.

McFadden, M. E., & Satorius, S. (1992b). Multiple system organ failure in the patient with cancer: Part II: Nursing implications. *Oncology Nursing Forum, 19*(5), 727–737.

Thelan, L., Davie, J., Urden, L., & Lough, M. (1994). *Critical care nursing: Diagnosis and management* (p. 800). St. Louis: Mosby-Year Book.

Weil, M., & Pakula, J. (1992, April 15). Urgent management of multiple organ failure. *Emergency Medicine,* 216 & 225–226.

24

Sepsis/Septic Shock

Lynn Rodgers, MSN, RNC, CCRN, CNRN

CASE PRESENTATION

Emergency Room

John Roberts, a 72-year-old man, arrived in the emergency department unconscious and with stab wounds to the right upper abdomen and right lower chest that were sustained in his home while fighting off a burglar. The paramedics secured two large-bore intravenous (IV) catheters in his right and left antecubital spaces and infused lactated Ringer's solution wide open in both sites. An endotracheal tube was inserted, and ventilation with a resuscitation bag with 100% oxygen was begun. Medical antishock trousers (MAST) were in place. Pressure dressings to both wounds were secured.

A 5 cm (2 in.) stab wound to his right lower chest and a 7.5 cm (3 in.) stab wound to his right upper abdomen were inspected. Chest tubes were inserted into the right upper and lower midaxillary region. Immediately, 500 ml of red drainage returned via the lower chest tube. His heart rate was 125 bpm, and the monitor showed sinus tachycardia without ectopy. His blood pressure was 70/50. Inserting a Foley catheter resulted in 400 ml clear dark yellow urine. After being infused with over 2000 ml of lactated Ringer's solution, Mr. Roberts was sent to surgery, still in a hypotensive state. Preoperative body weight was 74 kg (165 lb).

Surgical Intervention

During surgery a right thoracotomy and right abdominal laparotomy were performed. The right chest wound was explored, and a lacerated intercostal artery was ligated. Exploration of his right upper abdominal wound revealed more extensive damage. The liver and the duodenum were lacerated. Extensive hemorrhage and leaking of intestinal contents were apparent after opening the peritoneum. Mr. Roberts' injuries were repaired, the peritoneal cavity irrigated with antibiotic solution, and incisional sump drains were placed in the duodenum.

During the 4-hour surgery, Mr. Roberts received 6 U of blood and an additional 3 L of lactated Ringer's solution. A pulmonary artery catheter (PAC) and right radial arterial line were inserted.

ICU: Immediately After Surgery

Mr. Roberts arrived in the surgical intensive care unit (SICU) on a ventilator with the following settings:

Assist Mode
Rate 12
FIO_2 60%
V_T 800 ml

Vital signs and hemodynamic parameters immediately following surgery were

BP	92/52	PAP	20/8 mm Hg
HR	114 bpm	PCWP	6 mm Hg
Respirations	12/min	CVP	4 mm Hg
Temperature	36.2° C (97.2° F)	CO	5 L/min
		CI	2.9 L/min/m²
		SVR	1040 dynes/s/cm⁻⁵

Arterial blood gases (ABGs) were normal. Except for a white blood cell (WBC) count of $13.6 \times 10^3/mm^3$ and a hemoglobin of 10 g/dl, Mr. Roberts' other laboratory values were within normal limits.

ICU: Postoperative Day 1

Mr. Roberts remained drowsy but received ventilatory support for 24 days. His pain was controlled by IV morphine sulfate. The nasogastric tube (NGT) continued to drain large amounts of green fluid, and an incisional duodenal sump tube drained large amounts of greenish brown fluid. His chest and abdominal dressings remained dry. Breath sounds were diminished on the right but clear on the left. His chest tubes continued to drain small amounts of bloody fluid. Urine output was 40 to 60 ml/h. His abdomen was slightly firm and distended, and he had no bowel sounds.

ICU: Postoperative Day 2

Mr. Roberts remained stable until his second postoperative day. At this time, he became difficult to arouse but did respond to commands. His respirations were 28/min, shallow, and labored. His urine output dropped to 20 ml/h. His skin became warm, dry, and flushed. Other clinical data included

BP	80/50	PAP	14/7 mm Hg
HR	132 bpm	PCWP	4 mm Hg
Temperature	40° C (104° F)	CVP	2 mm Hg
WBCs	22,000/mm³	CO	8 L/min
Glucose	270 mg/dl	CI	4.7 L/min/m²
		SVR	560 dynes/s/cm⁻⁵

Culture and sensitivity reports from wound drainage indicated gram-negative bacilli. Appropriate IV antibiotics were administered, as well as IV hydrocortisone, nebacumab (Centoxin), and naloxone (Narcan) IV infusion. To prepare for the suspected hyperdynamic phase of septic shock, lactated Ringer's solution was increased to 150 ml/h, and dopamine at 5 µg/kg/min was started with a concentration of 200 mg/250 ml 5% dextrose in water (D_5W).

ICU: Postoperative Day 6

By the sixth postoperative day, Mr. Roberts' condition had deteriorated dramatically. His skin was cool, mottled, and moist. His sclerae were yellow tinged. He no longer responded to stimuli. A norepinephrine (Levophed) drip infused at 6 µg/min with a concentration of 4 mg/250 ml D_5W, along with a dopamine drip at 2 µg/kg/min. His monitor showed sinus tachycardia with short runs of ventricular tachycardia. ST segment elevation, T wave inversion, and Q waves had developed over most of the anterior V leads on his electrocardiogram (ECG). Lidocaine was started at 2 mg/min with a concentration of 2 g/500 ml D_5W. His breath sounds revealed crackles throughout his chest. Urinary output was only 3 to 5 ml/h. His abdomen was grossly enlarged and firm. His abdominal suture lines had dehisced, and the peritoneum could be seen. Further clinical data included

BP	70/52	PAP	44/26 mm Hg
HR	140 bpm	PCWP	24 mm Hg
Respirations	14/min	CVP	8 mm Hg
Temperature	35.8° C (96.4° F)	CO	2 L/min
		CI	1.1 L/min/m²
		SVR	2000 dynes/s/cm⁻⁵

Other abnormal laboratory results were

pH	7.14	Na⁺	152 mmol/L	FSP	39
Pco_2	49 mm Hg	K⁺	5.9 mmol/L	Platelets	75,000/mm³
Po_2	46 mm Hg	Creatinine	3.4 mg/dl	PT	22 s
Sao_2	85%	Amylase	290 U/L	PTT	98.5 s
HCO_3^-	12 mmol/L	AST	82 U/L	CK	640 U/L
		Lipase	3.9 U/L	ALT	100 U/L

Final Developments

Despite attempts to reduce afterload with sodium nitroprusside (Nipride) and increase contractility with dobutamine (Dobutrex), Mr. Roberts' hemodynamic status failed even further. When his cardiac rhythm deteriorated into ventricular fibrillation, resuscitation efforts were unsuccessful. An autopsy revealed several small abscessed areas in the lung, acute hepatic failure, and an acute myocardial infarction.

QUESTIONS

Sepsis/Septic Shock

1. Discuss the magnitude of bacteremia and sepsis in hospitalized patients and the relationship of these two diagnoses.

2. What are the risk factors for septic shock development? Identify those that Mr. Roberts displayed.

3. Discuss the rationale for a pulmonary artery catheter in monitoring septic shock.

4. What organisms most commonly cause septic shock?

5. What are the pathophysiologic effects of septic shock on the patient's vascular tank, volume, and pump?

6. Discuss clinical and laboratory changes that occurred on Mr. Roberts' second postoperative day.

7. What is the rationale for each of the following therapeutic modalities ordered for Mr. Roberts on the second postoperative day?

   - IV rate increased to 150 ml/h
   - dopamine 5 µg/kg/min
   - hydrocortisone IV
   - nebacumab (Centoxin)
   - naloxone (Narcan) IV infusion

8. Discuss the clinical changes that occurred during Mr. Roberts' sixth postoperative day.

9. What is the rationale for each of the following therapeutic modalities ordered on the sixth postoperative day? Calculate how many milliliters per hour should be infused for each drug listed.

   - norepinephrine 6 µg/min
   - dopamine 2 µg/kg/min
   - lidocaine 2 mg/min

10. What are the reasons for the changes in the following hemodynamic parameters noted on the sixth postoperative day?

    • SVR
    • CO and CI
    • PCWP

11. Interpret Mr. Roberts' blood gas levels on the sixth postoperative day.

12. Why are the renal, liver, and pancreatic laboratory values reported on the sixth postoperative day abnormal?

13. What complications do the hematologic laboratory values suggest?

14. What would account for the ECG changes described?

15. Mr. Roberts' liver was lacerated during the stabbing. What effect, if any, did this have on his eventual outcome?

16. Describe the differences in the parameters below between hyperdynamic or warm septic shock and hypodynamic or cold septic shock.

	Hyperdynamic	Hypodynamic
• LOC		
• BP		
• HR		
• Respirations		
• Pulse pressure		
• Skin		
• SVR		
• CO and CI		
• Urine output		

QUESTIONS AND ANSWERS

Sepsis/Septic Shock

1. **Discuss the magnitude of bacteremia and sepsis in hospitalized patients and the relationship of these two diagnoses.**

   Septic shock is the most common cause of death in today's ICUs (Bone, 1994). Lowry (1994) reports that each year 400,000 to 500,000 patients in the United States develop sepsis. Half of all patients diagnosed with sepsis/septic shock die (Russell, 1994). The Centers for Disease Control and Prevention estimate that over the past decade the incidence of sepsis has increased by 137% (Bone, 1994), and that 140,000 cases of gram-negative bacteremia occur annually. However, bacteremia does not always create systemic complications, and sepsis can be caused by pathogens other than bacteria. Regardless of the causative organism, systemic complications occur when circulating chemical mediators released by the inflammatory response compromise the patient's cardiovascular system.

   Sepsis is a physiologic response to a systematic inflammatory process. The probability of infection is related to the number of organisms present, their ability to cause disease, and the patient's degree of resistance. When the diagnosis of sepsis is followed by prompt therapy, mortality ranges from 40% to 60%. If management is delayed or ineffective, septic shock, which is associated with hypotension, develops, and mortality increases to 90% to 95% (Clochesy, Breu, Cardin, Rudy, & Whittaker, 1993).

2. **What are the risk factors for septic shock development? Identify those that Mr. Roberts displayed.**

   Clochesy et al. (1993) classified risk factors of septic shock development as host related and treatment related. Host-related risk factors include burns, trauma, malnutrition, leukemia, age over 70 years, and debilitating diseases (especially chronic lung disease, cardiovascular disease, diabetes mellitus, renal or liver failure), pregnancy, and immunocompromised states.

Treatment-related risk factors include foreign body insertion, drugs (especially immunosuppressives, cytotoxins, and antibiotics), artificial airways, surgery, and immobility.

Mr. Roberts had the following risk factors: IV infusion, endotracheal tube, chest tube, Foley catheter, PAC and right radial arterial line, abdominal trauma, age over 70 years, and leaking of gastrointestinal contents into the peritoneum.

3. Discuss the rationale for a pulmonary artery catheter in monitoring septic shock.

A pulmonary artery catheter is used to monitor septic shock because the cardiovascular and metabolic abnormalities involved in septic shock are readily determined by the patient's hemodynamic profile obtained from the PAC.

Vazquez, Lazear, and Larson (1992) described septic shock as having two distinct phases: hyperdynamic and hypodynamic. Initially a hyperdynamic response occurs. During this phase, systemic vascular resistance (SVR) is decreased. An increase in cardiac muscle contractility also develops as a compensatory mechanism. The decrease in SVR and increase in cardiac contractility result in an abnormally high cardiac output (CO) and cardiac index (CI). In addition, pulmonary artery and capillary wedge pressures (PAWP and PCWP, respectively) can be below normal because of the venous vasodilation and decreased venous return.

During the hypodynamic phase of septic shock, compensatory mechanisms begin to fail. Fluid escapes the vascular tree into the tissues because of an increase in capillary permeability. Sympathetic nervous system stimulation causes profound vasoconstriction. The heart muscle itself is depressed, and contractility decreases. Hypotension then results from decreased intravascular volume, increased SVR, and decreased cardiac contractility. CO and CI are decreased; however, PAWP and PCWP are increased. Treatment is guided by the hemodynamic information that a pulmonary artery catheter provides. With this information, the patient's chances of survival are increased.

4. What organisms most commonly cause septic shock?

The organisms that most commonly cause septic shock are the gram-negative bacteria, specifically *Escherichia coli, Klebsiella, Enterobacter, Serratia, Pseudomonas aeruginosa, Bacteroides,* and *Proteus* (Clochesy et al., 1993).

5. What are the pathophysiologic effects of septic shock on the patient's vascular tank, volume, and pump?

Clochesy et al. (1993) describe the three major effects of septic shock within the cardiovascular system as (1) vasodilation, (2) maldistribution of blood volume, and (3) myocardial depression. Dilation in the arterial and venous circulation decreases SVR and preload. Initially, compensation occurs by an increase in CO. However, tissue perfusion continues to decrease because of the maldistribution of blood flow and cardiac dysfunction.

Although septic shock is usually associated with vasodilation, pulmonary, renal, hepatic, splenic, and pancreatic vasoconstriction occurs. Maldistribution of blood flow develops as a consequence of blood volume displacement. Histamine and bradykinin increase capillary permeability, allowing serum to migrate into the interstitial spaces. This fluid shift depletes the circulating volume and increases blood viscosity. Blood flow becomes sluggish, white blood cells (WBCs) and platelets accumulate, and microemboli develop. Vascular occlusion and inadequate tissue perfusion progress. There is irreversible cellular dysfunction due to inadequate tissue perfusion (Brown, 1994b).

Although the exact mechanism of the septic inflammatory response is unclear, various mediators are thought to depress the function of the myocardium (Ognibene & Cunnion, 1993). Some findings suggest that microvascular and myocyte damage depresses the myocardial function. Other studies find evidence that the myocardium is hyporesponsive to catecholamines because of impaired β-adrenergic receptor stimulation of cyclic adenosine monophosphate (AMP). Still other researchers have found indirect evidence of specific myocardial depressant substances (Clochesy et al., 1993). Regardless of the mechanism, the depressed myocardium meets no resistance in the profoundly vasodilated systemic vascular bed. Thus CO and CI initially are maintained and often increased.

In summary, the common cardiovascular patterns demonstrated initially in septic shock consist of high CO, low SVR, decreased left ventricular ejection fraction (LVEF), a dilated left ventricle, and a normal or increased stroke volume. Death is usually a result of hypotension due to a perpetual decrease in CO, a progressively increasing SVR, and eventual multiple organ system failure.

6. **Discuss clinical and laboratory changes that occurred on Mr. Roberts' second postoperative day.**

Difficult to Arouse

This is an early cardinal sign of systemic infection and inflammatory response to circulating endotoxins. The septic patient's level of consciousness continues to deteriorate during an impending shock state as a result of decreased cerebral perfusion.

Respirations 28/min, Shallow and Labored

The lungs are a target organ throughout the progression of septic shock. Circulating endotoxins debilitate the pulmonary status of the patient. The initial pulmonary response to endotoxins creates bronchoconstriction. Pulmonary edema as a result of increased capillary permeability occurs. Tachypnea is also an early cardinal sign of systemic infection, hypoxemia, and physiologic stress.

Urine Output Decreased to 20 ml/h

As renal blood flow in the patient in septic shock is reduced, urine output decreases. Antidiuretic hormone (ADH) and aldosterone are released to increase intravascular water and sodium in an attempt to maintain CO and renal blood flow, often with no success. In addition, aminoglycoside antibiotics, frequently effective in sepsis, are nephrotoxic.

Warm, Dry, Flushed Skin

In the early stages of septic shock, vasoactive mediators create a flushed appearance because of peripheral vasodilation. This early stage is known as hyperdynamic or warm septic shock.

BP 80/50

Hypotension commonly is due to the vasodilation when cardiac compensation fails.

HR 132 bpm

Tachycardia is another early cardinal sign of a systemic infection and inflammatory response. An increase in heart rate is also a compensatory mechanism to maintain perfusion and CO.

Temperature 40° C (104° F)

The hypothalamus responds to bacteremia with an increase in temperature. As blood is shunted away from the skin during shock, the normal ability of the skin to disperse heat is decreased. Fever also is one of the cardinal signs of infection and inflammation.

CI 4.7 L/min/m², SVR 560 dynes/s/cm⁻⁵

The initial hyperdynamic pattern of septic shock consists of high CI as a result of low SVR. Toxic bacterial endotoxins are thought to decrease vasomotor tone of the blood vessels by activating the release of endorphins and histamine and the complement system.

WBCs 22,000/mm³

Leukopenia is an early finding in a septic immunocompromised patient. However, as sepsis progresses, the inflammatory response signals the bone marrow to accelerate leukocyte synthesis and release. Consequently, the WBC level will increase more than $10,000/mm^3$.

Glucose 270 mg/dl

The reaction of the adrenal cortex to shock is to release glucocorticoids. The glucocorticoids release glucagon. Glucagon stimulates the conversion of glycogen to glucose (glycolysis) and gluconeogenesis in the liver. Therefore the serum glucose level may be elevated.

Culture and Sensitivity Reports Indicate Gram-Negative Bacilli

Gram-negative bacteria are the organisms that most commonly cause septic shock (Brown, 1994b; Clochesy et al., 1993; Russell, 1994; Thelan, Davie, & Urden, 1994).

7. **What is the rationale for each of the following therapeutic modalities ordered for Mr. Roberts on the second postoperative day?**

IV Rate Increased to 150 ml/h

Restoration of adequate intravascular volume is an important aspect of patient care during episodes of hypotension. Vasodilation during sepsis dramatically decreases preload and afterload. The vascular tree is too large for the circulating volume. The circulating volume is also further decreased because increased capillary permeability allows fluid to escape into interstitial spaces (Thelan et al., 1994).

Dopamine 5 μg/kg/min

Low-dose dopamine increases renal blood flow, creates a moderate pressor effect, and improves cardiac performance.

Steroids

Corticosteroids are controversial and should be reserved for patients in septic shock who have a suspected or documented adrenal insufficiency. According to Littleton (1993), mortality of patients with sepsis or septic shock who received corticosteroids was not significantly reduced and in some cases was higher because of the development of secondary infections.

Nebacumab (Centoxin)

Centoxin is a monoclonal antiendotoxin antibody developed specifically to fight gram-negative sepsis. It binds to the circulating endotoxins, thus preventing the initiation of the mediator cascade thought to be responsible for the pathogenesis of septic shock. Antiendotoxin antibody therapy is still under investigation (Klein & Witek-Janusek, 1992; Suffredini, 1994).

Naloxone (Narcan) IV Infusion

Naloxone is a narcotic antagonist generally used to reverse the respiratory depression caused by narcotics. As described by Russell (1994), naloxone is now given to patients with severe septic shock before compensatory mechanisms cease. Its primary actions are to reverse the effects of endorphins and the myocardial depressant factor, thereby combating vasodilation and decreased contractility.

8. **Discuss clinical changes that occurred during Mr. Roberts' sixth postoperative day.**

As described by Gould (1990) the following clinical changes occur as septic shock progresses.

Cool, Mottled, Moist Skin

The skin indicates the change from hyperdynamic (warm) to hypodynamic (cold) septic shock. This is a poor prognostic sign for the patient, as it indicates failure of the compensatory mechanisms.

Yellow Sclerae

As chemical mediators continue to shunt blood to various organs, the patient's liver and kidneys become hypoperfused. Hyperbilirubinemia and jaundice are common clinical indicators that the liver is adversely affected. In addition, Mr. Roberts' liver was lacerated during his injury.

ECG Changes—Sinus Tachycardia with Short Runs of Ventricular Tachycardia

Sinus and ventricular tachycardias indicate further myocardial damage from the circulating endotoxins and the decreased CO. Because the kidneys are hypoperfused, the patient may be experiencing acute renal failure. The K^+ level of 5.9 mmol/L could suggest acute renal failure and is probably responsible for the ventricular tachycardia. The 12-lead ECG indicated a massive anterior wall myocardial infarction (MI).

BP 70/52, CO 2 L/min, CI 1.1 L/min/m², PAP 44/26 mm Hg, PCWP 24 mm Hg, SVR 2000 dynes/s/cm⁻⁵, CVP 8 mm Hg

Mr. Roberts' hemodynamic changes are classic indications of the hypodynamic phase of septic shock. Afterload is drastically increased, and contractility is decreased. Multisystem failure is imminent.

Respirations 14/min, Congested Breath Sounds

Mr. Roberts' respiratory assessment indicates further debilitation of the respiratory status due to circulating endotoxins, pulmonary edema, and left ventricular failure.

Temperature 35.8° C (96.4° F)

The low temperature is another indication that the patient has progressed from hyperdynamic to hypodynamic septic shock.

Abdomen Large and Firm, Wound Dehiscence

Because of increased capillary permeability, accumulation of inflammatory fluids, and cardiac failure, ascites is present. The increased intraabdominal pressure and poor healing produced wound dehiscence.

9. What is the rationale for each of the following therapeutic modalities ordered on the sixth postoperative day? Calculate how many
   milliliters per hour should be infused for each drug listed.

Norepinephrine 6 µg/min = 22.5 ml/h

Norepinephrine is indicated for hemodynamically significant hypotension unresponsive to other vasopressors.

Dopamine 2 µg/kg/min = 11.25 ml/h

Dopamine at 1 to 3 µg/kg/min dilates the renal and mesenteric vessels. Norepinephrine constricts the renal and mesenteric vessels, and
adding low doses of dopamine counteracts some of this effect.

Lidocaine 2 mg/min = 30 ml/h

Lidocaine was started to decrease the ventricular irritability, which is evidenced by the ventricular tachycardia and which most likely is caused
in part by the K^+ level of 5.9 mmol/L.

10. What are the reasons for the changes in the following hemody-
    namic parameters noted on the sixth postoperative day?

SVR

The SVR increased from 560 to 2000 dynes/s/cm^{-5}. Clinically the
SVR represents the resistance against which the left ventricle must
pump to eject its volume. This elevation indicates a change from hyperdynamic to hypodynamic septic shock.

CO and CI

The CO decreased from 8 to 4.7 L/min, and the CI decreased from
2 to 1.1 L/min/m^2 on the sixth postoperative day. Since CO represents the amount of blood pumped by the ventricle in 1 minute, it can
be concluded that an increase in SVR will decrease the CO and CI. A
drop in CO and CI indicates that hypodynamic septic shock has developed.

PCWP

The PCWP increased from 4 to 24 mm Hg, indicating an increase in
the pressure in the left side of the heart. This could be from the ventricular dilation and decreased ejection fraction that occurs in late sep-

tic shock as well as from the release of various chemical and hormonal mediators that depresss the myocardial function.

11. Interpret Mr. Roberts' blood gas levels on the sixth postoperative day.

Mr. Roberts' blood gas levels indicate metabolic and respiratory acidosis. Lactic acidosis due to increased oxygen debt from abnormal cellular metabolism is a common finding in patients with septic shock. During the progression of septic shock, a ventilation-perfusion mismatch also develops as chemical mediators create pulmonary interstitial edema and a maldistribution in pulmonic blood flow (Brown, 1994a).

pH 7.14 PCO_2 49 PO_2 46 SaO_2 65%   Bicarb 12

12. Why are the renal, liver, and pancreatic laboratory values reported on the sixth postoperative day abnormal?

As described by Gould (1990), the kidneys, liver, brain, and lungs are the organs most frequently affected by septic shock. As renal blood flow is reduced, urine output decreases, and the body is unable to eliminate waste products. Acute renal failure ensues. As chemical mediators continue to shunt blood to various organs, the liver and pancreas become hypoperfused.

13. What complications do the hematologic laboratory values suggest?

Possible complications based on the hematologic laboratory values include acute renal and hepatic failure, disseminated intravascular coagulation (DIC), adult respiratory distress syndrome (ARDS), and acute MI (Clochesy et al., 1993).

14. What would account for the ECG changes described?

Mr. Roberts' ECG changes could indicate an acute anterior wall MI. This diagnosis can be made by the ST segment elevation, T wave inversion, and diagnostic Q waves in the V anterior chest leads. The diagnosis was substantiated by his elevated CK and AST levels.

15. Mr. Roberts' liver was lacerated during the stabbing. What effect, if any, did this have on his eventual outcome?

According to Gould (1990), patients at greatest risk for development of septic shock are those who have sustained open wounds, open fractures, massive tissue injury, or significant head injury. The lacerated liver was directly related to the acute hepatic failure noted on the autopsy.

16. **Describe the differences in the parameters below between hyper-dynamic or warm septic shock and hypodynamic or cold septic shock.**

Vazquez et al. (1992) summarize the differences in the hyperdynamic and hypodynamic stages of septic shock as follows:

	Hyperdynamic	Hypodynamic
LOC	Mental cloudiness	Continued deterioration
BP	Normal to just below baseline	Profound hypotension
HR	Bounding pulses, tachycardia	Thready pulses, tachycardia
Respirations	Decreased rate or mild respiratory distress	Decreased rate with severe respiratory complications
Pulse pressure	Normal to wide	Narrow
Skin	Warm, dry	Cool, moist, mottled
SVR	Decreased	Increased
CO and CI	Increased	Decreased
Urine output	Normal	Decreased

Sepsis/Septic Shock

Bone, C. B. (1994). Sepsis and its complications: The clinical problem. *Critical Care Medicine, 22*(7), S8–S12.

Brown, K. K. (1994b). Septic shock: How to stop the deadly cascade. *American Journal of Nursing, 94*(9), 20–27.

Brown, K. K. (1994a). Critical interventions in septic shock. *American Journal of Nursing, 94*(10), 20–26.

Clochesy, J. M., Breu, C., Cardin, S., Rudy, E. B., & Whittaker, A. A. (1993). *Critical care nursing.* Philadelphia: Saunders.

Gould, K. A. (Ed.). (1990). *Critical care nursing clinics of North America.* Philadelphia: Saunders.

Klein, D. M., & Witek-Janusek, L. (1992). Advances in immunotherapy of sepsis. *Dimensions of Critical Care Nursing, 11*(2), 75–89.

Littleton, M. T. (1993). Trends in agents used for the management of sepsis. *Critical Care Nursing Quarterly, 15*(4), 33–46.

Lowry, S. F. (1994). Sepsis and its complications: Clinical definitions and therapeutic prospects. *Critical Care Medicine, 22*(7), S1–S2.

Ognibene, F. P., & Cunnion, R. E. (1993). Mechanisms of myocardial depression in sepsis. *Critical Care Medicine, 1*(1), 6–8.

Russell, S. (1994). Septic shock: Can you recognize the clues? *Nursing 94,* 40–46.

Thelan, L. A., Davie, J. K., & Urden, L. D. (1994). *Textbook of critical care nursing: Diagnosis and management.* St. Louis: Mosby–Year Book.

Suffredini, A. F. (1994). Current prospects for the treatment of clinical sepsis. *Critical Care Medicine, 22*(7), S12–S18.

Vazquez, M., Lazear, S. E., & Larson, E. L. (1992). *Critical care nursing.* Philadelphia: Saunders.

25

Burns

Ann H. White, MSN, MBA, RN, CNA

CASE PRESENTATION

Tony, a 21-year-old man, was involved in an industrial fire. Tony was welding a steel structure when a spark from his torch ignited a barrel of flammable material that was inadvertently placed in his work area. Tony sustained full-thickness burns over the upper half of his chest and circumferential burns to both arms. He also sustained superficial partial-thickness burns to his face, neck, and both hands. His entire abdomen, upper half of his back, and front of his upper legs sustained deep partial-thickness burns. It was calculated that 65% of Tony's total body surface area (TBSA) was burned.

He was transported to a small community hospital where two intravenous (IV) lines were started, a Foley catheter and nasogastric tube were inserted, and a nasal cannula with humidified oxygen at 3 L/min was started. He was given mannitol 12.5 g IV before being transported to a major burn center. Vital signs immediately before transport were

BP   136/84
HR   96 bpm
Respirations 24/min
Temperature 37.2° C (99° F) (oral)

Tony's preburn weight was established at 72 kg (160 lb). Tony was received in the burn unit 4 hours after sustaining the burn injury.

At admission to the burn unit, Tony was alert and oriented, and his vital signs were

BP   140/90
HR   110 bpm
Respirations 24/min
Temperature 36.1° C (97° F) (oral)

Tony's lungs were clear in all fields on auscultation, with an occasional productive cough of a small amount of carbon-tinged sputum. His voice was becoming hoarse. No bowel sounds were heard, and the nasogastric tube was draining dark yellow-green liquid. Peripheral pulses were obtained with a Doppler stethoscope, as they could not be palpated manually. The Foley catheter was draining a burgundy-colored urine. Urine output totaled 280 ml since the insertion of the Foley catheter 4 hours before. Fluid resuscitation efforts since the burn injury included 4 L of lactated Ringer's solution through the IV lines. The following laboratory results were determined after Tony's arrival in the burn unit:

WBCs	$12 \times 10^3/mm^3$
RBCs	$4.8 \times 10^6/mm^3$
Hgb	12.8 g/dl
Hct	52%

pH	7.37*
P_{CO_2}	35 mm Hg
P_{O_2}	105 mm Hg
HCO_3^-	18 mmol/L
Sa_{O_2}	99%

*On 3 L oxygen.

SMAC 20

Na^+	151 mmol/L
K^+	5.2 mmol/L
Cl^-	112 mmol/L
BUN	22 mg/dl
Creatinine	1.6 mg/dl
Myoglobin (RIA)	90 ng/ml
Carboxyhemoglobin	6%

Urinalysis

Specific gravity	1.040
Glucose	+ 1
Ketones	trace
Blood	trace
Protein	trace

The burn unit physician performed a fiberoptic bronchoscopy, which showed minimal redness of the glottis and no edema. Escharotomies were performed on Tony's arms immediately after admission to the burn unit. Tony was bathed, his scalp was shaved, and his burns were dressed in occlusive silver sulfadiazine (Silvadene) dressings. Tony's burns were then dressed twice a day with silver sulfadiazine. The following regimen was prescribed: ranitidine (Zantac) 150 mg IV push q12h; antacid 30 ml q1h instilled through a nasogastric tube and clamped for 15 minutes; and morphine sulfate 3 mg IV push q1h prn for pain.

Bowel sounds returned on day 3, and a high-calorie, high-protein diet was begun. On day 5 of the hospital stay, Tony was taken to surgery for the first of a series of surgical procedures to excise and graft the areas of full-thickness injury with split-thickness autografts. The donor sites included his buttocks and the backs of his legs. Tony was discharged from the hospital after a 65-day hospital stay with follow-up and rehabilitation scheduled.

Burns

1. Discuss the pathophysiology of burns, including the classification of burn depth and severity of burn injury.

2. Describe the three phases of burn physiology, including a discussion of the effects on the following systems during the emergent and acute phases:
   - cardiovascular
   - respiratory
   - immunologic
   - gastrohepatic
   - genitourinary

3. Based on the preburn weight, use the Parkland formula to calculate the fluid requirement to adequately resuscitate Tony.

4. What significance, if any, would the administration of mannitol have on fluid resuscitation?

5. What assessment findings would indicate myoglobinuria?

6. Describe the treatment protocol of myoglobinuria.

7. What assessment findings are critical to establish the presence of an inhalation injury? What assessment findings warrant concern with Tony?

8. Describe the treatment protocol of a burn patient with an inhalation injury or a suspected inhalation injury.

9. What is the purpose of escharotomies?

10. Discuss pain management in the treatment protocol of the burn-injured patient.

11. Using the Curreri formula for nutrition, calculate Tony's nutritional needs. Discuss the need for a high-calorie, high-protein diet.

12. Discuss burn wound care and dressing techniques. Include the types of topical antimicrobial agents commonly used in wound care, listing advantages and disadvantages of each.

13. Describe the types of biologic and synthetic dressings currently being used in wound care.

14. Discuss the use of autografts and the nursing care required.

15. Describe the appropriate care of donor sites.

16. Discuss the splinting and positioning required for Tony to maintain use of his extremities and upper body.

17. List the nursing diagnoses, outcomes, and interventions appropriate for the care of the burn patient during the emergent and acute phases of burn physiology.

18. Discuss the psychosocial aspects of caring for the burn patient and the impact on the patient's support system.

QUESTIONS AND ANSWERS

Burns

1. **Discuss the pathophysiology of burns, including the classification of burn depth and severity of burn injury.**

Thermal Burn

A thermal burn is a heat-related injury produced through exposure to hot liquids, steam, flames from a fire, or direct contact with some heat source. This exposure disrupts in the function of the skin and its appendages. The extent or severity of this disruption depends on the length of contact time with the heat source, extent of tissue exposed to the heat source, and ability of the heat source and tissue to dissipate the heat (Molter, Duncan, & DePew, 1993).

Classification of Burn Depth

Traditionally, burns have been classified as first, second, and third degree. Today, burns are described as superficial, partial thickness, and full thickness. Table 25–1 describes each type of burn and common characteristics of each.

Severity of Burn Injury

The severity of the burn injury is rated as minor, moderate, or major, depending on the areas of the body involved in the burn injury and the total body surface area (TBSA) burned (Caine & Lefcourt, 1993). A minor burn for adults usually has a small surface area (less than 15%) with no involvement of the face, hands, feet, or perineum and can be treated in the home environment. A moderate burn injury has a larger surface area (usually 15% to 25% of the TBSA), including partial- and full-thickness burns. A major burn has a TBSA of more than 25%, including partial- and full-thickness burns. Any burns involving parts of the face, hands, feet, or perineum are included in this category (Calistro, 1993). Moderate and major burn injuries should be treated in a burn center or a critical care area with expertise in the care of burn patients.

Table 25–1 Classification of Burn Depth

	Superficial	Partial Thickness Superfical	Deep	Full Thickness
Morphology	Destruction of epidermis (no other layers involved)	Destruction of epidermis and minimal dermis	Destruction of epidermis and dermis; skin appendages (hair follicles, etc) intact	Destruction of epidermis and dermis; loss of skin appendages and subcutaneous tissue
Skin function	Intact	Intact	Absent	Absent
Tactile and pain sensors	Intact	Intact	Diminished	Absent
Blisters	May be present after 24 h	Fluid-filled blisters appear immediately after injury	Usually not present, eschar formation	Not present; eschar formation
Appearance of wound	Redness of area with local edema	Moist, pink, or mottled red	Mottled with areas of waxy white, dry surface; absence of blanching	Thick, leathery eschar; white, cherry red, or brown-black; blood vessels may be thrombosed
Healing time	3 to 5 d	10 to 14 d	21+ d	Will not heal
Scarring	None	Low incidence; may be influenced by genetic predisposition	High incidence due to slow healing; may be influenced by genetic predisposition	High incidence; depends on time of grafting and surgical techniques used

Burgess (1991) describes three concentric zones of injury and their impact on the severity of the burn injury:

(1) Zone of hyperemia: the least damaged area, it typically heals in 3 to 5 days.

(2) Zone of stasis: area in which tissue perfusion is compromised. If resuscitative methods are effective in returning tissue perfusion, the tissue may survive.

(3) Zone of coagulation: area of permanent burn injury, which is characterized by cellular death.

2. **Descrbe the three phases of burn physiology, including a discussion of the effects on the following systems during the emergent and acute phases:**

- **cardiovascular**
- **respiratory**
- **immunologic**
- **gastrohepatic**
- **genitourinary**

The first phase of burn physiology is the emergent or shock phase. This phase typically lasts 48 hours and is a crucial period for the patient. The second phase begins when diuresis is noted and lasts until wound closure. This phase is referred to as the acute or fluid resuscitation phase. The third and last phase is the rehabilitation phase. This phase should begin immediately following the burn injury to help maintain or restore function and cosmetic appearance so the patient can function in society.

Emergent or Shock Phase

During the emergent phase the patient experiences a type of hypovolemic shock. This shock is the result of increased capillary permeability, which permits the shift of fluid from the plasma to the interstitial spaces. Direct cell damage increases capillary permeability, permitting the escape of large amounts of fluid, electrolytes, protein, and debris (Robins, 1990). Changes in capillary permeability begin within 30 minutes of the thermal injury, and fluid and electrolyte losses peak within 6 to 8 hours of the burn injury (Caine & Lefcourt, 1993). In addition, the fluid regulators, including the osmotic and hydrostatic pressures and the sodium pump, are lost. Again, these changes are due to direct cellular damage from the thermal injury. The cumulative effect of the loss of these regulatory mechanisms is hypovolemic shock, also referred to as burn shock. Rapid fluid shifts result in multisystem changes.

Cardiovascular System: The cardiovascular system responds to the hypovolemic shock by attempting to compensate for the massive loss of fluid. Catecholamines are released, decreasing cardiac output and increasing peripheral resistance in an attempt to increase the fluid volume in the vascular system. Ultimately, if fluid resuscitation efforts are not initiated, cardiac output is further decreased, and there is hemoconcentration of blood cells with diminished perfusion to major organs (Burgess, 1991).

Respiratory System: The respiratory system may sustain an inhalation injury (see Questions 7 and 8). Even if an inhalation injury is not sustained, lung compliance may decrease as a result of the extensive injury, and pulmonary care similar to that required for an inhalation injury may be necessary.

Immunologic System: In the immunologic system the mechanical barrier response and the cellular immune response are lost (Burgess, 1991). Loss of the mechanical barrier means a loss of the body's ability to protect itself from invading organisms. At the cellular level, a complex system of reactions occurs that has not been fully defined. Recent research suggests a relationship between postburn immunosuppression and prolonged exposure to burn eschar (Caine & Lefcourt, 1993). The final result is that the body loses powerful mechanisms to protect itself from invading organisms. Infection is one of the greatest concerns in a burn-injured patient. Because of colonization of bacteria on the burn wound itself and loss of the defense mechanisms to fight against this colonization, a burn-injured patient can be overcome by a massive infection.

Gastrohepatic System: The gastrohepatic system responds to a burn injury by shutting down. This response probably is due to the decrease in perfusion of this system and the endocrine response to the trauma (Burgess, 1991).

Genitourinary System: The genitourinary system responds by decreasing kidney function through secretion of antidiuretic hormone (ADH) and renal vasoconstriction. The body attempts to use compensatory mechanisms to offset the hypovolemia. In this case the kidneys may be compromised because of the extensive loss of fluid volume in the vascular system. Adequate fluid resuscitation to maintain effective kidney function is vital.

Acute or Fluid Resuscitation Phase

The second phase of burn physiology is the acute or fluid resuscitation phase. This phase begins when the return of fluid control mechanisms effects diuresis. The eschar begins to separate, and the focus of care turns to the preparation of the wound for healing or grafting. The cardiovascular system begins to stabilize because capillary permeability decreases and fluid shifts are less severe. Cardiac output and lymphatic system function return to normal. The respiratory system may be prone to pulmonary edema or pneumonia because of the massive fluid shifts and hospitalization. Patients with previous cardiovascular or pulmonary disease are more prone to respiratory problems. The patient remains immunosuppressed, and all efforts should continue to prevent any type of infection.

The gastrohepatic system begins to decrease its function, which leads to the concern for adequate nutritional intake. Along with this concern is the development of stress ulcers. Careful monitoring of the gastric contents, stool, and any emesis for blood is imperative. The use of antacids and histamine receptor antagonists to prevent the occurrence of stress ulcers is critical. Renal function should return. However, careful monitoring of kidney function is imperative as the body attempts to excrete waste products and debris from the burn injury. Renal failure is a possibility at this stage as well.

Rehabilitation Phase

The rehabilitation phase focuses on the return of the individual to his or her previous roles and responsibilities in society. With adequate fluid resuscitation efforts and care in the first two stages, the systems will have stabilized by the time the patient enters the third phase.

3. **Based on the preburn weight, use the Parkland formula to calculate the fluid requirement to adequately resuscitate Tony.**

The Parkland formula permits the calculation of fluid needs for the first 24 hours immediately after the burn injury. This particular formula calculates the fluid need of crystalloids only:

4 ml lactated Ringer's solution × kg body weight × %TBSA burned

Tony's fluid need based on 65% TBSA burned is

4 ml × 72 kg × 65% TBSA = 18,720 ml of fluid in the first 24 h

Half the fluid should be infused during the first 8 hours after the burn. This time is calculated from the *time of the actual burn injury* not from the time the patient is first seen by medical personnel. So it is essential for the critical care nurse to know the actual time of the injury and the amount of fluid that has been infused before the patient is received in the unit. (NOTE: 4 L has been infused thus far, and a total of 9.36 L must be infused. The nurse has 4 hours to infuse the remainder of the 9.36 L.) The remaining half of the fluid requirement is then infused over the remaining 16 hours.

Some experts use the modified Brooke formula, which is similar to the Parkland formula. The modified Brooke formula calculates the fluid needs as follows:

2 ml lactated Ringer's solution × kg body weight × %TBSA burned

In this case, Tony's fluid needs for the first 24 hours would be 9360 ml (Rue & Cioffi, 1991).

Lactated Ringer's solution without dextrose is the crystalloid solution most often used to provide a balanced salt solution. Because a burn injury affects the fluid and electrolyte balance of the body, the amount and type of IV fluid is important. In the first 24 hours after a burn injury, the capillary permeability is increased, and the selectivity is decreased (Caine & Lefcourt, 1993). Because of these physiologic changes in the capillary seal, large amounts of fluid shift from the intravascular space, leading to the loss of osmotic pressure and with it the body's ability to pull fluid back into the intravascular space. These changes lead to hypovolemic shock and massive edema (Caine & Lefcourt, 1993). Additional fluid is lost through the burn injury itself in the form of wound drainage and evaporation.

The destruction of the cells in a burn injury also leads to a loss of electrolytes during the first 24 hours. The loss of sodium and potassium is of greatest concern. The sodium loss is the result of the fluid shifts and the cellular destruction. Potassium is lost into the extracellular fluid because of the cellular destruction (Caine & Lefcourt, 1993).

Replacement therapy focuses on maintaining the patient until the capillary permeability and selectivity are restored. As stated earlier, lactated Ringer's solution is the IV solution of choice because the composition of lactated Ringer's solution closely resembles the composition of the fluid being lost. Table 25–2 compares the composition of lactated Ringer's solution and the extracellular fluid.

The use of colloids (albumin or fresh frozen plasma) during the first 24 hours continues to be controversial. As capillary integrity is restored,

Table 25-2 Comparison of Ringer's Lactated Solution and Extracellular Fluid

Electrolyte	Lactated Ringer's Solution (mmol/L)*	Extracellular Fluid (mmol/L)†
Na^+	130	135–145
K^+	4	3.2–4.5
Cl^-	109	95–105
HCO_3^-	28	24–28

Modified from Faldmo, L., & Kravitz, M. (1993). Management of acute burns and burn shock resuscitation. *AACN Clinical Issues in Critical Care Nursing, 4*(2), 351–366.
*Normal value ranges may differ slightly between clinical laboratories.
†Plus 80 to 100 ml free water per liter.

colloids may be infused to aid in the reestablishment of the fluid regulators, including osmotic and hydrostatic pressures. However, most burn units do not begin to infuse colloids until after the first 24 hours (Caine & Lefcourt, 1993). Each burn unit will have an accepted fluid resuscitation protocol to maintain the cardiovascular status.

An important consideration when calculating fluid requirements for the burn-injured patient is to understand these formulas as guidelines. The patient's urine output and vital signs must be monitored carefully, and age and response of the patient must be taken into consideration. The rate of fluid administration must be adjusted according to patient needs (Rue & Cioffi, 1991).

Hourly urine output is the most valuable parameter to assess the adequacy of fluid resuscitation and renal perfusion. Hourly outputs should range from 0.5 to 1 ml/kg of body weight per hour. Typically, this results in an hourly output of 30 to 50 ml of urine per hour. Hourly outputs below 0.5 ml/kg/h indicate hypovolemia if no prior renal disorder is present (Robins, 1990).

4. What significance, if any, would the administration of mannitol have on fluid resuscitation?

Mannitol functions as an osmotic diuretic to increase water excretion by osmotic action (Spencer, Nichols, Lipkin, Henderson, & West, 1993). Mannitol is administered to maintain urinary output adequate to prevent acute renal failure during trauma such as a burn injury. Also, osmotic diuretics are sometimes recommended when there is evidence of myoglobinuria, which necessitates the flushing of the kidneys to prevent sludging and possible acute tubular necrosis (Caine & Lefcourt, 1993). The major problem with this treatment approach is the absolute need for an accurate hourly urine output. As presented in Question 3, careful monitoring of the patient is required to ascertain the fluid resuscitation needs of a burn-injured patient. Hourly urine outputs are the major parameter in this monitoring. If an osmotic diuretic is administered, the burn unit staff treating the patient has no way of knowing if the urine output is due to adequate fluid resuscitation or from infusion of the osmotic diuretic.

Typically, osmotic diuretics should be used only as a last resort in an attempt to protect the kidneys. Adequate fluid resuscitation should maintain kidney functioning. If assessment findings support the presence of myoglobinuria, increasing the amount of IV fluids administered should be implemented first to flush out the kidneys and prevent the sludging of the myoglobin. If forced diuresis is attempted, the patient must be carefully monitored for fluid overload, especially in the elderly patient and those patients with previous cardiac or renal diseases.

5. What assessment findings would indicate myoglobinuria?

Myoglobin is a pigment released when muscle tissue is damaged. Myoglobin may be evident in large thermal and electrical burn injuries. Myoglobin is a fairly large molecule that the body attempts to excrete through the kidneys. However, myoglobin has a tendency to sludge in the kidneys. If inadequate amounts of urine are produced, sludging may occur, which can result in acute tubular necrosis.

Assessment findings that would indicate the presence of myoglobin in the urine include the TBSA of the burn, type of burn injury, and the color of the urine produced. Urine that contains myoglobin is usually a burgundy to rust color.

Tony has sustained a large (65%) TBSA thermal burn. Also on Tony's arrival at the burn unit the color of the urine is burgundy. Both assessment findings indicate a high possibility of the presence of myoglobin in the urine.

6. Describe the treatment protocol of myoglobinuria.

Two treatment protocols are available to assure adequate urine output to flush the myoglobin from the kidneys. The first option is adequate fluid resuscitation. The minimum urine output should remain somewhere around 30 ml/h. With a possibility of myoglobin in the urine the hourly urine output should be higher to ensure the flushing of the kidneys. The urine output may need to be somewhere between 40 and 50 ml/h. The patient's response to the fluid resuscitation must also be monitored. The patient must be able to withstand the amount of fluids required to sustain the target hourly urine output.

A second option is the use of osmotic diuretics. Mannitol is usually the drug of choice, administered intravenously based on body weight. The decision to administer an osmotic diuretic must be made cautiously, since it destroys the validity of the hourly urine output (Caine & Lefcourt, 1993).

7. **What assessment findings are critical to establishing the presence of an inhalation injury? What assessment findings warrant concern with Tony?**

The extent of pulmonary injury depends on the anatomic location of the insult, the agent inhaled such as steam or smoke, the toxic substances in the agent inhaled, and the length of exposure to the agent (Carrougher, 1993).

Inhalation injuries can result from two forms of toxic exposure and should be suspected if there are obvious burns to the face, neck, or upper chest. The first form of exposure is smoke inhalation, which is often the cause of death in burn-related injuries. Smoke inhalation injuries typically result in carbon monoxide or cyanide toxicity (Demling, 1993).

A second type of exposure is a direct burn to the glottis as a result of inhaling heated air or steam. Edema formation leads to airway obstruction and respiratory distress. The edema may be the result of an actual burn to the tissues in the airway or may result from fluid resuscitation efforts, especially if the face, neck, and chest are involved in the burn.

An inhalation injury below the glottis is rare because of the ability of the trachea to dissipate heat and the reflex action of the vocal cords to close off the lower airway when they are exposed to toxic air (Caine & Lefcourt, 1993; Demling, 1993).

Caine and Lefcourt (1993) and Carrougher (1993) have reported the following indications of possible inhalation injury:

- a burn injury sustained in an enclosed space
- burns to the face, neck, and chest*
- singed nasal hair or eyebrows
- carboniferous material in mouth
- carboniferous sputum*
- carboxyhemoglobin more than 10%
- wheezing
- hoarseness of the voice*
- deep, labored respirations
- altered level of consciousness
- cough
- tachypnea

According to Carrougher (1993), pertinent historical information includes the following:

- burn injury sustained in an enclosed space
- documented exposure to smoke
- presence of noxious chemicals*
- alteration in mental status

*Seen in the assessment of Tony.

8. **Describe the treatment protocol of a burn patient with an inhalation injury or a suspected inhalation injury.**

Monitoring of the respiratory status of a burn–injured patient is critical and should take priority over all other concerns. The basic ABCs of survival (airway, breathing, and circulation) must be met first, as with any trauma patient. Monitoring of the respiratory system and the treatment protocols include the following:

- frequent assessment of the respiratory rate, rhythm, and quality.
- periodic testing of arterial blood gases (ABGs) and carboxyhemoglobin.
- delivery of humidified oxygen. The type of delivery system used depends on the extent of the inhalation injury. It can vary from a nasal cannula to intubation and ventilator support if the inhalation injury is severe. Some advocate starting 100% oxygen through a tight, nonrebreather mask for all burn-injured patients suspected of sustaining an inhalation injury (Carrougher, 1993).
- pulmonary hygiene efforts including positioning, coughing and deep breathing, incentive spirometry, or ultrasound nebulizers.
- head of the bed elevated at least 30 to 40 degrees unless contraindicated by another condition.
- chest x–rays.
- fiberoptic bronchoscopy to directly visualize the airway.
- xenon 133 ventilation-perfusion lung scan: Xenon 133 is injected intravenously with serial scans done to monitor the clearance of the xenon by the lungs. Xenon is usually washed out of the alveoli within 90 seconds (Carrougher, 1993).
- possible escharotomies if chest expansion is compromised.

Initially, the chest x–ray, ABGS, and carboxyhemoglobin findings may appear normal. The initial results become baseline data for comparison with subsequent laboratory results. Serial studies can identify deterioration of the pulmonary function. A xenon 133 lung scan and fiberoptic bronchoscopy can accurately diagnose 93% of inhalation injuries (Carrougher, 1993).

9. **What is the purpose of escharotomies?**

Escharotomies are incisions made through the eschar to allow for swelling without compromising tissue perfusion. An eschar is typically thick and leathery, allowing for little expansion if there is swelling below the eschar. If the burn is circumferential, the swelling from the burn injury itself and the swelling associated with fluid resuscitation can compromise the arterial blood flow to the area. Escharotomies may be necessary if there is extensive burn injury to the anterior or posterior trunk. If eschar is present, the respiratory effort and therefore ventilation may be compromised. Escharotomies on both sides of the chest through the midaxillary line may aid in decreasing the respiratory effort (Burgess, 1991; Rue & Cioffi, 1991).

The incisons should extend through the eschar down to the subcutaneous fat to allow for adequate separation of the edges of the incision and relieve the pressure of the swelling. Incisions are made in the mid-lateral or midmedial line, moving from the proximal to the distal end of the involved extremities. The incisions may be performed at the bedside because there is no pain sensation in these types of burn injuries. Antimicrobial agents should be applied after the incisions are performed to delay colonization of bacteria (Rue & Cioffi, 1991).

10. Discuss pain management in the treatment protocol of the burn-injured patient.

A major concern is pain management in the care of the burn-injured patient. Continual assessment should be completed to monitor both the physical and emotional pain experienced by these patients during all phases of the burn injury. Many believe that anyone experiencing a full-thickness burn does not have pain because of the loss of pain sensors in the burned tissue. However, total full-thickness burns are rare. There is actually a mixture of partial-thickness and full-thickness burns. Because the pain sensors are intact with partial-thickness burns, the patient may experience severe pain. Initially, because of the massive edema resulting from the burn and fluid resuscitation efforts, only IV pain medication such as morphine should be administered. Massive edema compromises the absorption of the pain medication if given intramuscularly or subcutaneously. Once the patient enters the acute and rehabilitation phases, other routes of pain medication administration can be considered. Alternative methods of pain management should also be considered. For example, guided imagery has been used very successfully for some burn-injured patients.

11. Using the Curreri formula for nutrition, calculate Tony's nutritional needs. Discuss the need for a high-calorie, high-protein diet.

The Curreri formula is used to establish the number of calories required by the burn-injured patient. The formula only estimates the number of calories and does not address the percentage of proteins, fats, and carbohydrates the patient requires.

$$(25 \text{ kcal} \times \text{weight [kg]}) + (40 \times \text{TBSA}) = \text{total calories}$$

For Tony, his caloric need per day would be calculated as follows:

$$(25 \text{ kcal} \times 72 \text{ kg}) + (40 \times 65\%) = 4400 \text{ kcal}$$

Some experts believe that the Curerri formula overestimates the caloric requirements for the burn-injured patient (Carlson & Jordan,

1991). They advocate the use of several parameters such as indirect calorimetry to estimate nutritional needs.

Nutritional support becomes paramount once the burn-injured patient's condition has stabilized. Hypermetabolism that is directly proportional to the extent of the burn injury results. The basal metabolic rate may increase as much as 100% in a patient with a 50% or greater TBSA burn injury (Caine & Lefcourt, 1993).

Because of the high metabolic rate and the need for a positive nitrogen balance to promote healing, a diet high in calories and protein is essential. Once the patient's condition is stabilized, nutritional intake must begin. If the patient cannot consume enough calories orally, enteral feedings may be required to meet the extensive nutritional needs. This includes oral supplements or continuous feedings through a nasoenteric (intestinal) tube. Specific types of feedings and tubes used for enteral therapy depend on the condition of the patient, the anticipated time of nutritional support required to meet the metabolic needs, and the risk of aspiration.

The protein intake per day ranges from 1.5 to 4 g/kg body weight. For Tony, this would result in an intake of 108 to 288 g of protein per day.

12. **Discuss burn wound care and dressing techniques. Include the types of topical antimicrobial agents commonly used in wound care, listing advantages and disadvantages of each.**

Bayley (1990, p. 210) lists five goals of burn wound care:

(1) closing the wound as soon as possible
(2) fostering the development of granulation tissue
(3) preparing the wound for grafting
(4) reducing scarring and contractures
(5) providing patient comfort

The first step in the process of burn wound care is wound cleansing. Hydrotherapy is begun as soon as possible to promote meticulous cleansing and wound debridement. The type of hydrotherapy completed depends on infection control policies of the unit and the condition of the patient. Some patients are placed in a Hubbard tank or are given a shower. Typically, hydrotherapy is completed at least daily but may be given more often if ordered by the burn unit team. The goal is to wash all areas carefully, being sure to thoroughly remove all antimicrobial agents previously placed on the burn wound. Also, any eschar that is beginning to separate may be removed with forceps and scissors. All hair should be shaved around the burn wound to decrease the chance of infection.

Hydrotherapy can be a painful ordeal for the patient. Adequate premedication is required. The actual time of the hydrotherapy (usually 20 minutes) should be carefully monitored to prevent hypothermia. Heat lamps may be used to decrease the amount of heat lost by the patient.

During hydrotherapy the wound must be continually assessed for color and appearance: presence of eschar and healing as seen by budding of the skin; presence of drainage including odor, color, and amount; and any exposed deep tissue such as tendons and bone (Walter, 1993).

Once the wound is cleansed, an antimicrobial agent is applied. These agents have been found to be the best method to control burn wound sepsis (Bayley, 1990). These antimicrobial agents reduce the number of bacteria colonizing in the wound and ideally will restrain colonization of bacteria to a level that the body can control through its internal defense mechanisms. Four of the most commonly used antimicrobial agents are listed in Table 25–3 (Molter et al., 1993). Selection of an antimicrobial agent depends on the wound depth, location, condition, and specific organism isolated, which is established by wound culture (Walter, 1993).

There are two methods of dressing a burn wound. The first method is the open method. An antimicrobial cream is applied with a sterile glove with no dressing applied. This approach allows for direct visualization of the wound, less discomfort for the patient during wound care, and simplicity in wound care. However, the patient may experience hypothermia, may further traumatize the wound, or may have difficulty looking at the wound psychologically (Bayley, 1990).

A second method is the closed method in which dressings are applied to the wound. Antimicrobial cream is applied to the wound using a sterile glove or coated on a gauze and laid on the wound, which is then covered with an additional dressing. If a solution is used, the dressing is saturated and placed on the wound and covered with additional dressings. These dressings should be wrapped distal to proximal with no two burn surfaces touching each other. The advantages of this type of dressing are limitation of fluid loss through evaporation, debridement of the wound when the dressings are removed, absorption of the exudate from the wound, and patient comfort. Disadvantages of this type of dressing are the discomfort experienced by the patient during dressing changes and the warm moist environment created under the dressings.

13. **Describe the types of biologic and synthetic dressings currently being used in wound care.**

Biologic dressings are used as temporary wound coverings until autografts are available. Duncan and Driscoll (1991, p 210) list several reasons why biologic dressings aid in the management of burn wounds:

- decreasing bacterial proliferation on the wound
- preventing necrosis of viable elements in the dermis
- preventing wound desiccation

Table 25-3   Commonly Used Antimicrobial Agents

Agent	Indications	Nursing Considerations
Clotrimazole cream	Fungal colonization of wounds	Apply thin coat of agent to wound and wait 20 min before applying any dressings; make use of an antibacterial agent in addition to the antifungal agent; painless; may cause skin irritation and blistering
Mafenide acetate (Sulfamylon)	Active against most gram–positive and gram–negative wound pathogens; drug of choice for electrical and ear burn	Apply once or twice daily with sterile glove; do not use dressings that reduce effectiveness and cause maceration; monitor respiratory rate, electrolyte values, and arterial pH for evidence of metabolic acidosis; painful on application to partial thickness burns for about 30 min
Silver nitrate	Effective against a wide spectrum of common wound pathogens and fungal infections; used in patients with sulfa allergy or toxic epidermal neurolysis; poor penetration of eschar	Apply 0.5% solution wet dressings two or three times a day; ensure that dressings remain moist by wetting every 2 h; preserve solution in a light–resistant container; protect walls, floors, etc., with plastic to prevent black staining that occurs; monitor for hyponatremia and hypochloremia
Silver sulfadiazine (Silvadene)	Active against a wide spectrum of microbial pathogens; use with caution in patients with impaired renal or hepatic function	Apply once or twice a day with sterile gloved hand; leave wounds exposed or wrap lightly with gauze dressing; painless

Modified from Molter, N. C., Duncan, D. J., & DePew, C. L. (1993). Burns. In J. Hartshorn, M. Lamborn, & M. L. Noll (Eds.), *Introduction to critical care nursing* (pp. 470–501). Philadelphia: Saunders.

- assisting in control of evaporation of fluid and heat loss through the open wound
- decreasing protein loss in fluid exudate
- decreasing the pain experienced by patients
- protecting exposed structures such as blood vessels, tendons, and nerves
- stimulating healing and preparing the wound bed for autograft skin
- facilitating joint motion

The most commonly used biologic and synthetic dressings are described in Table 25–4.

14. Discuss the use of autografts and the nursing care required.

With a full-thickness burn, healing and reepithelialization are not possible. As a result, an autograft using viable skin from the burn patient is the only option for covering the wound (Bayley, 1990).

For the autograft to "take," the wound itself must be pink, firm, and free of exudate or eschar, which is accomplished through wound cleansing and debridement. Once the wound is ready for the graft, the patient is taken to surgery, where the autograft is obtained. Autografts may be split thickness, full thickness, pedicle flaps, or free flaps, depending on the area of the body requiring the autograft. Most autografts are split–thickness grafts to cover the wound early. If the area requiring coverage is large, the autograft is meshed so that it can cover a larger surface area. The autograft can be meshed by a ratio of 1:1.5 to 1:4. This means that the autograft can cover one and a half to four times its own surface area. Meshed grafts have a tendency to adhere better to the wound and allow exudate and debris to ooze through the open meshed

Table 25–4   Common Biologic and Synthetic Dressings

Type of Dressing	Definition
Biologic dressing	Temporary wound cover of human or animal species tissue
Allograft (homograft)	Temporary wound cover composed of a graft of skin transplanted from another human, living or dead
Xenograft (heterograft) skin	Used as a temporary wound cover to promote healing; a graft of skin, usually pigskin, transplanted between animals of different species
Biosynthetic dressing	A wound covering composed of both biologic and synthetic materials
Temporary skin substitute (Biobrane)	A bilaminar wound dressing composed of nylon mesh enclosed in a collagen derivative with a silicone rubber outer membrane; permeable to some antibiotic ointments
"Artificial skin" (Integra)	A wound dressing composed of two layers: (1) a "dermal" layer made of animal collagen that interfaces with an open wound surface; (2) an "epidermal" layer made of polymeric silicone (Silastic) that controls water loss from the dermis and acts as a bacterial barrier; the dermal layer biodegrades within several months and is reabsorbed; the epidermal layer may be removed and replaced with autograft skin when appropriate

Modified from Molter, N. C., Duncan, D. J., & DePew, C. L. (1993). Burns. In J. Hartshorn, M. Lamborn, & M. L. Noll (Eds.), *Introduction to critical care nursing* (pp. 470–501). Philadelphia: Saunders.

areas (Bayley, 1990). The graft is laid on the wound and stapled or sutured in place. Some burn units use a fibrin glue to hold the autograft in place. Further investigation of this approach is needed. Once the autograph is secured to the wound, a dressing is applied, and the patient is returned to the burn unit.

The nurse must take special care not to disrupt the autograft. The patient may be confined to bed rest or the extremity may be immobilized with splints to promote proper positioning and to prevent disruption of the graft. The nurse must ensure proper positioning while being fully aware of the potential for other complications, such as respiratory infection and skin breakdown as a result of the immobility.

An autograft "takes" when it becomes a permanent part of the wound. Blood flow through capillaries growing into the autograft is established by the third to fifth postgraft day. Wound closure is anticipated within 7 to 10 days after graft placement (Bayley, 1990).

15. Describe the appropriate care for donor sites.

Selection of autograft skin donor sites is based on the location and the extent of the burn. Once the autograft skin is obtained, the donor site must be monitored because of the creation of a partial-thickness injury. In surgery a fine mesh gauze (either dry or impregnated with a substance such as scarlet red or a synthetic material) is placed over the donor site to promote healing and prevent further injury. On the patient's return to the burn unit the donor site should be exposed to air. Some burn units apply a radiant heat source to the area to increase drying. Once the donor site begins to heal, which usually is 7 to 14 days after the graft is obtained, the gauze or synthetic material will begin to separate from the wound. As this separation occurs, the material can be trimmed from the wound with scissors.

The nurse must be careful to keep the donor site clean, dry, and trimmed. A donor site can be used more than once if there are no complications such as an infection. If the donor site becomes infected, it should be treated as the burn wound.

16. Discuss the splinting and positioning required for Tony to maintain use of his extremities and upper body.

Most burn units have physical therapists and occupational therapists available to assist burn patients. In collaboration with the nursing staff, their goal is to maintain as much function as possible so the patient can return to society. All joints should be placed in a neutral position if possible. Splints must be applied correctly. If necessary, the therapist should apply the splints or provide inservice training for nurses on the application of splints. Footboards or shoes are used to prevent foot drop. Early ambulation requires coordination of the nursing staff and physical therapist to provide the optimal environment for the patient to accomplish this goal. Pain management that allows the patient to ambulate and participate in exercises becomes an important issue.

17. List the nursing diagnoses, outcomes, and interventions appropriate for the care of the burn patient during the emergent and acute phases of burn physiology.

Molter et al. (1993) created a nursing care plan identifying the most common nursing diagnoses for a burn-injured patient. Although many nursing diagnoses may be important for this type of patient, this care plan presents the most common interventions (Table 25–5).

18. Discuss the psychosocial aspects of caring for the burn patient and the impact on the patient's support system.

Burn injuries are one of the most devastating injuries to sustain. An individual's identity and self-image are directly related to his or her appearance. Disfigurement from burns to the face can be especially difficult.

The nurse must constantly assess the patient and the support system available through family or friends. This assessment includes identifying feelings of guilt, abandonment, pain, loss, and fear. The nurse can encourage the patient, family, and friends to verbalize their concerns and provide them with appropriate information. Also, a referral to a social worker, psychologist, or chaplain may be necessary to provide additional psychosocial or spiritual support.

Table 25–5 Nursing Care Plan for Resuscitative and Acute Care Phase of the Patient with Major Burn Injury

Nursing Diagnosis	Outcome	Interventions
Ineffective airway clearance or impaired gas exchange related to tracheal edema or interstitial edema secondary to inhalation injury and manifested by hypoxemia and hypercapnia	$Po_2 > 90$ mm Hg, $Pco_2 < 40$ mm Hg, O_2 saturation > 95% Respirations 16–20/min Clear mentation Ability to mobilize secretions Clear to white secretions Absence of dyspnea and increased work of breathing with appropriate positioning	Assess respiratory rate and character q1h, breath sounds q4h, level of consciousness q1h, evaluate need for chest escharotomy during fluid resuscitation. If not intubated, assess for stridor, hoarseness q1h. Monitor oxygen situation q1h, obtain and evaluate arterial blood gases prn. Administer humidified oxygen as ordered. Cough, deep breathe q1h while awake. Suction q1–2h or prn, monitor sputum characteristics and amount.

Table 25–5   Nursing Care Plan for Resuscitative and Acute Care Phase of the Patient with Major Burn Injury *Continued*

Nursing Diagnosis	Outcome	Interventions
		Elevate head of bed to facilitate line expansion. Schedule activities to avoid fatigue, dyspnea. Turn q2h to mobilize secretions. Assist with obtaining chest x-ray as ordered.
Fluid volume deficit secondary to fluid shifts to the interstitium and evaporate loss of fluids from the injured skin	Weight gain based on volume of fluids administered in first 48 h followed by moderate diuresis over next 8–10 d with a weight loss rate of no more than 10%–12% of weight gain per day Hourly urine output: 30–50 ml/h; 1 ml/kg/h—children < 30 kg body weight; 75–100 ml/h—electric injury Normal specific gravity except during diuresis, when it may be slightly decreased; negative urine sugar and acetone Heart rate: 80–120 bpm, blood pressure adequate in relation to pulse and urine output Clear sensorium Laboratory values; Na$^+$ approaches that of resuscitation fluid initially then returns to normal with diuresis; K$^+$ initially high, hematocrit 50–55% until adequate resuscitation established; all other values WNL	Titrate calculated fluid requirements in first 48 h to maintain acceptable urinary output. Obtain and evaluate urine specific gravity and sugar and acetone q2h. Monitor vital signs q1h until hemodynamically stable. Monitor mental status q1h for at least 48 h. Obtain and record daily or b.i.d. weights. Record hourly intake and output measurements and evaluate trends. Monitor electrolytes, hematocrit, serum glucose, BUN, creatinine at least b.i.d. for first 48 h and then as required by patient status.
High risk for impaired vascular perfusion in extremities with circumferential burns manifested by decreased or absence peripheral pulses	Absence of tissue injury in extremities secondary to inadequate perfusion related to vascular compression from edema	Check peripheral pulses q1h for 72 h by palpation or ultrasonic flowmeter; evaluate sensation of pain and capillary refill in extremities. Notify physician of changes in pulses, capillary refill, or pain sensation; be prepared to assist with escharotomy or fasciotomy. Evaluate upper extremities.
Alteration in comfort: acute pain related to burn trauma	Able to identify factors that contribute to pain Verbalizes improved comfort level Physiologic parameters return to normal Adequate respirations and hemodynamic stability after administration of narcotic analgesia	Medicate before bathing, dressing changes, major procedures, prn. Reduce anxiety; explain all activities before initiating them; talk to patient while performing activities; assess need for analgesic or anxiolytic medication; use nonpharmacologic pain-reducing methods as appropriate.

Table continued on following page

Table 25–5 Nursing Care Plan for Resuscitative and Acute Care Phase of the Patient with Major Burn Injury *Continued*

Nursing Diagnosis	Outcome	Interventions
		Monitor and document response to analgesics or other interventions.
High risk for infection related to loss of skin, impaired immune response, invasive therapies	Absence of inflamed burn wound margins Negative results from sputum, blood, and urine cultures Absence of evidence from wound biopsy of burn wound invasion Body temperature of 37.2° and 38.3° C (99° and 101° F) Absence of glucosuria, vomiting, ileus, or change in mentation Acceptable white blood cell and platelet counts, coagulation times, and serum glucose levels Clean, dry invasive catheter sites with normal skin color and temperature Autograft or allograft skin adherence to granulation tissue	Assess burn wound and invasive catheter sites b.i.d. and prn. Assess and document characteristics of urine and sputum q8h. Obtain wound, sputum, urine, and blood cultures as ordered. Assess and record temperature and vital signs q1–4h as appropriate. Provide protective isolation appropriate to method of wound care. Provide wound care with antimicrobial topical agents as ordered.
Impaired skin integrity related to burn wound, or consequences of immobility	No evidence of decubitus ulcers or other injury in unburned skin No evidence of progressive burn wound or donor site injury Burn wound or donor site healing and skin graft adherence within appropriate time frames	Assess b.i.d. and document: skin over pressure areas, burn wounds, donor sites, pressure points under splints, dependent area of unburned skin. Pad pressure areas; heels, elbows, sacrum, scapulas, and burned ears. Assess need for special beds such as low-air-loss and air-fluidized beds; at a minimum, provide extra padding to mattress. Remove blood pressure cuff from area of burn skin after each reading. Check circulation distal to restraints q1h; check circulation of digits in splinted extremities. Loosen securing devices for facial tube to accommodate changes occurring with edema; ensure that devices do not put pressure on ears. Promote drying of donor sites as appropriate; keep heat lamps at a safe distance to prevent injury.

Table 25–5   Nursing Care Plan for Resuscitative and Acute Care
Phase of the Patient with Major Burn Injury *Continued*

Nursing Diagnosis	Outcome	Interventions
		Immobilize skin graft sites for 5–7 d postgrafting to promote graft adherence.
		Moisten meshed graft dressings as ordered or roll sheet grafts as ordered to promote skin graft adherence.
High risk for aspiration R/T; hypoactivity of gastrointestinal tract	No aspiration of gastric contents No respiratory complications from aspirations	Insert and maintain nasogastric tube to low suction until bowel sounds return. Auscultate for bowel sounds q4h. Test stools and gastric contents for pressure of blood. Administer histamine blockers and antacids as ordered.
High risk for nutritional deficit related to increased metabolic demands secondary to wound healing	Consumption of daily requirement of nutrients, based on formulas for appropriate calorie calculation Positive nitrogen balance Progressive wound healing	Monitor weights every day or biweekly. Assess abdomen, bowel sounds q8h. Record all oral intake. Activate enteral, parenteral feeding protocol as appropriate prn. Provide adaptive devices to facilitate self–feeding. Have family assist at mealtime.
High risk for hemorrhage related to presence of a stress ulcer	No occurrence of stress ulcer while in hospital	Assess all stools, emesis, and residual of the tube feedings for blood. Monitor hemoglobin and hematocrit levels. Administer histamine blockers and antacids as ordered. Auscultate abdomen and monitor for bowel sounds and pain. Encourage oral diet as soon as possible.
Impaired mobility and self-care deficit related to therapeutic splinting and post–skin graft immobilization requirements	No evidence of permanent decreased joint function from preburn status unless directly related to trauma Return to vocation without functional limitations or adjustment to new vocation based on functional limitations	Perform range of motion exercises for all extremities q4h. Increase patient's activity as tolerated. Promote the use of adaptive devices to decrease dependency. Provide pain relief measures before physical therapy.
High risk for hypothermia related to loss of skin or external cooling	Rectal and core temperature is 37.2° to 37.8° C (99° to 100° F)	Monitor and document rectal and core temperature q1–2h. For temperature < 37.2° C (99° F): warm with heat lamps or shield; warm solutions used for dressing changes; cover patient with foil blanket or other substance to conserve heat.

Table continued on following page

Table 25–5 Nursing Care Plan for Resuscitative and Acute Care
Phase of the Patient with Major Burn Injury *Continued*

Nursing Diagnosis	Outcome	Interventions
High risk for ineffective patient and family coping related to acute stress of critical injury and potential life-threatening crisis; alteration in family processes related to critical injury	Patient or family verbalize goals of treatment regimen Patient or family demonstrate knowledge of support systems that are available Patient or family able to express concerns and fears Patient or family coping functional and realistic for phase of hospitalization, family processes at precrisis level	Support adaptive and functional coping mechanisms. Use interventions to reduce patient fatigue and pain. Promote use of group support session for patients and families. Orient patient and family to unit and support services and reinforce information frequently. Involve patient and family in treatment goals and plan of care.

Modified from Molter, N. C., Duncan, D. J., & DePew, C. L. (1993). Burns. In J. Hartshorn, M. Lamborn, & M. L. Noll (Eds.), *Introduction to critical care nursing* (pp. 470–501). Philadelphia: Saunders.

Burns

Bayley, E. W. (1990). Wound healing in the patient with burns. *Nursing Clinics of North America, 25*(1), 205–222.

Burgess, M. (1991). Initial management of a patient with extensive burn injury. *Critical Care Nursing Clinics of North America, 3*(2), 165–179.

Caine, R. M., & Lefcourt, N. D. (1993). Patients with burns. In J. M. Clochesy, C. Breu, S. Cardin, E. B. Ruby, & A. A. Whittaker (Eds.), *Critical care nursing* (pp. 1188–1215). Philadelphia: Saunders.

Calistro, A. M. (1993). Burn care basics and beyond. *RN, 56*(3), 26–31.

Carlson, D. E., & Jordan, B. S. (1991). Implementing nutritional therapy in the thermally injured patient. *Critical Care Nursing Clinics of North America, 3*(2), 221–235.

Carrougher, G. (1993). Inhalation injury. *AACN Clinical Issues in Critical Care Nursing, 4*(2), 367–377.

Demling, R. H. (1993). Smoke inhalation injury. *New Horizons: The Science and Practice of Acute Medicine, 1*(3), 422–434.

Duncan, D. J., & Driscoll, D. M. (1991). Burn wound management. *Critical Care Nursing Clinics of North America, 3*(2), 199–220.

Faldmo, L., & Kravitz, M. (1993). Management of acute burns and burn shock resuscitation. *AACN Clinical Issues in Critical Care Nursing, 4*(2), 351–366.

Molter, N. C., Duncan, D. J., & DePew, C. L. (1993). Burns. In J. Hartshorn, M. Lamborn, & M. L. Noll (Eds.), *Introduction to critical care nursing* (pp. 470–501). Philadelphia: Saunders.

Robins, E. V. (1990). Burn shock. *Critical Care Nursing Clinics of North America, 2*(2), 299–307.

Rue, L. W., & Cioffi, W. G. (1991). Resuscitation of the thermally injured patient. *Critical Care Nursing Clinics of North America, 3*(2), 181–189.

Spencer, R. T., Nichols, L. W., Lipkin, G. B., Henderson, H. S., & West, F. M. (1993). *Clinical pharmacology and nursing management* (4th ed.). Philadelphia: J. B. Lippincott.

Walter, P. (1993). Burn wound management. *AACN Clinical Issues in Critical Care Nursing, 4*(2), 378–387.

26

Acquired Immunodeficiency Syndrome

Connie Cooper, MSN, RN

CASE PRESENTATION

John Michael, a 35-year-old white man, came to the local mental health hospital complaining of impaired concentration, withdrawal from family and friends, mood swings, difficulty with his memory, fatigue, and suicidal ideation. Two months before coming to the hospital he had moved to the area from San Francisco to be with his family.

On admission, Mr. Michael's assessment revealed he had lost 4.5 to 7 kg (10 to 15 lb) since coming to his parent's home. He has not been able to read or concentrate. His suicidal ideas involve harming himself but no specific plan. Mr. Michael's psychosocial history revealed that he was gay and in the mid-1980s had visited several bath houses in San Francisco before settling down with his one close friend. Mr. Michael stated he returned home to tell his family that he had tested positive for human immunodeficiency virus (HIV). His family told him they would stand by him. He denied the use of intravenous (IV) drugs but has used marijuana on occasion. His medical history included having had diarrhea for the past 3 weeks, night sweats, and enlarged glands in his neck and under his arms. Mr. Michael revealed that before moving to the area he was told he was HIV positive. Two of his friends recently had been diagnosed as HIV positive, and two other friends have died from AIDS. He fears he has become depressed, believes he is losing his mind, and is becoming more confused. He told the nurse he was having difficulty with tremors in his legs, which occasionally have given him problems with walking.

His admitting diagnosis was major depression—single episode; rule out AIDS dementia complex (ADC).

After Mr. Michael's psychiatrist was informed of his history, the following medication orders were given: fluoxetine (Prozac) and nortriptyline (Pamelor).

Current vital signs and laboratory results are

BP	134/88
HR	90 bpm
Respirations	20/min
Temperature	37.2° C (98.9° F) (Oral)

ELISA	positive for HIV antigens (confirmed by Western blot test)
CXR	within normal limits

RBCs	$3.5 \times 10^6/mm^3$
WBCs	$6.6 \times 10^3/mm^3$
Hgb	12.9 g/dl
Hct	36.8%
Lymphocytes	13%

After 1 week of psychotherapy and medication therapy, Mr. Michael did not show any improvement in mood, affect, or neurologic deficits. He began falling when attempting to walk, had difficulty with the Mini–Mental Health Exam, and became more confused. The psychiatrist made a medical referral. Two physicians refused to accept the referral. Finally an oncologist accepted Mr. Michael's case. Two days later Mr. Michael was transferred to the oncology unit. More tests were ordered. The results were

CBC with Differential

RBCs	$5.5 \times 10^6/mm^3$
WBCs	$4.4 \times 10^3/mm^3$
Hgb	12.7 g/dl
Hct	38.9%
Lymphocytes	11%
Monocytes	3%

Lymphocyte Subset Results

Total lymphocyte count	$411/mm^3$
Absolute B cell	$99/mm^3$
Absolute T cell	$206/mm^3$
Helper:suppressor ratio	0.07

Routine Chemistry

Na^+	137 mmol/L
Glucose	120 mg/dl
Creatinine	0.8 mg/dl
Albumin	2.6 g/dl
BUN	9 mg/dl
Total protein	6.3 g/dl
K^+	3.7 mmol/L
Cl^-	100 mmol/L
CO_2	26 mmol/L

Other

VDRL	negative
Hepatitis B serology	negative
Stool culture	*Salmonella*
CT scan	mild brain atrophy and white matter changes

Once Mr. Michael was transferred to a medical floor, treatment with zidovudine (Retrovir) and ampicillin (Ampicin) for *Salmonella* infection was begun. During Mr. Michael's hospitalization, his assessment revealed no previous opportunistic diseases. He reported that his first symptoms were night sweats, diarrhea, and difficulty with his memory. Difficulty walking began shortly thereafter. His respiratory status began to change. Day 9 he developed a nonproductive cough, dyspnea, chills, and a few crackles in the base of his lungs. The physician was informed of changes, and orders included oxygen per mask at 40%, chest x-ray, and a second CD4 count. Chest x-ray revealed bilateral infiltrates. A flexible fiberoptic bronchoscopy revealed *Pneumocystis carinii* pneumonia (PCP). Mr. Michael was treated with IV pentamidine. On day 13 his respiratory status worsened. There were indications of respiratory failure, and a decision had to be made about intubation and mechanical ventilation. Mr. Michael had difficulty with decision making and also exhibited some psychomotor slowing. His family was kept informed of his physical condition. Mr. Michael wanted his family to help him make this difficult decision. Considering the quick onset of John's symptoms and change in condition, the family chose admission to the intensive care unit (ICU) and mechanical ventilation. Mr. Michael was admitted to the ICU. Treatment with IV ampicillin and IV hydrocortisone was initiated.

Within 2 days Mr. Michael was afebrile and was weaned from the ventilator. His respiratory rate had fallen from 40/min to 25/min, and his respiratory distress had lessened. Mr. Michael was then transferred back to the medical unit, receiving oxygen via nasal cannula. A third CD4 cell count was 190/mm³. Tables 26–1 and 26–2 show diagnostic data at Mr. Michael's return to the medical unit.

Following his return to the medical unit Mr. Michael was treated for oral candidiasis with nystatin (Nyaderm) and ketoconazole (Nizoral). His skin tests indicated complete failure of delayed hypersensitivity reactions. Mr. Michael was diagnosed with acquired immunodeficiency syndrome (AIDS). After 1½ weeks of IV sulfamethoxazole-trimethoprim (Bactrim), Mr. Michael was weaned from oxygen and discharged.

Following discharge from the hospital, Mr. Michael was treated with zidovudine (formerly azidothymidine [AZT]) and aerosol pentamidine for secondary PCP.

Table 26–1   Vital Signs

Day:	4	7	9	13	14	15
BP	112/72	154/82	132/84	132/62	112/72	130/84
HR (bpm)	112	112	112	120	112	90
Respirations (/min)	20	22	26	36	40	25
Temperature						
(°C)	36.7–37.2	36.7–37.2	37.2–37.8	37.8–38.9	38.9–39.4	36.7–37.2
(°F)	98–99	98–99	99–100	100–102	102–103	98–99

Table 26–2   Laboratory Results

Day:	7 (room air)	9 (40% O₂)	13 (100% O₂)	14 (40% O₂)	15 (room air)
pH	7.48	7.49	7.45	7.48	7.46
P_{CO_2} (mm Hg)	36	32	35	28	32
Pa_{O_2} (mm Hg)	49	44	104	93	85
Sa_{O_2}	89%	83%	97%	97%	96%
HCO_3^- (mmol/L)	27	25	24	20	23
Mode			A/C	A/C	
Ventilation rate			17	17	
V_T (ml)			900	900	
PEEP (cm H_2O)			14	12	

QUESTIONS

Acquired Immunodeficiency Syndrome

1. What factors put Mr. Michael at risk for AIDS?

2. What tests are used to screen for HIV infection?

3. What clinical indicators would classify Mr. Michael as having major depression or ADC?

4. What is the difference between HIV infection and AIDS?

5. What clinical indicators classified Mr. Michael as having AIDS rather than being HIV positive?

6. Describe the symptoms of PCP.

7. What symptoms and pulmonary diagnostics in Mr. Michael's case indicated the need for transfer to the ICU?

8. Mechanical ventilation and ICU admission for a person with AIDS is controversial. Why was Mr. Michael admitted to the ICU?

9. What treatments were done for Mr. Michael to ensure a successful outcome from the ICU?

10. Are the ICU nurses at an increased risk of acquiring AIDS from patients who receive mechanical ventilation?

11. What are some of the nursing interventions that will help Mr. Michael with his psychosocial and physiologic needs?

12. When assigned to an HIV–infected patient, what personal feelings or concerns should be acknowledged?

QUESTIONS AND ANSWERS

Acquired Immunodeficiency Syndrome

1. What factors put Mr. Michael at risk for AIDS?

Mr. Michael's history revealed that he was gay and had many sexual partners. Researchers have agreed that the greatest risk of exposure to HIV in the homosexual man comes from anal sexual intercourse and sexual practices with multiple sexual partners (Flaskerud & Ungvarski, 1995). Such sexual practices cause trauma to the rectal mucosa, which increases the chances of transmission of the HIV virus and other sexually transmitted diseases.

2. What tests are used to screen for HIV infection?

Two tests are used to screen for HIV infection: enzyme-linked immunosorbent assay (ELISA) and Western blot. Exposure to HIV elicits an antigen-antibody reaction and creates antibodies. These antibodies are then detected by the screening tests.

The presence of the antibody indicates that the person is infected and is infectious. The incubation period for AIDS is wide. The incubation period can vary from 6 months to 5 years. The average is 2.5 to 4.5 years (Alspach, 1991; Oskins, 1990).

The ELISA was first developed to protect the blood supply before transfusion. The Western blot is more specific than the ELISA. It confirms that the antibody in question is specifically reactive with HIV by detecting antibody reactivity to individual components of the virus (Flaskerud & Ungvarski, 1992).

Lymphocyte subset enumeration is used in combination with cultures for confirmation of opportunistic infection to help diagnose AIDS. Skin tests with known antigens for the person with mumps or *Candida* infection can demonstrate normal results until later stages of the disease (Chernecky, Krech, & Berger, 1993).

3. **What clinical indicators would classify Mr. Michael as having major depression or ADC?**

A patient with major depression usually complains of depressed mood, diminished interest or pleasure in activities, appetite changes with weight changes (up or down), insomnia or hypersomnia, fatigue or loss of energy, inability to concentrate, feelings of worthlessness or guilt, psychomotor agitation or retardation, and thoughts of death or suicide. Any five of these symptoms lasting for at least 2 weeks are clinically significant for a major affective disorder requiring intervention (Thompson, Novak, Pursell, & Swift, 1993). It is important to take a careful history to determine symptoms and situational crises that could precipitate the symptoms. Assessment of suicidal ideation is important at the time of the initial interview. Any precipitating factors such as bereavement, medication reaction, or thyroid problems should be ruled out. Nurses in acute care or mental health settings must be aware of the psychosocial and neuropsychiatric aspects of HIV disease. It may be necessary to manage the case of a patient who has anxiety or depression associated with a new diagnosis of HIV infection or AIDS or a patient who may be manifesting dementia associated with AIDS (Flaskerud & Ungvarski, 1992).

The HIV virus is capable of invading brain tissue. Neurologic symptoms have been reported in approximately 40% to 70% of all AIDS patients, with 10% of these patients having demonstrated neurologic involvement at the time of diagnosis (Beckman, 1990; Flaskerud & Ungvarski, 1992). According to Thompson et al. (1993), the early manifestations of ADC are memory loss, impaired concentration, apathy, depressed mood, agitation, unsteady gait, tremor, clumsiness, motor weakness, and psychotic features. HIV-positive patients are often aware of the changes in their neurologic well-being, which may lead to an adjustment disorder with fear, anxiety, or depression.

Mr. Michael presented with symptoms that fit both categories. The most significant symptom that precipitated the transfer to a medical unit was the change in his walking abilities. It is important to avoid medications that have anticholinergic side effects because these can cause delirium, including hallucinations, confusion, and sometimes agitation. The medications of choice include zidovudine, psychostimulants, and antidepressants (Thompson et al., 1993). ADC is considered a fatal illness. It has been difficult to find a proven treatment for HIV encephalopathy, which has a survival time reported of 90 days from diagnosis to death (Beckman, 1990). Cognitive and motor faculties decline further in people with CD4+ cell counts below 200/mm^3 (Scherer, 1990). Clinical symptoms have improved with combinations of zidovudine and psychostimulants (Clochesy, Breu, Cardin, Rudy, & Whittaker, 1993).

4. What is the difference between HIV infection and AIDS?

The terms *HIV infection* and *AIDS* are not synonymous. AIDS is used to indicate only the most severe diseases or clinical conditions observed in the continuum of illness related to infection with the retrovirus human immunodeficiency virus type 1 (HIV-1) (Flaskerud & Ungvarski, 1995).

The definition and classification system for HIV infection was revised and published in December 18, 1992, by the Centers for Disease Control and Prevention (CDC). The CDC classify HIV infection according to $CD4^+$ T-lymphocyte count and clinical conditions associated with HIV infection (CDC, 1992). The $CD4^+$ T-lymphocyte cell is affected by the HIV virus. The $CD4^+$ T-lymphocyte (helper) cells are often called the "quarterback" of the immune system. "The destruction of $Cd4^+$T-cells creates an imbalance in the ratio of T4 to T8 (suppressor) cells; suppressor cells turn off the immune response when it is no longer needed" (Alspach, 1991). The reduction of the $CD4^+$ T-cell count compromises the immune system. The compromised immune system allows opportunistic organisms to invade the body, which normally would be able to defend itself from these invaders.

The HIV/AIDS classification system emphasizes the clinical importance of the $CD4^+$ lymphocyte count in the categorization of HIV-related clinical conditions (CDC, 1992). The definition includes all infected persons with $CD4^+$ counts of less than $200/mm^3$ and patients diagnosed with three additional opportunistic infections: pulmonary tuberculosis, invasive cervical cancer, and recurrent bacterial pneumonia (Thompson et al., 1993).

According to the CDC (1992) Revised Classification System, $CD4^+$ T lymphocytes are placed in three categories.

- Category 1: $\geq 500/\mu l$
- Category 2: 200 to $499/\mu l$
- Category 3: $\leq 200/\mu l$

These categories guide clinical and therapeutic management of HIV-infected adolescents and adults. The $CD4^+$ T-cell count classification presents a continuum for HIV disease. The continuum ranges from an asymtomatic stage to advanced HIV disease.

The asymptomatic stage is manifested by an acute primary HIV infection, an asymptomatic condition, or persistent generalized lymphadenopathy (PGL) (CDC, 1992). As many as 90% of HIV-infected persons have severe flulike symptoms 1 to 3 weeks after infection. These symptoms may last 1 to 2 weeks. During this time their HIV antibody test results are usually negative, although they do have a steady decline in their $CD4^+$ T-lymphocyte count (Flaskerud & Ungvarski, 1995). The HIV antibody test results usually become positive 2 to 18 weeks after infection.

The early symptomatic stage develops when CD4+ T-cell counts drop to around 500/μl (Flaskerud & Ungvarski, 1995). Clinical conditions that could occur at this stage include candidiasis, herpes zoster, pelvic inflammatory disease, and peripheral neuropathy (CDC, 1992).

The late symptomatic stage begins when a patient's CD4+ T-lymphocyte cell count drops below 200/μl (Flaskerud & Ungvarski, 1995). A patient may develop life-threatening infections and cancers. The infections usually remain treatable. At this point the stage of infection reflects the CDC criteria for AIDS. The last stage of HIV infection is the advanced HIV disease stage. The patient's CD4+ T-cells have dropped to less than 50/μl (Flaskerud & Ungvarski, 1995). Once this level has been reached, death is likely within 1 year.

5. What clinical indicators classified Mr. Michael as having AIDS rather than as being HIV positive?

Laboratory findings in the diagnosis of AIDS include a positive HIV antibody test, decreased white blood cell (WBC) and lymphocyte counts, depressed CD4+ T-cell count, and an abnormal CD4-CD8 ratio (Jones, 1993). According to the CDC's definition and classification of the disease, Mr. Michael converted from being HIV positive to having AIDS when his CD4 count went below 200/μl. Mr. Michael also had three opportunistic diseases. He was diagnosed with PCP, *Candida* of the oral mucosa, and *Salmonella* of the gastrointestinal tract.

6. Describe the symptoms of PCP.

Individuals infected with HIV eventually have at least one episode of PCP. The statistics are as high as 75% to 80% of patients diagnosed with AIDS will have PCP. PCP is a simple fungus and is found in the lungs of humans, rats, cats, dogs, and several other animals (Flaskerud & Ungvarski, 1992). Most children by age 4 years have developed antibodies to *Pneumocystis carinii* (Thompson et al., 1993). PCP is not considered a serious pathogenic organism unless a person is severely immunocompromised. In PCP the alveoli fill with proteinaceous material that contains cysts and trophozoites. Air distribution into alveoli filled with PCP is impaired.

Symptoms associated with PCP include fever, high respiratory rate (>30/min) usually dyspnea on exertion then at rest, normal or abnormal chest examination results, normal breath sounds or minimal rales, cyanosis around the mouth, nailbeds, and mucous membranes, nonproductive cough (unless patient is a smoker), and thrush, which indicates immunosuppression (Flaskerud & Ungvarski, 1992; Thompson et al., 1993).

7. **What symptoms and pulmonary diagnostics in Mr. Michael's case indicated the need for transfer to the ICU?**

Mr. Michael's symptoms following his transfer to the medical unit included dyspnea, fever, and nonproductive cough. His chest x-ray showed minimal infiltrates in both lobes. Oxygen was necessary for his hypoxia. His vital signs were within normal limits except for his temperature. He required admission to the ICU when his respiratory status became life threatening. Because of his diminished respiratory status, Mr. Michael required intubation and mechanical ventilation.

8. **Mechanical ventilation and ICU admission for a person with AIDS is controversial. Why was Mr. Michael admitted to the ICU?**

The primary reason for patients with PCP to be admitted to the ICU is for mechanical ventilation related to respiratory failure. Early studies indicated an 87% to 100% mortality rate for patients with PCP requiring mechanical ventilation (Henry & Holzemer, 1992). Later studies indicate survival rate is better for a first episode of PCP than for subsequent episodes. PCP is being diagnosed earlier and is being treated more effectively (Singer, Askanazi, Akiva, Bursztein, & Kvetan, 1990). With this early treatment, 72% of patients with AIDS and PCP survive their first bout (Clochesy et al., 1992).

This episode of PCP for Mr. Michael was his first. His CD4 count was below 200/μl but not significantly. According to Hall, Schmidt, and Wood (1992), there are two fundamental issues determining ICU eligibility for patients with AIDS: the patient's prognosis and the patient's wishes regarding life support (Hall et al., 1992). Hall et al. (1992) also suggest a prognostic staging system for patients with AIDS. They suggest the presence of each of the following abnormalities be scored as one point:

- severe diarrhea or serum albumin <2 g/dl
- any neurologic deficit
- PaO_2 <50 mm Hg
- hematocrit <30%
- lymphocyte count <2500/mm^3
- WBC count <2500/mm^3
- platelet count <140,000/mm^3

Patients are divided into stages I to III according to their scores (0 points, 1 point, and 2 to 7 points, respectively). In the original study 1-year survivals were 50%, 30%, 8% for stages I to III, respectively (Hall et al., 1992).

In addition to assessment based on a staging system, the patient and family must be involved in the decision process, and their wishes taken into consideration. It is important that the patient make his or her wishes known to the nurse, physician, and significant others. Rigid policies regarding ICU admission are undesirable, and it is necessary to make a detailed evaluation of each situation on a case-by-case basis (Hall et al., 1992).

9. **What treatments were done for Mr. Michael to ensure a successful outcome from the ICU?**

The results from the flexible fiberoptic bronchoscopy indicated PCP. This in turn alerted the physician to begin IV pentamidine. When Mr. Michael's status did not improve, additional medications were used: ampicillin and hydrocortisone. His oral candidiasis was treated with ketoconazole.

10. **Are the ICU nurses at an increased risk of acquiring AIDS from patients who receive mechanical ventilation?**

The statistics of medical personnel contracting AIDS from patients are quite low. The use of universal precautions by all medical personnel lessens the risk of infection. It is important to handle blood and body fluids properly. It is important to follow the CDC recommendations for prevention of HIV transmission in health care settings and to follow the Occupational Safety and Health Administration's (OSHA's) blood and body fluid precautions.

The risk of acquiring HIV infection from patients in health care settings is less than 1% at a 95% confidence level (Oskins, 1990). From a recent study over a 6-year period, 76 ICU employees were exposed to 56 mucosal splashes and 25 needle-sticks. None of the health care personnel seroconverted for HIV (Hall et al., 1992). It is important that ICU staff take precautions to avoid blood and body fluids from all patients. In a survey published in an article by Scherer, Haughey, Wu, and Kuhn (1992), 59% of nurses were fearful of contracting AIDS from patients; 67% stated a major concern was not knowing a patient's HIV status.

11. **What are some of the nursing interventions that will help Mr. Michael with his psychosocial and physiologic needs?**

Mr. Michael's initial admission assessment demonstrated several psychosocial needs. It is important to assess his safety both through necessary suicidal precautions and assistance with ambulation. Mr. Michael's safety should be a priority. It is also very important to maintain the patient's support systems.

Potential nursing diagnoses for ADC include the following:

➤ anxiety related to unknown progression of HIV/AIDS
➤ ineffective coping related to depression and AIDS dementia

> ➤ ADC related to unknown progression of HIV/AIDS
> ➤ fear related to the unknown progression of HIV/AIDS

It is necessary to design a plan of care according to assessment data and expected outcomes. For example, since Mr. Michael will have perceptual alterations, including diminishing memory, it is important to have him keep a calendar to help him follow treatment regimens. Instructions should be simple and concise.

During the time that Mr. Michael has PCP, it is important to follow care according to developed nursing diagnoses and expected outcomes.

Nursing diagnoses developed by Henry and Holzemer (1992, pp. 247–248) include the following:

> ➤ hyperthermia related to human responses to the disease responses to PCP
> ➤ impaired gas exchange related to the disease process of PCP
> ➤ high risk for altered respiratory function: dyspnea related to the disease process of PCP
> ➤ alteration in comfort: nausea or vomiting related to administration of pentamidine or sulfamethoxazole-trimethoprim

The nursing care of a patient with ADC and PCP in the critical care unit depends not only on the nurses' knowledge of the physiology of the disease process but also on the psychosocial needs of the critically ill patient (Henry & Holzemer, 1992).

12. When assigned to an HIV-infected patient, what personal feelings or concerns should be acknowledged?

According to Bradley–Springer, Schwanberg, and Frank (1994), in a quantitative study assessing nurses' reactions to the possibility of caring for HIV-infected patients, nurses held a wide variety of opinions and concerns. In the area of caring, the nurses expressed sadness, empathy, and compassion. They wanted to give the best care possible, would trust precautions, and would not refuse to care for HIV-positive patients. In the area of avoidance, the authors found that nurses were concerned for themselves and their families. Forty–two percent of the nurses felt that they were not properly prepared to care for HIV-infected patients.

Acquired Immunodeficiency Syndrome

Alspach, J. G. (1991). *Core curriculum for critical care nursing* (pp. 699 & 735–739). Philadelphia: Saunders.

Beckman, M. (1990). Neurologic manifestations of AIDS. *Critical Care Nursing Clinics of North America, 2*(1), 29–32.

Bradley-Springer, L., Schwanberg, S., & Frank, B. (1994). Anticipating care for HIV-infected clients: Nurse's reaction. *Journal of the Association of Nurses in AIDS Care, 5*(1), 29–38.

Centers for Disease Control and Prevention. (1992, December, 18). *1993 revised classification system for HIV infection and expanded surveillance case definition for AIDS among adolescents and adults. Morbidity and Mortality Weekly Report, 41*(RR-17), 1–19.

Chernecky, C. C., Krech, R. L., & Berger, B. J. (1993). *Laboratory tests and diagnostic procedures* (pp. 147–150). Philadelphia: Saunders.

Clochesy, J. M., Breu, C., Cardin, S., Rudy, E. B., & Whittaker, A. A. (1993). *Critical care nursing.* Philadelphia: Saunders.

Flaskerud, J. H., & Ungvarski, P. J. (1992). *HIV/AIDS: A guide to nursing care* (2nd ed.). Philadelphia: Saunders.

Flaskerud, J. H., & Ungvarski, P. J. (1995). *HIV/AIDS: A guide to nursing care* (3rd ed.).. Philadelphia: Saunders.

Hall, J., Schmidt, G., & Wood, L. (1992). AIDS in the intensive care unit. In *Principles of critical care* (pp. 1227–1228). St. Louis: McGraw–Hill.

Henry, S. B., & Holzemer, W. L. (1992). Critical care management of the patient with HIV infection who has *Pneumocystis carinii* pneumonia. *Heart & Lung, 21*(3), 243–249.

Jones, A. M. (1993). Hematology/immunology. In J. Hartshorn, M. Lamborn, & M. L. Noll (Eds.). *Introduction to critical care nursing* (pp. 378–384). Philadelphia: Saunders.

Oskins, S. L. (1990). Acquired immune deficiency syndrome. In B. C. Mims (Ed.), *Case studies in critical care nursing* (pp. 432–445). Baltimore: Williams & Wilkins.

Scherer, P. (1990). How AIDS attacks the brain. *American Journal of Nursing, 90*(1), 44–53.

Scherer, Y. K., Haughey, B. P., Wu, Y. B., & Kuhn, M. M. (1992). AIDS: What are critical care nurses' concerns? *Critical Care Nurse, 12*(7), 23–29.

Singer, P., Askanazi, J., Akiva, L., Bursztein, S., & Kvetan, V. (1990). Re-assessing intensive care for patients with the acquired immunodeficiency syndrome. *Heart & Lung, 19*(4), 387–394.

Thompson, S., Novak, R., Pursell, K., & Swift, R. Y. (Eds.). (1993). Neuropsychiatric protocols. In *Clinical management of the HIV-infected adult: A manual for mid-level clinicians* (2nd ed., pp. 74–75 & 79–80). Chicago: U.S. Public Health Service Grant 5 D35 PE00104-03.

Abbreviations

A-a	Alveolar-arterial
ABCs	Airway, breathing, and circulation
ABGs	Arterial blood gases
A-c	Alveolar-capillary
A/C (mode)	assist/control
ACE	Angiotensin converting enzyme
ac	before meals
ACTH	Adrenocorticotropic hormone
ADC	Acquired immunodeficiency syndrome dementia complex
ADH	Antidiuretic hormone
AIDS	Acquired immunodeficiency syndrome
ALT	Alanine aminotransferase
AMI	Acute myocardial infarction
AMP	Adenosine monophosphate
ANH	Atrial natriuretic hormone
APD	Acid phosphate dextrose
ARDS	Adult respiratory distress syndrome
ARF	Acute renal failure
AST	Aspartate aminotransferase
ATG	Lymphocyte immune globulin
ATN	Acute tubular necrosis
ATP	Adenosine triphosphate
AV	Atrioventricular; arteriovenous
BE	Base excess
BGM	Blood glucose monitoring
b.i.d.	Two times a day
BP	Blood pressure
bpm	Beats per minute
BUN	Blood urea nitrogen
C	Celsius
CABG	Coronary artery bypass graft
CAD	Coronary artery disease
CaO_2	Oxygen content, arterial blood
CAPD	Continuous ambulatory peritoneal dialysis

CAVH	Continuous arteriovenous hemofiltration
CAVHD	Continuous arteriovenous hemofiltration dialysis
CBC	Complete blood count
CDC	Centers for Disease Control and Prevention
CHF	Congestive heart failure
CI	Cardiac index
CK	Creatine kinase
cm	Centimeter
CMV	Controlled mechanical ventilation; cytomegalovirus
CNS	Central nervous system
CO	Cardiac Output
COMT	Catechol-O-methyltransferase
COPD	Chronic obstructive pulmonary disease
CPAP	Continuous positive airway pressure
CPD	Citrate phosphate dextrose
CPK	Creatine phosphokinase
CPR	Cardiopulmonary resuscitation
CRH	Corticotropin-releasing hormone
CRRT	Continuous renal replacement therapy
CSF	Cerebrospinal fluid
CT	Computed tomography, computed tomographic
CVA	Cerebrovascular accident
Cvo_2	Oxygen content, venous blood
CVP	Central venous pressure
Cx	Circumflex artery
CXR	Chest x-ray
DAI	Diffuse axonal injury
DI	Diabetes insipidus
DIC	Disseminated intravascular coagulation
DKA	Diabetic ketoacidosis
2,3-DPG	Diphosphoglycerate
DTR	Deep tendon reflexes
DVT	Deep venous thrombosis
D_5LR	5% dextrose in lactated Ringer's solution
D_5NS	5% dextrose in normal saline
D_5W, $D_{10}W$	5% dextrose in water, 10% dextrose in water, etc.
E	Epinephrine
ECG	Electrocadiogram
ECMO	Extracorporeal membrane oxygenation
ED	Emergency department
EDH	Epidural hematoma
EGD	Esophagogastroduodenoscopy
ELISA	Enzyme-linked immunosorbent assay
ERCP	Endoscopic retrograde cholangiopancreatography
F	Fahrenheit

FEV	Forced expiratory volume
FFA	Free fatty acid
FiO$_2$	Fraction of inspired oxygen
FRC	Functional residual capacity
FSP	Fibrin split products
GAS	General adaptation syndrome
GH	Growth hormone
GI	Gastrointestinal
h	Hour
HBV	High biologic value
HCG	Human chorionic gonadotropin
HCO$_3^-$	Becarbonate
Hct	Hematocrit
Hgb	Hemoglobin
HIV	Human immunodeficiency virus
HOB	Head of bed
HR	Heart rate
hs	bedtime
IABP	Intraaortic balloon pump
ICP	Intracranial pressure
ICU	Intensive care unit
IDDM	Insulin-dependent diabetes mellitus
IGF	Insulin-like growth factor
IIR	Inflammatory immune response
IM	Intramuscular
IMV	Intermittent mandatory ventilation
IRV	Inverse ratio ventilation
IU	International unit
IV	Intravenous
IVP	Intravenous push
JG	Juxtaglomerular
JGA	Juxtaglomerular apparatus
JVD	Jugular venous distension
kcal	Kilocalorie
kg	Kilogram
KUB	Kidneys, ureters, and bladder (x-ray)
L	Liter
LAD	Left anterior descending (coronary artery)
lb	Pound
LDH	Lactate dehydrogenase
LDL	Low-density lipoprotein
LR	Lactated Ringer's solution
LV	Left ventricle, left ventricular
LVEF	Left ventricular ejection fraction
LVEDP	Left ventricular end-diastolic pressure
LVF	Left ventricular failure

MAP	Mean arterial pressure
MAST	Medical antishock trousers
mEq	Milliequivalent
mg	Milligram
µg	Microgram
MHC	Major histocompatibility complex
MI	Mycardial infarction
min	Minute (time)
ml	Milliliter
mm	Millimeter
mm³	Cubic millimeter
MMFR	Maximal midexpiratory flow rate
mmol/L	Millimolar; millimole per liter
MODS	Multiple organ dysfunction syndrome
mol/L	Molar; mole per liter
mOsm	Milliosmole
MRI	Magnetic resonance imaging
MSH	Melanocyte-stimulating hormone
MSOF	Multisystem organ failure
NE	Norepinephrine
ng	Nanogram
NGT	Nasogastric tube
NPO	Nothing by mouth
NS(S)	Normal saline (solution)
NSAID	Nonsteroidal antiinflammatory drug
NSR	Normal sinus rhythm
NTG	Nitroglycerin
OM_1	First obtuse marginal artery
OSHA	Occupational Safety and Health Administration
OTC	Over the counter
PA	Pulmonary artery
$PA\text{-}aO_2$	Alveolar-arterial oxygen difference
PAC	Pulmonary artery catheter
$Paco_2$	Carbon dioxide pressure (tension), arterial
PACU	Postanesthesia care unit
PAD	Pulmonary artery diastolic (pressure)
Pao_2	Oxygen pressure (tension), arterial
PAP	Pulmonary artery pressure
PAS	Pulmonary artery systolic (pressure)
PAWP	Pulmonary artery wedge pressure
PCA (pump)	Patient-controlled analgesia
Pco_2	Carbon dioxide pressure (tension)
PCP	*Pneumocystis carinii* pneumonia
PCWP	Pulmonary capillary wedge pressure
PE	Pulmonary embolism
PEEP	Positive end expiratory pressure

PERRLA	Pupils equal, round, reactive to light, and accommodate
pg	Picogram
PGL	Persistent generalized lymphadenopathy
pH	Hydrogen ion concentration
PIP	Peak inspiratory pressure
pm	Picometer
PMI	Point of maximal impulse
PMN	Polymarphonuclear neutrophil leukocyte
PO	By mouth
PO_2	Oxygen pressure (tension)
PO_4	Phosphate
POMC	Proopiomelanocortin
prn	As necessary
PT	Prothrombin time
PTCA	Percutaneous transluminal coronary angioplasty
PTT	Partial thromboplastin time
PVC	Premature ventricular contraction
Pvo_2	Oxygen pressure (tension), venous
q.i.d.	Four times a day
q6h, q8h	Every 6 hours, every 8 hours, etc.
RA	Airway resistance
RAAS	Renin-angiotensin-aldosterone system
RAP	Right atrial pressure
RBC	Red blood cell
RCA	Right coronary artery
RCEA	Right carotid endarterectomy
REM	Rapid eye movement
RIA	Radioimmunoassay
RIND	Reversible ischemic neurologic deficit
RV	Residual volume
RVEDP	Right ventricular end-diastolic pressure
s	Second
Sao_2	Saturation with oxygen, arterial blood
SCUF	Slow continuous ultrafiltration
SDH	Subdural hematoma
SGOT	Serum glutamic-oxaloacetic transaminase
SGPT	Serum glutamate pyruvate transaminase
SIADH	Syndrome of inappropriate antidiuretic hormone
SICU	Surgical intensive care unit
SIMV	Synchronized intermittent mandatory ventilation
SIRS	Systemic inflammatory response system
Svo_2	Saturation with oxygen, venous blood
SVR	Systemic vascular resistance
T_3	Triiodothyronine
T_4	Tetraiodothyronine, thyroxine
TB	Tuberculosis

TBSA	Total body surface area
TCDB	Turn, cough, and deep breathe
TIA	Transient ischemic attack
t.i.d.	Three times a day
TIPS	Transjugular intrahepatic portosystemic shunt
TPA	Tissue plasminogen activation
TPN	Total parenteral nutrition
TRH	Thyrotropin-releasing hormone
TSH	Thyroid-stimulating hormone
U	Unit
VC	Vital capacity
VDRL	Venereal Disease Research Laboratories (test)
$\dot{V}/\dot{Q}$	Ventilation-perfusion ratio
VT	Ventricular tachycardia
V_T	Tidal volume
WBC	White blood cell
wk	Week
y	Year

Index

Note: Page numbers followed by t refer to tables.